# The Toxicant Induction of Irritant Asthma, Rhinitis, and Related Conditions

William J. Meggs
Editor

# The Toxicant Induction of Irritant Asthma, Rhinitis, and Related Conditions

Springer

*Editor*
William J. Meggs
East Carolina University
Greenville, NC, USA

ISBN 978-1-4899-7949-0 ISBN 978-1-4614-9044-9 (eBook)
DOI 10.1007/978-1-4614-9044-9
Springer New York Heidelberg Dordrecht London


Softcover reprint of the hardcover 1st edition 2013


Printed on acid-free paper

Springer is part of Springer Science+Business Media (www.springer.com)

# Contents

1 **Introduction: Irritant Asthma, Irritant Rhinitis, and Related Conditions** ........ 1
William J. Meggs

2 **Airway Anatomy, Physiology, and Inflammation** ........ 19
Michael R. Van Scott, Joyce Chandler, Stephen Olmstead, Jared M. Brown, and Mark Mannie

3 **Reactive Airways Dysfunction Syndrome (RADS) and Irritant-Induced Asthma** ........ 63
Stuart M. Brooks

4 **Acute Toxicity of Respiratory Irritant Exposures** ........ 83
Susan Ney Miller

5 **Particulate Exposure and Cardiovascular Inflammation** ........ 103
Christopher J. Wingard, Emily Cozzi, Michael R. Van Scott, and Robert M. Lust

6 **Products of Tobacco Combustion** ........ 131
Rebecca Bascom, Anne E.F. Dimmock, and Judie Ann Howrylak

7 **Irritant and Airborne Contact Dermatitis** ........ 193
Payton A. Kuhlenbeck and Tanner J. Parrent

8 **Exposure Limits** ........ 207
Grace Ziem

9 **Occupational Issues Related to Respiratory Irritants** ........ 219
Ricky Langley and David Lipton

10 **The Brain as a Target Organ for Allergic and Irritant Sensitivity: A Review and Suggestions for Research** ........ 231
William J. Meggs, Richard M. Bloch, and Kori L. Brewer

**11 An Approach to Treating Irritant Airway Inflammation** .................... 247
Grace Ziem

**12 Summary and Research Needs** .................................................. 277
William J. Meggs

**Index** .................................................................................... 287

# Chapter 1
# Introduction: Irritant Asthma, Irritant Rhinitis, and Related Conditions

**William J. Meggs**

**Abstract** Inhaled substances produce airway inflammation by two well-defined and distinct mechanisms. Aeroallergens are proteins on airborne particles that induce IgE antibodies with a high affinity for mast cells and basophils. Exposure causes degranulation and the release of inflammatory mediators. Respiratory irritants are chemicals that bind to chemoreceptors on sensory nerve fibers, leading to the release of mediators of neurogenic inflammation. Clinical manifestations are independent of the mechanism, have intra- and interindividual variability, and range from rhinorrhea and congestion in the upper airway to bronchospasm and bronchorrhea in the lower airway. Acute exposures to respiratory irritants are known to induce persistent upper and lower airway inflammation that have been termed reactive airways dysfunction syndrome and reactive upper-airway dysfunction syndrome, respectively. The mechanism is a remodeling of the structure of the airway mucosa, leading to pathological changes that lower the threshold for irritant sensitivity, so that chronic inflammation is induced by ongoing previously tolerated exposures.

**Keywords** Asthma • Rhinitis • Reactive airways dysfunction syndrome • Reactive upper-airways dysfunction syndrome • Respiratory irritants

## Introduction

Several decades ago asthma was classified as extrinsic or intrinsic. Rhinitis was likewise classified as allergic or non-allergic. Extrinsic asthma was allergic asthma. Both allergic asthma and rhinitis are well understood as a characteristic lower

W.J. Meggs, M.D., Ph.D., F.A.C.M.T., F.A.C.E.P. (✉)
Division of Toxicology, Department of Emergency Medicine, Brody School of Medicine at East Carolina University, 600 Moye Boulevard, Greenville, NC, USA
e-mail: meggsw@ecu.edu

W.J. Meggs (ed.), *The Toxicant Induction of Irritant Asthma, Rhinitis, and Related Conditions*, DOI 10.1007/978-1-4614-9044-9_1,

airway inflammation induced by inhaled allergens in the environment. The mechanism is production of antibodies of the IgE class directed against proteins found on pollen grains and mold spores and arising from animals such as dust mites and cat. The IgE antibodies are found on the surfaces of mast cells and basophils. When environment proteins interact with these antibodies, a number of substances are released that lead to inflammation of the airway. Clinical manifestations include varying degrees of rhinorrhea, congestion, sinus headaches, dyspnea, bronchospasm, bronchorrhea, and cough. Allergy skin tests, in vitro measurements of specific IgE antibodies, inhalational challenges, and correlation of symptoms with exposures can be used to diagnose allergy asthma. Allergy immunotherapy is efficacious and cost effective to prevent exacerbations of allergic asthma, rhinitis, and conjunctivitis resulting from exposures (Simoens 2012).

Those with asthma but negative evaluations for allergy were classified as having intrinsic asthma. Their asthma was thought to be internal with no external triggers. Over time, it was realized that environmental exposures other than allergens can trigger asthma attacks in individuals with susceptibility to a particular exposure. These range from exposure to cold dry air, exercise, and emotional stress. It has also been established that there is another mechanism through which airborne exposures trigger exacerbations of asthma, rhinitis, and conjunctivitis. A class of chemical inhalants termed *respiratory irritants* can induce an exacerbation of asthma and rhinitis in susceptible individuals. Examples of respiratory irritants that can exacerbate asthma, rhinosinusitis, or conjunctivitis are given in Table 1.1.

There has been an increasing recognition of the role of irritants in exacerbating the airway inflammation of asthma (Brooks et al. 1990, Nordin et al. 2004) and rhinitis (Bernstein 2012; Millqvist et al. 2005). It is generally true that more attention is given to asthma than to rhinitis, even though rhinitis is more prevalent than asthma. Deaths from rhinitis are virtually unknown, while asthma can be devastating and fatal. Rhinitis would be more deadly than asthma except for anatomical redundancy with an alternative path for the upper airway; that is, the alimentary canal provides an alternative airway to the nasal passages. Significant blockage of the nasal passages by congestion is common and would be a major emergency except an afflicted person can bypass nasal airway obstruction by opening the mouth.

Rhinitis is sometimes regarded as a trivial disease, but this is not the case. Quality of life studies document the devastating impact rhinitis can have on the quality of life (Rudmik and Smith 2011). To quote from the Joint Task Force on Practice Parameters, representing the American Academy of Allergy, Asthma & Immunology; the American College of Allergy, Asthma and Immunology; and the Joint Council of Allergy, Asthma and Immunology (Wallace et al. 2008): "Although sometimes mistakenly viewed as a trivial disease, symptoms of allergic and non-allergic rhinitis may significantly affect a patient's quality of life and can be associated with conditions such as *fatigue, headache, cognitive impairment, and sleep disturbance*." (Italics added). Asthma, rhinitis, and sinusitis are terms denoting airway inflammation in different parts of the airway, with overlapping pathophysiology, exacerbating causes, and treatments. Rhinitis and sinusitis are so similar that the American

**Table 1.1** Examples of irritants associated with exacerbations of asthma, rhinosinusitis, or conjunctivitis

| Substance | Selected references |
|---|---|
| *Products of combustion* | |
| Environmental tobacco smoke | Al-Sayed and Abrahim 2012, Bascom 1991, Bascom et al. 1991, Willes et al. 1998 |
| Diesel exhaust | Hussain et al. 2012 |
| Wood smoke | Van Miert et al. 2012, Henderson and Johnston 2012 |
| Vehicle exhaust | Gasana et al. 2012 |
| *Dusts* | |
| Cement dust | Baur et al. 2012 |
| Grain dust | Baur et al. 2012 |
| Cotton dust | Yerpude and Jogdand 2010 |
| *Fragrances and perfumes* | Elberling et al. 2005, 2007, Heydorn et al. 2003, Kumar et al. 1995, Millqvist and Lowhagen 1998, Millqvist et al. 1999, Opiekun et al. 2003, Steinemann 2009, Steinemann et al. 2011 |
| *Pesticides* | Senthilselvan et al. 1992, Hernandez et al. 2011 |
| *Noxious gases* | |
| Sulfur dioxide | Deger et al. 2012, Kim et al. 2012 |
| Ozone | Youssefagha et al. 2012 |
| Chlorine | Bougault and Boulet 2012, Bougault et al. 2012 |
| Oxides of nitrogen | Youssefagha et al. 2012 |
| Chlorine dioxide | Meggs 1995 |
| Ammonia | Baur et al. 2012 |
| Chloramine | D'Alò et al. 2012 |
| Bleach (sodium hypochlorite) | Arif and Delclos 2012 |
| *Complex mixtures* | Banauch et al. 2003 |

Academy of Otolaryngology has proposed using the diagnosis rhinosinusitis rather than the separate terms.

Accompanying our increasing knowledge of the role irritants play in human disease has been the recognition that irritant exposures can induce permanent and lifelong asthma and/or rhinitis. Soldiers who survived the irritant gas exposures such as chlorine and mustard gas in the trenches of World War I developed chronic asthma (Ghanei and Harandi 2007). The classic description of asthma induced by irritant exposures as described by Brooks and his collaborators has been termed reactive airways dysfunction syndrome (RADS) (Brooks, Brooks). This syndrome is discussed in detail in Chap. 3. Persistent rhinitis can also occur after an irritant exposure (Meggs and Cleveland 1993; Meggs et al. 1996b; Leroyer et al. 1999; Moscato et al. 2008; Hellgren et al. 2003; Gautrin et al. 2006; Castano and Malo 2010). Extension to rhinitis induced by an acute exposure to irritants has been termed reactive upper-airway dysfunction syndrome (RUDS) (Meggs and Cleveland 1993; Meggs et al. 1996b).

## Mechanism of Irritant Asthma and Irritant Rhinitis

In a classic set of experiments a century ago, the German physiologist A. N. Bruce demonstrated that the inflammatory response to an irritant was dependent upon sensory innovation. Mustard oil was instilled into the conjunctiva in experimental models. Bruce proved that the inflammatory response was blocked by cutting the sensory nerves to the conjunctiva (Bruce 1910, 1913). Since that time, literally thousands of studies have established the role of sensory nerve stimulation in inflammatory processes in the skin, airway, conjunctiva, gastrointestinal tract, synovial lining of joints, and genitourinary tract. There have been many reviews that summarize our knowledge in this area (Jansco 2008; Veronesi and Oortgiesen 2001; Nielsen 1991; Barnes 2001; Meggs 1995; Stahl 1999; Spampinato and Ferri 1991; Groneberg et al. 2004). The subject is so vast that we will not be able to reference and credit the many investigators who have made contributions to this important area of research, from identification and synthesis of neuropeptides and their receptors, mechanisms of action, and interactions with other systems. The mechanism will be summarized here. Receptors on nerve cells that identify external stimuli and initiate a reaction are termed nociceptors. Nociceptors can be stimulated by chemical irritants, mechanical stimulation such as stretch, and thermal stimuli. Nociceptors that respond to chemical irritants are sometimes termed chemoreceptors or irritant receptors. Respiratory irritants are chemicals that bind to nociceptors on sensory nerve fibers in the airway and initiate an inflammatory response. The nerve cells release inflammatory mediators termed neurokinins. These include substance P, vasopressin, and calcitonin gene-related peptide.

Many mast cells have receptors for substance P on their surface, so mast cells can be stimulated to add to the inflammatory process, with the release of histamine and chemotactic factors. Immune cells are recruited to the site. Blood vessels dilate and can leak fluid into the tissues, producing congestion. Mucus glands are stimulated, leading to bronchorrhea and rhinorrhea. There can be burning of the nasal passages and secondarily itching from histamine release. Coughing and bronchospasm can occur. The end result is an exacerbation of asthma and/or rhinosinusitis. A schematic of this process is given in Fig. 1.1.

## Induction of Irritant Asthma and Rhinitis

A distinction must be made between exacerbation of asthma and/or rhinosinusitis in an individual with preexisting airway inflammation and the induction of chronic airway inflammation from irritant exposures. RADS describes a chronic asthma-like syndrome following irritant exposures (Brooks et al. 1985). RADS is discussed in detail in Chap. 3. Chronic rhinitis following irritant exposures (Meggs et al. 1996b) has been termed RUDS. Exacerbations from exposures represent hyperreactivity, occur at low doses generally tolerated by healthy individuals, and are not

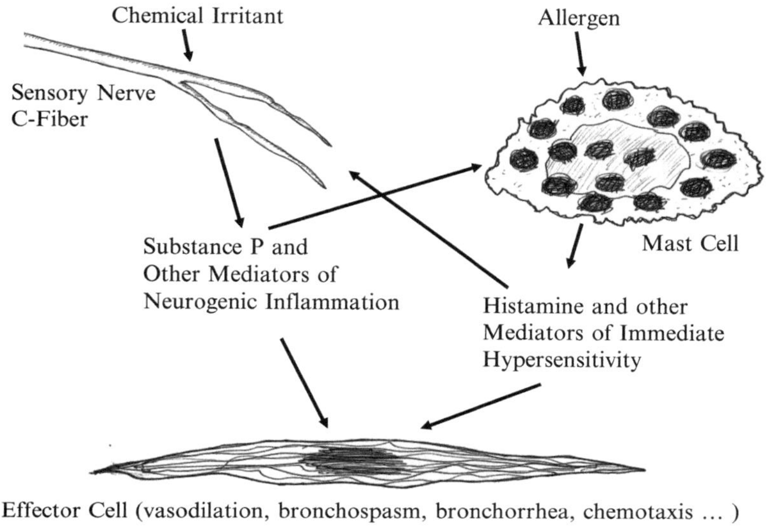


**Fig. 1.1** Schematic showing the mechanisms by which allergens and chemical irritants act on effector cells. Allergens bind to immunoglobulins (IgE) on mast cells, triggering the release of allergic mediators. Chemical irritants bind to chemoreceptors on sensory nerve fibers, triggering the release of neurokinins. The crossover network between allergic and irritant reactions is depicted, with histamine binding to receptors on nerve fibers and substance P binding to receptors on mast cells. The clinical manifestations can be similar, with rhinorrhea, bronchorrhea, bronchospasm, etc.

dose dependent, though there might be a threshold dose below which the inflammatory cascade is not activated. The induction of chronic airway inflammation from an irritant exposure is thought to be a toxic event that follows a dose–response curve. The higher the dose, the more likely the effect is to occur.

Historically, induction of chronic airway inflammation from irritant exposures was described in veterans who were exposed to irritant gases such as chlorine in the trenches of World War One (US Army). Asthma, rhinitis, emphysema, and chronic obstructive pulmonary disease are related conditions that can all result from irritant exposures.

Chronic airway inflammation results from an irritant exposure because irritants induce inflammation. The effects of the irritant and resulting inflammation lead to a remodeling of the airway. Remodeling refers to the pathological changes that occur in the airway that changes the anatomy and physiology. An important change is a proliferation of sensory nerves in the airway that respond to respiratory irritants, as demonstrated by increases in nerve growth factor in the airways of subjects with rhinitis (Sanico et al. 1999, 2000; Millqvist et al. 2005). These can be verified by light microscopy and electron microscopy of biopsy specimens (Meggs 1992) as well as changes in the composition of interstitial and bronchial fluids. Figure 1.2 depicts these changes graphically.

Electron micrographs of nasal biopsies from individuals who developed chronic airway inflammation after an irritant exposure are depicted in Figs. 1.3 and 1.4.

Fig. 1.2 Mechanism of chronic airway inflammation and hyper-reactivity to respiratory irritants resulting from an irritant exposure. (**a**) Schematic of normal airway epithelium. (**b**) Schematic of changes in airway epithelium in individuals with remodeling secondary to irritant exposures. Reprinted from Meggs (1997) with permission

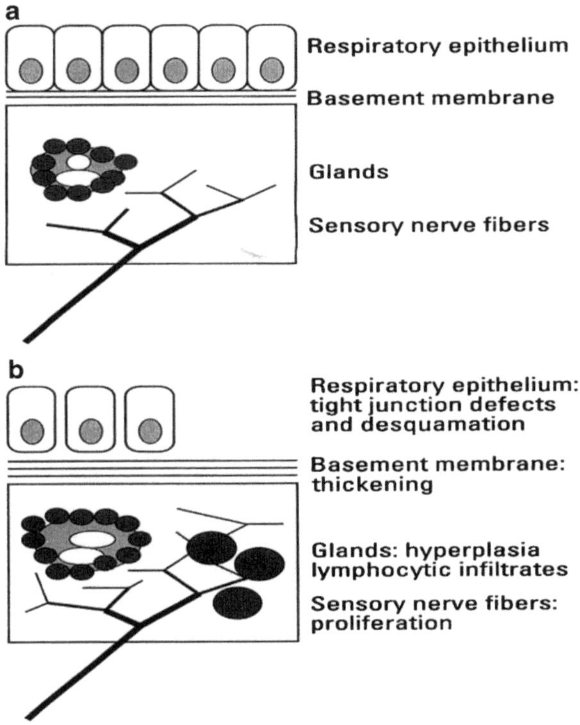


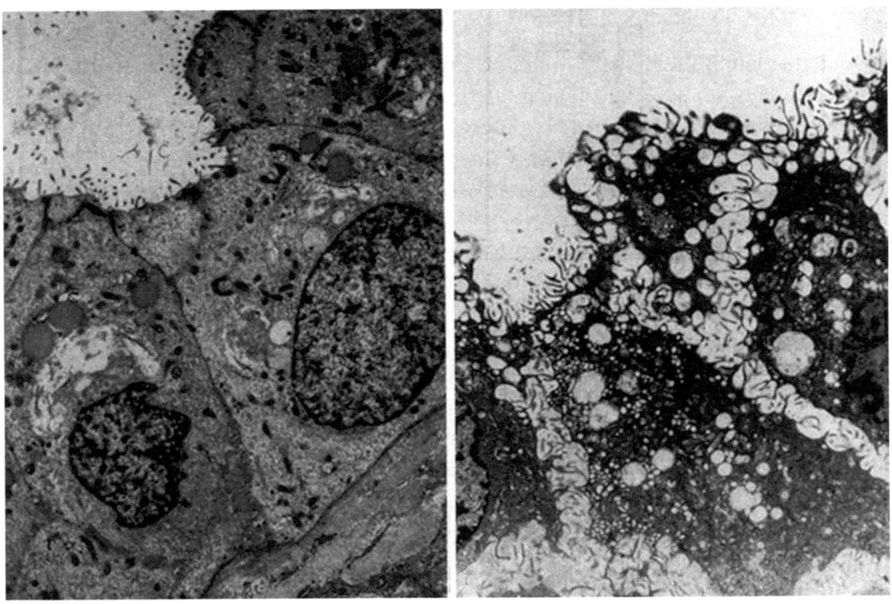

**Fig. 1.3** Electron micrograph of nasal mucosa biopsy of an individual with irritant rhinitis (*right*), compared to a normal mucosa (*left*). Note the defects in tight junctions. Reprinted from Meggs (1996b) with permission

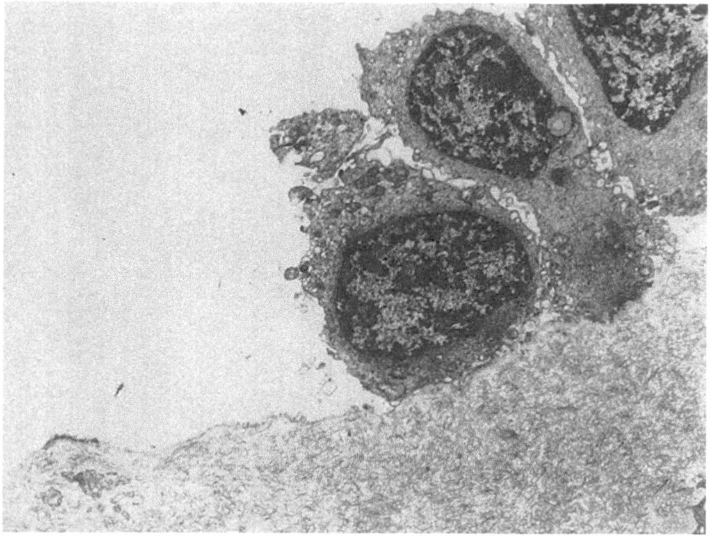

**Fig. 1.4** Electron micrograph of an individual with irritant rhinitis. Note the defects in the tight junctions between epithelial cells, the defects in the junctions between respiratory epithelial cells and the basement membrane, and the loss of respiratory epithelial cells. Reprinted from Meggs (1996b) with permission

Figure 1.3 compares the findings in a normal biopsy, in which there are tight junctions between respiratory epithelial cells and those of an individual with RUDS, with defects in tight junctions between adjacent cells. Tumor necrosis factor has been shown to disrupt tight junctions (Shen 2012), and the abnormal lymphocytic infiltrates in the airway of affected individuals may be the source of tumor necrosis factor, though further work is needed to verify this hypothesis. In Fig. 1.4, one sees disruption of the tight junctions not only between adjacent respiratory epithelial cells but also between epithelial cells and the basement membrane, with loss of epithelial cells (desquamation).

Individuals with irritant rhinitis have characteristic findings on visualization of the upper airway that are best appreciated with rhinolaryngoscopy. Figure 1.5 is a photograph of the nasal passages of an individual who developed chronic irritant rhinitis after an acute high-dose exposure to respiratory irritants. There is a patchy loss of the normal uniform rose coloration of the upper airway, with pale-to-yellow coloration. In the areas of discoloration, blood vessels are clearly visible. These changes are often seen on the uvula and soft pallet. Biopsies of the discolored areas in comparison to the areas of normal coloration in individuals with irritant rhinitis revealed no difference in light microscopy, with chronic inflammation being seen at both sites (Meggs and Cleveland 1993).

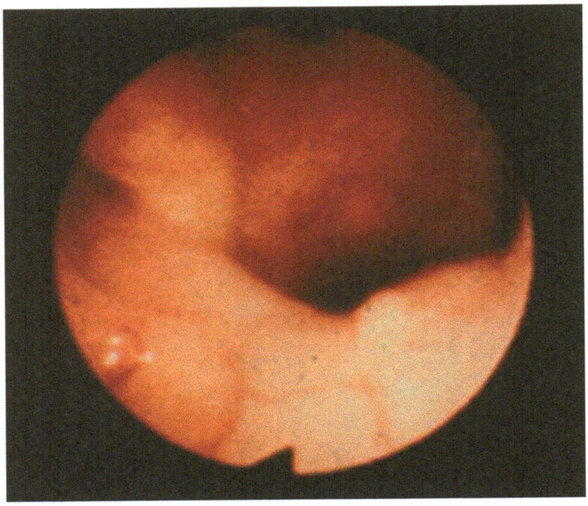

**Fig. 1.5** Nasal airway of an individual with irritant rhinitis. Note the area of discoloration with loss of the uniform coloration seen in a normal airway. There are also prominent blood vessels in the areas of discoloration. This pattern can be seen in the nasal mucosa, soft pallet, and uvula

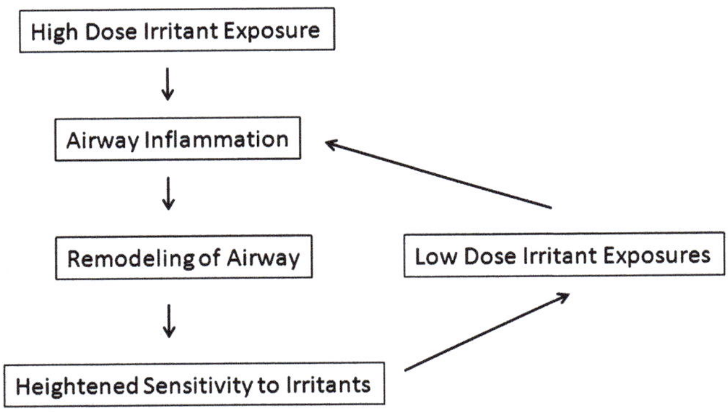


**Fig. 1.6** A positive feedback loop is set up when a high-dose irritant exposure initiates airway inflammation which leads to remodeling of the airway. The remodeled airway has a heightened sensitivity to irritants so that exposures to lower levels that were previously tolerated produce inflammation, which in turn prevents normalization of the remodeled airway

One of the consequences of remodeling is a decreased threshold for irritants to trigger airway inflammation. An individual who develops RADS or RUDS will have susceptibility to irritant exposures at lower concentrations than that were tolerated before the onset of illness. In situations where exposures to respiratory irritants are unavoidable, inflammation becomes chronic and remodeling becomes permanent. In effect, a positive feedback loop is established, as depicted in Fig. 1.6.

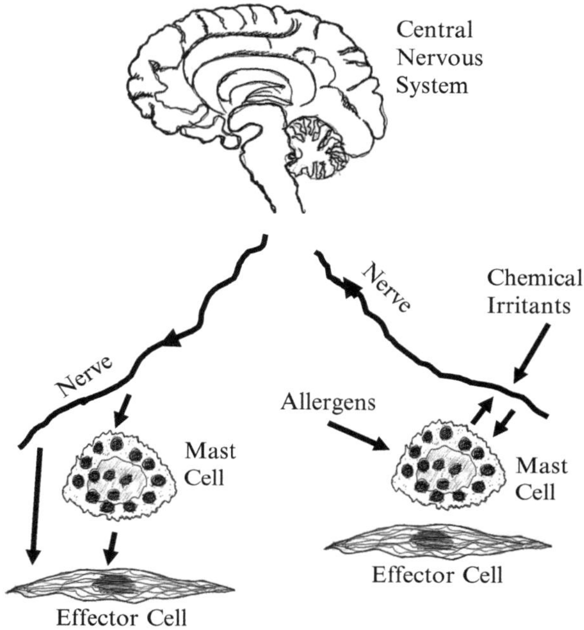


**Fig. 1.7** Neurogenic switching in allergic and irritant reactions. Initiating event sends nerve pulse upward, with retrograde propagation of the nerve signal to another site

## Relationship of Allergy and Irritant Sensitivity

### *Site Switching*

Allergens and irritants generally induce inflammation at the site of inoculation. There are well-documented situations where inflammation can develop at other sites. This is best established for allergic reactions. Examples include urticaria and asthma attacks from food allergy, a condition known as gustatory rhinitis, and even systemic anaphylaxis. Site switching to the central nervous system may underlie cognitive dysfunction, mood disturbance, chronic fatigue, and sleep disturbances associated with allergic and irritant rhinitis (Wallace). A discussion of the brain as a target organ for both allergic and irritant reactions is given in Chap. 10.

There are several mechanisms for site switching. Polyclonal activation occurs when stimulation of a clone of immune cells to one antigen or irritant results in the activation of other unrelated clones. The release of cytokines from one site of infection may enhance inflammation at other sites of preexisting inflammation. This phenomenon may underlie the clinical observation that viral infections including influenza infections can lead to exacerbations of conditions such as asthma (Yamaya 2012). The critical role of the nervous system in site switching has been termed *neurogenic switching* (Meggs 1995). This process, in which a nerve signal is transmitted to the central nervous system from the site of inoculation, followed by retrograde propagation (Hinsey and Gasser 1930; Chahl 1988) to another site, is depicted in Fig. 1.7.

A positive allergy skin test consists of two components, wheal and flare. Wheal is a palpable swelling about the site of inoculation. Flare is a larger area of erythema about the site of inoculation. The flare is an example of neurogenic switching. Inoculation of the skin with antigen induces mast cell degranulation. Histamine induces capillary leak, with edema of the dermis (wheal) at the site of inoculation. Histamine binds to receptors on sensory nerve c-fibers so that an electrical pulse travels toward the central nervous system. The pulse flows in a retrograde fashion down the neighboring nerve fibers leading to substance P release at their terminal ends. Substance P in turn binds to vessels to increase blood flow to the area, resulting in hyperemia (flare).

Systemic anaphylaxis may be a manifestation of neurogenic switching. Cutaneous inoculation with an antigen, such as a bee sting, or gut inoculation, as in the ingestion of a food or a drug, can affect multiple organ systems immediately. Respiratory involvement with bronchospasm, bronchorrhea, and laryngeal edema; gastrointestinal symptoms; skin involvement away from the site of inoculation with diffuse flushing or urticaria; and cardiovascular symptoms with hypotension from diffuse vasodilation can all arise. A role for the nervous system in systemic anaphylaxis has been demonstrated in experimental models. It is known that vagotomy protects rats from lethal anaphylaxis without changing the production of antibody or histamine release (Levy et al. 1976). Experimental lesions of the anterior hypothalamus lessen the anaphylactic reaction in a guinea pig model (Leslie and Mathe 1989). Neurogenic switching may be the mechanism for this observed modulation of anaphylaxis by the nervous system.

Gustatory rhinitis is known to be an example of neurogenic switching based on pharmaceutical studies. In this syndrome, rhinorrhea, nasal congestion, and facial sweating develop after the ingestion of spicy foods. Ingested irritants such as capsaicin, the active ingredient in chili peppers, interact with branches of the trigeminal nerve innervating the oral cavity. The efferent signal is switched to the nose and face (Raphael et al. 1989). That atropine, an antagonist of the neurotransmitter acetylcholine at muscarinic receptors, blocks the effect is convincing evidence of the role of the nervous system in site switching.

Site switching has been rigorously demonstrated in experiments by Dr. Eva Millqvist and her collaborators in Sweden. Instilling fragrance in the lateral conjunctival sac, away from the lacrimal duct and without sensations of odor or taste, of subjects with sensitivity to irritants resulted in respiratory symptoms even though a mask was used to isolate the respiratory and conjunctival systems (Millqvist et al. 1999). Millqvist developed the capsaicin cough challenge that demonstrates that subjects with irritant sensitivity develop increased coughing relative to controls with inhalation of nebulized capsaicin (Ternesten-Hasséus et al. 2002). That remodeling of the airway in response to neuroinflammatory activation is a role in irritant sensitivity was further demonstrated by increased levels of nerve growth factor in this patient population relative to controls after inhalation of capsaicin (Millqvist et al. 2005).

## Environmental Adjuvants

The concept of environmental adjuvants closes the loop relating allergic and irritant sensitivity. In immunology, an adjuvant is a substance that potentiates the immune response to other substances. Environmental adjuvants are substances in the environment that induce immune reactivity to other environmental substances. The prevalence of asthma, atopy, and rhinitis, both allergic and nonallergic, is increasing in many countries (Tang et al. 2008). One possible reason for this increase is that environmental exposures both initiate and exacerbate airway inflammation. It is reasonable to assume that inflamed tissue will process antigens so that an immune response develops to allergens that are present concurrently. It has been demonstrated that inhalation of irritant gases can induce production of IgE antibody to concomitant exposures. A notable example is diesel exhaust particles that can induce IgE responses to a co-administered aeroallergen (Nel et al. 1998). Other irritant exposures that can enhance immunity to other substances include ozone (Biagini et al. 1986; Matsumura et al. 1972), nitrogen dioxide (Matsumura et al. 1972), and sulfur dioxide (Reidel; Matsumura et al. 1972). Hence, air polluted with irritants is a possible explanation for increases in allergic diseases. The notable rise in allergy to Japanese cedar in Japan, from a rare condition to the most common immunological disease, after the introduction of motor vehicles, illustrates the remarkable effects irritants can have in a population (Matsumura et al. 1972).

## Related Conditions

A number of conditions and/or terminologies are related to irritant airway inflammation. These include atherosclerosis, sick building syndrome, world trade center syndrome, chronic fatigue syndrome, office eye syndrome, irritable bowel syndrome, irritant contact dermatitis, airborne contact dermatitis, multiple chemical sensitivity syndrome, idiopathic environmental intolerances, and fibromyalgia.

Atherosclerosis is an inflammatory process of arterial walls that can lead to heart attacks and strokes. It has long been recognized that both active and passive exposures to cigarette smoke can accelerate atherosclerosis. There is increasing recognition that other forms of air pollution are associated with atherosclerosis and in particular traffic fumes (Berglind et al. 2009). It has been found that transient exposure to traffic fumes can increase the risk of myocardial infarction in susceptible individuals (Peters et al. 2004). Small particulates from fossil fuel combustion are associated with myocardial infarction (Murakami and Ono 2006). Particulate exposure and cardiovascular inflammation are discussed in detail in Chap. 5.

Sick building syndrome is a term introduced by a World Health Organization Committee to describe widespread complaints in poorly ventilated buildings. These occurred after the energy crisis of the 1970s, when ventilation in buildings was reduced to save heating and cooling costs. Symptoms were most commonly respiratory. A comparison of a poorly ventilated building to a traditional building found a marked increase in respiratory complaints.

Irritant-associated vocal cord dysfunction syndrome: Vocal cord dysfunction syndrome, in which there is a paradoxical adduction of the vocal cords during inspiration, can be associated with irritant exposures, from both extrinsic chemical irritant exposures and intrinsic causes (acid reflux in gastroesophageal reflux disease, rhinitis and sinusitis, and laryngopharyngeal reflux) (Morris and Christopher 2010).

Chronic fatigue syndrome is defined by the Centers for Diseases Control as severe chronic fatigue for 6 or more consecutive months that is not due to ongoing exertion or other medical conditions associated with fatigue, significantly interferes with daily activities and work, and has four or more of the eight symptoms: post-exertion malaise lasting more than 24 h; unrefreshing sleep; significant impairment of short-term memory or concentration; muscle pain; pain in the joints without swelling or redness; headaches of a new type, pattern, or severity; tender lymph nodes in the neck or armpit; and a sore throat that is frequent or recurring (http://www.cdc.gov/cfs/case-definition/index.html). Fatigue is commonly seen in chronic rhinitis (Bhattacharyya 2003). Chronic rhinitis should be ruled out before a diagnosis of chronic fatigue syndrome is made, recognizing that individuals with chronic rhinitis may present with complaints of face pain, headache, fatigue, or other associated symptoms while minimizing or denying symptoms of rhinitis. Individuals with perennial allergic rhinitis or irritant rhinitis who are chronically exposed to allergens or irritants suffer from chronic fatigue.

*Irritable bowel syndrome (IBS).* This chronic condition characterized by crampy abdominal pain, nausea, emesis, and diarrhea alternating with constipation is reportedly induced after both chemical and infectious exposures. Post-infectious IBS is common, with the onset of IBS after an episode of acute gastroenteritis (Thabane and Marshall 2009). In analogy to RADS, the term reactive intestinal dysfunction syndrome (RIDS) has been introduced to describe individuals who develop IBS after irritant exposures (Lieberman and Craven 1998). IBS shares mechanistic aspects with irritant rhinitis and related conditions, including the roles of substance P, neurogenic inflammation, nociceptors, and central nervous system modulation and associated co-morbidities (Hunt and Tougas 2002; Stasi et al. 2012).

*Multiple chemical sensitivity syndrome (MCS).* This syndrome was defined as a condition of self-reported intolerance to environmental chemicals. In one description, it is an acquired condition in association with a chemical exposure, with symptoms involving multiple organ systems that are exacerbated by exposure to chemicals of diverse classes (Cullen 1987). This syndrome differs from RADS and RUDS with exacerbations when exposed to some of the irritants given in Table 1.1 in that reported symptoms involve more than one organ system. Hence, someone with airway inflammation exacerbated by irritant exposures who also experienced fatigue, headaches, rashes, and sleep disturbances—conditions known to be associated with rhinitis—would meet a case definition of MCS. Individuals with somatic disorders, odor aversion, chemophobia, anxiety attacks triggered by odors, and other psychological conditions would likewise meet these case definitions. Idiopathic environmental intolerances (IEI) is a term introduced to describe patients with no diagnosable medical condition and reported chemical intolerances (Anonymous 1996). IEI should only be used as a diagnosis for individuals without diagnosable medical conditions that can be caused or exacerbated by environmental exposures. Subjects who develop RADS and/or RUDS after a chemical exposure meet case definitions for MCS (Meggs 1992).

As our knowledge of the brain as a target organ for irritant and allergic reactions advances, diagnostic methods for irritant sensitivity improve, and understanding of the neuroscience of conditions such as depression and anxiety matures, some individuals now classified as IEI may have better descriptors.

The concept of MCS is in a sense flawed because it confuses diagnosis with etiology. Further, there are many conditions known to be caused by or exacerbated by chemical exposures, including irritant asthma and rhinitis, dermatitis, and so forth. Physicians would better serve their patients by diagnosing the conditions such as rhinitis or asthma and headaches than labeling them as having MCS. Case definitions of MCS do not specify the symptoms that are exacerbated by chemical exposures. Despite these challenges, the burden in the population of individuals who meet case definitions is huge. A study conducted by the California Department of Health found that 15.9 % of the population meet the criteria for MCS and that 7 % of the population had been diagnosed with MCS by a physician (Kreutzer et al. 1999). A prevalence of 15 % was found in New Mexico (Voorhees 1998) and 12.6 % in Georgia (Caress and Steinemann 2004a).

A population-based study in the United States found the prevalence of hypersensitivity to common chemical products such as perfume, fresh paint, pesticides, and other petrochemical-based substances to be 11.2 % (Caress and Steinemann 2004b). Further, 2.5 % reported that they had been medically diagnosed with MCS. Additionally, 31.1 % of those sampled reported adverse reactions to fragranced products, and 17.6 % experienced breathing difficulties and other health problems when exposed to air fresheners. Although chemical hypersensitivity was more common in women, it affected individuals in all demographic groups studied.

A study in North Carolina of the prevalence of allergies and chemical sensitivity that was more general—the screening questions would capture individuals with conditions such as asthma and/or rhinitis exacerbated by irritants but did not meet more stringent criteria for MCS—found a prevalence of 33 % for chemical sensitivity, comparable to the 35 % reporting allergy, with a 50 % overlap between the two groups (Meggs 1996a). These studies indicate that the burden of chemical sensitivity in the population is significant.

The burden of airway inflammation is also significant. In the United States, 20 % of the population suffers from allergic rhinitis, but the burden of nonallergic rhinitis is even greater, with 25 % suffering from nonallergic rhinitis and 50 % with mixed rhinitis (Bernstein 2010, Molgaard et al. 2007, Settipane and Lieberman 2001; Settipane and Charnock 2007).

## References

Al-Sayed EM, Abrahim KS. Second-hand tobacco smoke and children. Toxicol Ind Health. 2012; (Epub ahead of print).

Anonymous. International Programme on Chemical Safety/World Health Organization (IPCS/WHO). Conclusions and recommendations of a workshop on multiple chemical sensitivity (MCS). Regul Toxicol Pharmacol 1996;24:S188–S189.

Arif AA, Delclos GL. Association between cleaning-related chemicals and work-related asthma and asthma symptoms among healthcare professionals. Occup Environ Med. 2012;69(1):35–40. doi:10.1136/oem.2011.064865.

Banauch GI, Alleyne D, Sanchez R, Olender K, Cohen HW, Weiden M, Kelly KJ, Prezant DJ. Persistent hyperreactivity and reactive airway dysfunction in firefighters at the World Trade Center. Am J Respir Crit Care Med. 2003;168(1):54–62.

Barnes PJ. Neurogenic inflammation in the airways. Respir Physiol. 2001;125:145–54.

Bascom R. Differential susceptibility to tobacco smoke: possible mechanisms. Pharmacogenetics. 1991;1(2):102–6.

Bascom R, Kulle T, Kagey-Sobotka A, Proud D. Upper respiratory tract environmental tobacco smoke sensitivity. Am Rev Respir Dis. 1991;143(6):1304–11.

Baur X, Bakehe P, Vellguth H. Bronchial asthma and COPD due to irritants in the workplace – an evidence-based approach. J Occup Med Toxicol. 2012;7(1):19.

Bernstein DI. Diesel exhaust exposure, wheezing and sneezing. Allergy Asthma Immunol Res. 2012;4(4):178–83.

Bernstein JA, Levin LS, Al-Shuik E, Martin VT. Clinical characteristics of chronic rhinitis patients with high vs low irritant trigger burdens. Ann Allergy Asthma Immunol. 2012;109(3):173–8.

Bernstein JA. Allergic and mixed rhinitis: epidemiology and natural history. Allergy Asthma Proc. 2010;31:365–9.

Berglind N, Bellander T, Forastiere F, von Klot S, Aalto P, Elosua R, Kulmala M, Lanki T, Löwel H, Peters A, Picciotto S, Salomaa V, Stafoggia M, Sunyer J, Nyberg F, HEAPSS Study Group. Ambient air pollution and daily mortality among survivors of myocardial infarction. Epidemiology. 2009;20(1):110–8.

Bhattacharyya N. The economic burden and symptom manifestations of chronic rhinosinusitis. Am J Rhinol. 2003;17(1):27–32.

Biagini RE, Moorman WJ, Lewis TR, Bernstein IL. Ozone enhancement of platinum asthma in a primate model. Am Rev Respir Dis. 1986;134(4):719–25.

Bougault V, Boulet LP. Airway dysfunction in swimmers. Br J Sports Med. 2012;46(6):402–6. doi:10.1136/402 bjsports-2011-090821.

Bougault V, Loubaki L, Joubert P, Turmel J, Couture C, Laviolette M, Chakir J, Boulet LP. Airway remodeling and inflammation in competitive swimmers training in indoor chlorinated swimming pools. J Allergy Clin Immunol. 2012;129(2):351–8. 385 e1.

Brooks SM, Weiss MA, Bernstein IL. Reactive airways dysfunction syndrome (RADS). Persistent asthma syndrome after high level irritant exposures. Chest. 1985;88:376–84.

Brooks SM, Bernstein IL, Raghuprasad PK, Maccia CA, Mieczkowski L. Assessment of airway hyperresponsiveness in chronic stable asthma. J Allergy Clin Immunol. 1990;85:17–26.

Bruce AN. Vaso-dilatory axon reflexes. QJ Exp Physiol. 1913;6:339–54.

Bruce AN. Uber die beziehung der sensiblen nervenendigungen zum Enzundungsvorgang. Arch Exp Pathol Pharmakol. 1910;63:424.

Caress SM, Steinemann AC. Prevalence of multiple chemical sensitivities: a population-based study in the southeastern United States. Am J Public Health. 2004a;94(5):746–7.

Caress SM, Steinemann AC. A national population study of the prevalence of multiple chemical sensitivity. Arch Environ Health. 2004b;59(6):300–5.

Castano R, Malo JL. Occupational rhinitis and asthma: where do we stand, where do we go? Curr Allergy Asthma Rep. 2010;10:135–42.

Chahl LA. Antidromic vasodilation and neuro-genic inflammation. Pharmacol Ther. 1988;37: 275–300.

Cullen MR. The worker with multiple chemical sensitivities: an overview. In: Cullen MR, editor. Workers and Multiple Chemical Sensitivities. Philadelphia: Hanley & Belfus; 1987. p. 655–62.

D'Alò S, De Pasquale T, Incorvaia C, Illuminati I, Mistrello G, Roncarolo D, Pucci S. Chloramine-induced anaphylaxis while showering: a case report. J Med Case Rep. 2012;6(1):324. doi:10.1186/1752-1947-6-324.

Deger L, Plante C, Jacques L, Goudreau S, Perron S, Hicks J, Kosatsky T, Smargiassi A. Active and uncontrolled asthma among children exposed to air stack emissions of sulphur dioxide from petroleum refineries in Montreal, Quebec: a cross-sectional study. Can Respir J. 2012;19:97–102.

Elberling J, Skov PS, Mosbech H, Holst H, Dirksen A, Johansen JD. Increased release of histamine in patients with respiratory symptoms related to perfume. Clin Exp Allergy. 2007;37:1676–80.

Elberling J, Linneberg A, Dirksen A, Johansen JD, Frolund L, Madsen F, Nielsen NH, Mosbech H. Mucosal symptoms elicited by fragrance products in a population-based sample in relation to atopy and bronchial hyper-reactivity. Clin Exp Allergy. 2005;35:75–81.

Gasana J, Dillikar D, Mendy A, Forno E, Ramos Vieira E. Motor vehicle air pollution and asthma in children: a meta-analysis. Environ Res. 2012;117:36–45.

Gautrin D, Desrosiers M, Castano R. Occupational rhinitis. Curr Opin Allergy Clin Immunol. 2006;6:77–84.

Ghanei M, Harandi AA. Long term consequences from exposure to sulfur mustard: a review. Inhal Toxicol. 2007;19:451–6.

Groneberg DA, Quarcoo D, Frossard N, Fischer A. Neurogenic mechanisms in bronchial inflammatory diseases. Allergy. 2004;59(11):1139–52.

Hellgren J, Karlsson G, Torén K. The dilemma of occupational rhinitis: management options. Am J Respir Med. 2003;2:333–41.

Henderson SB, Johnston FH. Measures of forest fire smoke exposure and their associations with respiratory health outcomes. Curr Opin Allergy Clin Immunol. 2012;12(3):221–7.

Hernandez AF, Parron T, Alarcon R. Pesticides and asthma [review]. Curr Opin Allergy Clin Immunol. 2011;11(2):90–6.

Heydorn S, Johansen JD, Andersen KE, Bruze M, Svedman C, White IR, et al. Fragrance allergy in patients with hand eczema—a clinical study. Contact Dermatitis. 2003;48:317–23.

Hinsey JC, Gasser HS. The component of the dorsal root mediating vasodilation and the Sherrington contracture. Am J Physiol. 1930;92:679.

Hunt RH, Tougas G. Evolving concepts in functional gastrointestinal disorders: promising directions for novel pharmaceutical treatments. Best Pract Res Clin Gastroenterol. 2002;16(6):869–83.

Hussain S, Laumbach R, Coleman J, Youssef H, Kelly-McNeil K, Ohman-Strickland P, Zhang J, Kipen H. Controlled exposure to diesel exhaust causes increased nitrite in exhaled breath condensate among subjects with asthma. J Occup Environ Med. 2012;54(10):1186–91.

Jansco G. Neurogenic Inflammation in Health and Disease, Volume 8 (NeuroImmune Biology). Elsevier Science 2008.

Kim S, Kim Y, Lee MR, Kim J, Jung A, Park JS, Jang AS, Park SW, Uh ST, Choi JS, Kim YH, Buckley T, Park CS. Winter season temperature drops and sulfur dioxide levels affect on exacerbation of refractory asthma in South Korea: a time-trend controlled case-crossover study using soonchunhyang asthma cohort data. J Asthma. 2012;49:679–87.

Kreutzer R, Neutra RR, Lashuay N. Prevalence of people reporting sensitivities to chemicals in a population-based survey. Am J Epidermol. 1999;150:1–12.

Kumar P, Caradonna-Graham VM, Gupta S, Cai X, Rao PN, Thompson J. Inhalation challenge effects of perfume scent strips in patients with asthma. Ann Allergy Asthma Immunol. 1995;75: 429–33.

Leroyer C, Malo JL, Girard D, Dufour JG, Gautrin D. Chronic rhinitis in workers at risk of reactive airways dysfunction syndrome due to exposure to chlorine. Occup Environ Med. 1999;56(5):334–8.
Leslie CA, Mathe AA. Modification of guinea pig lung anaphylaxis by central nervous system. (CNS) perturbations. J Allergy Clin Immunol. 1989;83:94–101.
Levy RM, Rose JE, Johnson JS. Effect of vagotomy on anaphylaxis in rat. Clin Exp Immunol. 1976;24:96–101.
Lieberman AD, Craven MR. Reactive intestinal dysfunction syndrome (RIDS) caused by chemical exposures. Arch Environ Health. 1998;53:354–8.
Matsumura Y, Mizuno K, Miyamoto T, Suzuki T, Oshima Y. The effects of ozone, nitrogen dioxide, and sulfur dioxide on experimentally induced allergic respiratory disorder in guinea pigs. IV. Effects on respiratory sensitivity to inhaled acetylcholine. Am Rev Respir Dis. 1972;105(2):262–7.
Meggs WJ, Cleveland Jr CH. Rhinolaryngoscopy findings in patients with the multiple chemical sensitivity syndrome. Arch Environ Health. 1993;48:14–8.
Meggs WJ, Dunn KA, Bloch RM, Goodman PE, Davidoff AL. Prevalence and nature of allergy and chemical sensitivity in a general population. Arch Environ Health. 1996a;51:275–82.
Meggs WJ, Elsheik T, Metzger WJ, Albernaz M, Bloch RM. Nasal pathology and ultrastructure in patients with chronic airway inflammation (RADS and RUDS) following an irritant exposure. J Toxicol Clin Toxicol. 1996b;34(4):383–96.
Meggs WJ. Hypothesis for induction and propagation of chemical sensitivity based on biopsy studies. Environ Health Perspect. 1997;105 Suppl 2:473–8.
Meggs WJ. Neurogenic inflammation and sensitivity to environmental chemicals. Environ Health Perspect 1993;101:1–6.
Meggs WJ. Neurogenic switching: a hypothesis for a mechanism for shifting the site of inflammation in allergy and chemical sensitivity. Environ Health Perspect. 1995;103(1):54–6.
Millqvist E, Ternesten-Hasséus E, Ståhl A, Bende M. Changes in levels of nerve growth factor in nasal secretions after capsaicin inhalation in patients with airway symptoms from scents and chemicals. Environ Health Perspect. 2005;113(7):849–52.
Millqvist E, Bengtsson U, Löwhagen O. Provocations with perfume in the eyes induce airway symptoms in patients with sensory hyperreactivity. Allergy. 1999;54(5):495–9.
Millqvist E, Lowhagen O. Methacholine provocations do not reveal sensitivity to strong scents. Ann Allergy Asthma Immunol. 1998;80:381–4.
Molgaard E, Thomsen SF, Lund T, Pedersen L, Nolte H, Backer V. Differences between allergic and nonallergic rhinitis in a large sample of adolescents and adults. Allergy. 2007;62:1033–7.
Morris MJ, Christopher KL. Diagnostic criteria for the classification of vocal cord dysfunction. Chest. 2010;138:1213–23.
Moscato G, Vandenplas O, Van Wijk Gerth R, Malo JL, Quirce S, Walusiak J, Castano R, De Groot H, Folletti I, Gautrin D, Yacoub MR, Perfetti L, Siracusa A. Occupational rhinitis. EAACI Task Force on Occupational Rhinitis. Allergy. 2008;63:969–80.
Murakami Y, Ono M. Myocardial infarction deaths after high level exposure to particulate matter. J Epidemiol Community Health. 2006;60(3):262–6.
Nielsen GD. Mechanisms of activation of the sensory irritant receptor by airborne chemicals. Crit Rev Toxicol. 1991;21:183–208.
Nel AE, Diaz-Sanchez D, Ng D, Hiura T, Saxon A. Enhancement of allergic inflammation by the interaction between diesel exhaust particles and the immune system. J Allergy Clin Immunol. 1998;102(4 Pt 1):539–54.
Nordin S, Millqvist E, Lowhagen O, Bende M. A short chemical sensitivity scale for assessment of airway sensory hyperreactivity. Int Arch Occup Environ Health. 2004;77:249–54.
Opiekun RE, Smeets M, Sulewski M, Rogers R, Prasad N, Vedula U, Dalton P. Assessment of ocular and nasal irritation in asthmatics resulting from fragrance exposure. Clin Exp Allergy. 2003;33:1256–65.
Peters A, von Klot S, Heier M, Trentinaglia I, Hörmann A, Wichmann HE, Löwel H. Exposure to traffic and the onset of myocardial infarction. N Engl J Med. 2004;351:1721–30.

Raphael G, Raphael MH, Kaliner M. Gustatory rhinitis: a syndrome of food-induced rhinorrhea. J Allergy Clin Immunol. 1989;83(1):110–5.
Rudmik L, Smith TL. Quality of life in patients with chronic rhinosinusitis [Review]. Curr Allergy Asthma Rep. 2011;11(3):247–52.
Sanico AM, Koliatsos VE, Stanisz AM, Bienenstock J, Togias A. Neural hyperresponsiveness and nerve growth factor in allergic rhinitis. Int Arch Allergy Immunol. 1999;118(2–4):154–8.
Sanico AM, Stanisz AM, Gleeson TD, Bora S, Proud D, Bienenstock J, Koliatsos VE, Togias A. Nerve growth factor expression and release in allergic inflammatory disease of the upper airways. Am J Respir Crit Care Med. 2000;161(5):1631–5.
Senthilselvan A, McDuffie HH, Dosman JA. Association of asthma with use of pesticides. Results of a cross-sectional survey of farmers. Am Rev Respir Dis. 1992;146(4):884–7.
Settipane RA, Charnock DR. Epidemiology of rhinitis: allergic and nonallergic. Clin Allergy Immunol. 2007;19:23–34.
Settipane RA, Lieberman P. Update on nonallergic rhinitis. Ann Allergy Asthma Immunol. 2001;86:494–507.
Shen L. Tight junctions on the move: molecular mechanisms for epithelial barrier regulation. Ann N Y Acad Sci. 2012;1258:9–18.
Simoens S. The cost-effectiveness of immunotherapy for respiratory allergy: a review. Allergy. 2012;67(9):1087–105. doi:10.1111/j.1398-9995.2012.02861.x.
Spampinato S, Ferri S. Pharmacology of spinal peptides affecting sensory and motor functions: dynorphins, somatostatins and tachykinins. Pharmacol Res. 1991;23:113–27.
Stahl SM. Substance P and the neurokinins: novel peptide neurotransmitters in psychopharmacology. J Clin Psychiatry. 1999;60:77–8.
Stasi C, Rosselli M, Bellini M, Laffi G, Milani S. Altered neuro-endocrine-immune pathways in the irritable bowel syndrome: the top-down and the bottom-up model. J Gastroenterol. 2012;47:1177–85.
Steinemann AC. Fragranced consumer products and undisclosed ingredients. Environ Impact Assess Rev. 2009;29:32–8.
Steinemann AC, MacGregor IC, Gordon SM, Gallagher LG, Davis AL, Ribeiro DS, et al. Fragranced consumer products: chemicals emitted, ingredients unlisted. Environ Impact Assess Rev. 2011;31:328–33.
Tang EA, Matsui E, Wiesch DG, Samet JM. Epidemiology of asthma and allergic diseases (chapter 42). In: Adkinson NF et al., editors. Middleton's allergy: principles and practice. 7th ed. St Louis: Mosby; 2008.
Ternesten-Hasséus E, Bende M, Millqvist E. Increased capsaicin cough sensitivity in patients with multiple chemical sensitivity. J Occup Environ Med. 2002;44(11):1012–7.
Thabane M, Marshall JK. Post-infectious irritable bowel syndrome. World J Gastroenterol. 2009;15(29):3591–6.
US Army. Medical aspects of chemical and biological warfare. Volume 14. World War I.
Van Miert E, Sardella A, Nickmilder M, Bernard A. Respiratory effects associated with wood fuel use: a cross-sectional biomarker study among adolescent. Pediatr Pulmonol. 2012;47(4): 358–66.
Veronesi B, Oortgiesen M. Neurogenic inflammation and particulate matter (PM) air pollutants. Neurotoxicology. 2001;22:795–810.
Voorhees RM. Memorandum from New Mexico Deputy State Epidemiologist to Joe Thompson, Special Council, Office of the Governor. 13 March 1998.
Wallace DV, Dykewicz MS, Bernstein DI, Blessing-Moore J, Cox L, Khan DA, Lang DM, Nicklas RA, Oppenheimer J, Portnoy JM, Randolph CC, Schuller D, Spector SL, Tilles SA, Joint Task Force on Practice, American Academy of Allergy, Asthma & Immunology, American College of Allergy, Asthma and Immunology, Joint Council of Allergy, Asthma and Immunology. The diagnosis and management of rhinitis: an updated practice parameter. J Allergy Clin Immunol. 2008;122(2 Suppl):S1–84.
Weed FW, Editor. Medical Aspects of Gas Warfare. Vol 14 of The Medical Department of the United States Army in World War. Washington DC: Government Printing Office, 1926.

Willes SR, Fitzgerald TK, Permutt T, Proud D, Haley NJ, Bascom R. Acute respiratory response to prolonged, moderate levels of sidestream tobacco smoke. J Toxicol Environ Health A. 1998;53(3):193–209.

Yamaya M. Virus infection-induced bronchial asthma exacerbation. Pulm Med. 2012;2012:834826.

Yerpude PN, Jogdand KS. Morbidity profile of cotton mill workers. Indian J Occup Environ Med. 2010;14(3):94–6.

Youssefagha AH, Jayawardene WP, Lohrmann DK, El Afandi GS. Air pollution indicators predict outbreaks of asthma exacerbations among elementary school children: integration of daily environmental and school health surveillance systems in Pennsylvania. J Environ Monit. 2012;14(12):3202–10.

# Chapter 2
# Airway Anatomy, Physiology, and Inflammation

**Michael R. Van Scott, Joyce Chandler, Stephen Olmstead, Jared M. Brown, and Mark Mannie**

**Abstract** Approximately 10,000 l of air and 8,000 l of blood transit the respiratory system each day driven by small pressure gradients developed in response to rhythmic contraction and relaxation of striated muscle under both voluntary and involuntary control of the central nervous system. Matching of air- and blood flow results from central and local reflexes responding to both internal and external stimuli and subsequently controlling the pumps, as well as the smooth muscle in walls of the airways and blood vessels. A wide range of neural and immune mechanisms protect the lungs against environmental insults, and many are adaptive in nature, resulting in memory that increases sensitivity and responsiveness upon repeated exposure to stimuli. In over 10 % of the population, the responses to environmental stimuli become pathological, resulting in excessive sensitivity and aberrant responses to both specific and nonspecific stimuli, and culminate in physical remodeling of the airways and lungs. Prevention, definitive diagnosis, and effective treatment of the disorders require a better understanding of the mechanisms underlying excessive responses to environmental stimuli.

**Keywords** Pulmonary anatomy and physiology • Innervations of the respiratory tract • Airway remodeling

M.R. Van Scott, Ph.D. (✉) • J. Chandler, D.V.M. • S. Olmstead
Department of Physiology, Brody School of Medicine, East Carolina University,
600 Moye Blvd, Room 6N98, Greenville, NC 27858-4353, USA
e-mail: VANSCOTTMI@ecu.edu

J.M. Brown, Ph.D.
Department of Pharmacology and Toxicology, East Carolina University, Greenville, NC USA

M. Mannie, Ph.D.
Department of Microbiology and Immunology, East Carolina University, Greenville, NC USA

W.J. Meggs (ed.), *The Toxicant Induction of Irritant Asthma, Rhinitis, and Related Conditions*, DOI 10.1007/978-1-4614-9044-9_2,

An average adult at rest moves over 10,000 l of air through the respiratory tract and exchanges over 400 l of $O_2$ and $CO_2$ across the alveolar surface each day. Toxins and pathogens in the ambient air can damage the lung tissue, interfere with respiratory mechanics, and limit gas exchange. Both passive and active processes protect the lungs against environmental insults by filtering the inspired air; altering airflow and blood flow to limit alveolar and systemic exposure; capturing, killing, and rapidly clearing pathogens; and efficiently repairing damaged tissues to restore the mucosal barrier. Some of the defense mechanisms are adaptive, increasing the sensitivity of the system and intensity of responses to future insults. Dysregulation of defense pathways can increase sensitivity to nonspecific stimuli and lead to responses that are out of proportion to the insult. This chapter provides a brief overview of the anatomy and physiology of the respiratory tract in relation to development of hypersensitivity and hyperresponsiveness of the respiratory tract.

## Functional Anatomy of the Respiratory Tract

Flow of air through the respiratory tract is driven by small pressure gradients, and both the work of breathing and partitioning of airflow to different regions of the lungs are impacted by the resistance to airflow in each segment of the airways. The resistance to laminar flow of air through a rigid tube is related to its length and diameter. But most airways are deformable, not rigid; and are affected by mechanical forces and pressures impinging on the wall. Muscle, blood vessels, and glands in the airway wall are under local and reflex control, and actively respond to changes in the internal and external environments.

The respiratory tract is divided into two broad divisions: the upper and lower airways. The upper airways consist of the extrathoracic structures from the nares and mouth down to, and including, the larynx. Being extrathoracic, these airways are impacted by barometric pressure impinging on their external surface. The lower airways include the extrathoracic and intrathoracic portions of the trachea; the extrapulmonary and intrapulmonary bronchi; and the bronchioles, alveolar ducts, and alveoli, which are intrathoracic and intrapulmonary. Intrathoracic extrapulmonary airways are impacted by pressure that develops in the pleural space, which is normally negative, but becomes positive during forced expiration. Intrapulmonary airways are surrounded by alveoli, and their diameter is affected by changes in tension in the lung tissue impinging on their surface, as well as pressure of the alveolar gas, which oscillates from negative to positive during the respiratory cycle. Airways proximal to the respiratory bronchioles lack alveoli and are therefore classified as conducting airways, whereas the respiratory bronchioles, alveolar ducts, and alveoli constitute the gas exchange region of the lungs. With the exception of the pharynx, the walls of the airways become less rigid distally, with the walls of the upper airways containing bone and cartilage, the large lower airways containing cartilage rings or plates, and the small lower airways lacking bone and cartilage.

The nose and mouth represent two parallel pathways by which air enters and leaves the system. The nasal cavity and nasopharynx have a large surface area and tortuous path of airflow that is conducive to filtering, warming, and humidifying ambient air. The nares open into a vestibule, which leads to a constricted region called the nasal valve (Rhee and Kimbell 2012). Inferior, middle, and superior turbinates posterior to the nasal valve protrude into the airstream from each side of the central septum, increasing the surface area for exchange of heat and moisture. An olfactory region with a high density of olfactory receptors is located high in the nasal cavity. The majority of air passes through the nasal cavity along the floor, between the hard palate and inferior turbinate, and is forced to make a near 90° bend in the nasopharynx. Air flowing through the upper regions of the nasal cavity is forced to flow around the turbinates, but enters the nasopharynx at a less acute angle (Kelly et al. 2000). Both pathways are conducive to removal of large particles by impaction with the airway surface. Airflow through the nose is laminar at velocities up to 200 ml/s, which includes resting conditions; but the velocity is not uniform throughout the nose (Kelly et al. 2000). The olfactory region has a relatively low airflow velocity, which is presumed to protect the delicate olfactory receptors as well as keep the air in contact with the receptors for a longer period of time, allowing for detection of scents within the airstream (Kelly et al. 2000). At flow rates greater than 200 ml/s, turbulence develops, which increases resistance and work of breathing. The nasal cavity has fairly rigid walls, and the main factors that impact resistance to airflow in this region are physical obstructions such as polyps and septal deviation, swelling of the mucosa, and accumulation of secretions in the airway lumen.

The pharynx is posterior to the turbinates and separated into the nasopharynx, oropharynx, and laryngopharynx. The nasopharynx passes over the soft palate before opening into the oropharynx. Right and left Eustachian tubes open into the nasopharynx and connect the middle ear with the upper airway. In contrast to the nasal cavity, the pharynx in humans is deformable. The hyoid bone and soft tissue comprising the airway wall in this region are not directly attached to the surrounding skeletal structures, making the wall of the pharynx deformable (Dempsey et al. 2010; Susarla et al. 2010). In humans, there is a relatively large distance between the soft palate and epiglottis, and the face is flattened, resulting in a long, narrow oropharynx upon which the tongue encroaches. Another unique feature is that adipose tissue accumulates in the surrounding tissue and can apply pressure to the outside of the airway, affecting lumen diameter. As discussed later, all of these factors predispose the pharynx to collapsing late in expiration and during inspiration. The tendency to collapse is offset by two factors, neural reflexes that activate pharyngeal muscles and stiffen the wall, and by traction developed in the pharyngeal wall as the lung inflates (Dempsey et al. 2010; Susarla et al. 2010).

The epiglottis and larynx play major roles in protecting the lower airways. The epiglottis deflects solids and liquids traveling through the oropharynx airway from entering the larynx, directing them down the esophagus. The larynx has a high density of receptors for diverse chemical entities, that when stimulated evoke a cough reflex that expels solids and liquids from airway.

Humans have two lungs, which are divided into three lobes on the right—superior, middle, and inferior—and two lobes on the left—superior and inferior. The inner surface of the chest wall and outer surface of the lung are covered by parietal and visceral pleura, respectively, which are separated by a thin fluid-filled space. Anatomical and functional tracer studies indicate that drainage of the pleural space is via the superior mediastinal, intercostals, paraesophageal, and intra-abdominal lymph nodes, with the superior mediastinal lymph nodes being the sentinel nodes (Parungo et al. 2004, 2005).

The trachea, bronchi, and terminal bronchioles are conducting airways that lack alveoli. The trachea extends from the larynx in the cervical region to the carina in the thoracic cavity. Like the larynx, the carina is sensitive to tactile stimulation, which evokes cough. The wall of the trachea is supported by 15–20 C-shaped rings of cartilage interspersed with soft tissue. The posterior membrane connecting the ends of cartilaginous rings contains smooth muscle that can shorten the distance between the ends of the cartilage, decreasing the diameter of the trachea. Smooth muscle is also located between the cartilaginous rings allowing at least a small degree of active regulation of tracheal length. Shortening of the trachea can reduce resistance to airflow by both decreasing the length of the airway and increasing traction on the pharynx, stiffening the wall and opposing collapse.

In contrast to the trachea, the bronchial wall is supported by plates of cartilage with a higher degree of deformability than the tracheal rings. The bronchioles lack cartilage, with the wall consisting of epithelium attached to its basement membrane, a lamina propria, and a smooth muscle layer. Alveolar septa attach to the outside of the bronchioles, and changes in alveolar pressure and tension in the lung tissue have large effects on the diameter of the bronchioles. The bronchioles branch into alveolar ducts that terminate in alveolar sacs.

Dichotomous branching of the airways leads to an increase in the number of airways in parallel. The diameter of each airway decreases; but the aggregate, or total cross-sectional diameter of the airspace increases distally, which has two prominent functional impacts. First, the velocity of airflow diminishes, decreasing turbulence. Second, total resistance to airflow decreases exponentially with the increase in the effective/aggregate radius of the airways. Only about 2 % of the total airway resistance is accounted for by the bronchioles and alveolar ducts; and likewise only a small decrease in lumen pressure occurs along normal distal airways during exhalation. The relatively small pressure drop along the intrapulmonary airways minimizes the tendency for dynamic compression of the airways induced by the differential between a positive alveolar pressure surrounding the airways and reduced luminal pressure due the resistive drop during exhalation. Partial obstruction of distal airways due to contraction of smooth muscle or accumulation of secretions in the airway lumen leads to increased resistance and a greater-than-normal decrease in luminal pressure, predisposing the airways to close earlier than normal during exhalation.

The airways terminate in alveolar sacs, which are polygonal structures covered largely by a simple squamous Type 1 alveolar epithelial cells. Cuboidal alveolar Type II cells that produce and secrete surface active alveolar surfactant localize to the corners of the alveoli. The barrier between the blood in the capillaries and the air in the each alveolus is less than 1 μm thick. The thinness of the barrier is in part due to the alveolar epithelium and alveolar capillary endothelium sharing the same basement membrane, thereby eliminating excess interstitial tissue. This extremely thin barrier facilitates rapid diffusion of gas between the alveolar air and blood while maintaining an intact barrier between the external and internal environments.

Collagen and elastin fibers run through the lung tissue, interconnecting proteoglycans and glycosaminoglycans of the ground substance with the cells making up the lung surface, alveolar walls, blood vessels, and airways. This fibrous matrix results in interdependence of lung structures (i.e., airways, blood vessels, alveoli) (Faffe and Zin 2009). The elastin fibers are largely responsible for the elastance of the lung tissue and its tendency to return to its original shape after being deformed. Collagen fibers are stiffer than elastin fibers, and at low lung volumes are thought to be slack. As lung volumes increase, collagen fibers become taut and provide tissue rigidity and opposition to over-stretching of the lung tissue.

In addition to the tissue properties that affect expansion and contraction of the lungs, the air–liquid interface at the alveolar surface impacts lung mechanics and function. Surface tension pulls on surface of curved air–liquid interfaces, tending to reduce the surface area of the interface. The pressure developed by surface tension adds to the tissue recoil force, facilitating exhalation but resisting lung expansion. The pressure developed by surface tension promotes the transfer of air from alveoli with small radii into larger alveoli, which can result in collapse of small alveoli and development of atelectasis if surface tension is too great. Surface tension also induces a pressure differential between fluid in the interstitial compartment and the airway surface, which acts to pull water out of capillaries and the alveolar wall and into the airspace, leading to alveolar edema.

Surface tension in normal lungs is reduced by surfactant released from Type II pneumocytes. Surfactant is comprised of phospholipid, mainly dipalmitoylphosphatidylcholine (DPPC), neutral lipids including cholesterol, and proteins (Perez-Gil and Weaver 2010). When released from Type II cells, the lipids form a complex tubular structure, tubular myelin, in the liquid layer on the alveolar surface. During lung inflation, surfactant apoproteins B and C (SP-B and SP-C) facilitate the insertion of the lipid into the interfacial film to maintain a relatively uniform concentration of the surface-active material at the interface. Compression of the surface during exhalation leads to regeneration of the tubular myelin. The insertion of the hydrophilic heads of the phospholipid molecules into the water layer is thought to disrupt the intermolecular attraction of the water molecules that give rise to surface tension.

Both SP-B and SP-C are produced as proproteins in Type II cells. SP-B is also produced by Clara cells, but unlike Type II cells that process the proprotein to produce mature SP-B, Clara cells cannot produce the mature protein. Of the two proteins, SP-B appears to be of greater importance on an acute basis, and a 75 % reduction in SP-B levels in the airspaces is fatal (Perez-Gil and Weaver 2010). In contrast, SP-C deficiency leads to chronic, progressive lung disease in both humans and animals (Perez-Gil and Weaver 2010).

Two other surfactant-associated proteins, SP-A and SP-D, belong the collectin family of proteins with collagen-like lectin domains. SP-A has some ability to facilitate formation of tubular myelin and adsorption of surfactant on the alveolar surface, but also enhances killing, aggregation, and phagocytosis of microorganisms (Orgeig et al. 2010). The antimicrobial activity of SP-A is a result of direct opsonization of pathogens, as well as upregulation of pattern recognition receptors on phagocytes that mediate uptake and elimination of the foreign bodies. SP-D has similar functional properties to SP-A, but in addition, modulates macrophage, dendritic cell, and T-cell functions (Orgeig et al. 2010; Forbes and Haczku 2010). Deficiency in SP-D leads to increased numbers of myeloid dendritic cells in the lungs that promote Th2 responses. Treatment with recombinant SP-D can reduce allergen-induced eosinophilic inflammation and antigen-specific IgE production (Orgeig et al. 2010).

Separate circulations supply blood to the nose, larynx, trachea, and lungs. The nasal mucosa is perfused by the sphenopalatine branches of the maxillary artery, the anterior and posterior ethmoidal branches of the ophthalmic artery, and the superior labial artery, a branch of the facial artery (Osborn 1978). The larynx is perfused by the superior and inferior branches of the laryngeal artery, which stem from superior and inferior thyroid arteries, and run to the larynx alongside the superior and inferior laryngeal nerves (Weir 1997). Blood flow to the trachea is via the inferior thyroid, supreme intercostal, subclavian, internal mammary, innominate, and bronchial arteries. The branching from these arteries connects with one another to form longitudinal tracheal anastomoses that give rise to intercartilaginous submucosal capillary plexuses (Salassa et al. 1977). The bronchial circulation provides oxygenated blood to the bronchi and walls of the intrapulmonary airways, and the pulmonary circulation delivers mixed venous blood to the alveolar capillaries for gas exchange.

An extensive lymphatic system drains the lungs and thoracic cavity (Gray 2000; Carati and Gannon 2006). The lymph vessels are divided into parietal and visceral components. Plexuses of parietal lymphatic vessels drain into sternal, intercostals, diaphragmatic, and axillary nodes. The visceral lymph nodes are located along the mediastinum in associated with the esophagus, large veins and arteries, and pericardium and along the trachea and bronchi. Drainage of the lungs is via two plexuses: superficial and deep. The superficial plexus is located beneath the visceral pleura and drains to nodes at the hilus. The deep plexus consists of vessels surrounding airways and blood vessels. In the bronchioles, there is a single plexus, but in the bronchi there are two plexuses, submucosal and peribronchial. The deep plexus drains into tracheobronchial nodes. The lymphatic vessels terminate at the alveolar ducts, and fluid from the alveolar wall moves to the vessels in response to the "pumping" action of respiration.

## Airway Musculature

Muscles of the upper airways are striated under autonomous, and in some cases, conscious control. Pharyngeal muscles are separated into four muscle groups based on the structures they control: the tongue, palate, hyoid bone, and wall of the pharynx (Edwards and White 2011). The extrinsic muscles of the tongue include the genioglossus, styloglossus, and hypoglossus. The genioglossus pulls the tongue forward and down, keeping the tongue from occluding the oropharynx. The genioglossus exhibits phasic activity during inspiration, tonic activity during expiration, and responds to hypoxia, hypercapnia, and negative pressure in the larynx, indicating that it is controlled in least in part through the respiratory centers in the brain stem. Both the styloglossus and hypoglossus retract the tongue. When activated in concert with the genioglossus muscle, they help stiffen the tongue and oppose collapse of the oropharynx.

The palate is controlled by five muscles: the tensor palatini, levator palatini, palatoglossus, palatopharyngeus, and muscular uvula. The tensor palatine stiffens the soft palate. The levator palatini and palatoglossus raise and lower the soft palate, respectively, either closing or opening the nasal and oral air passages, respectively. The palatopharyngeus lifts and moves the soft palate anteriorly, and the muscular uvula raises the uvula. The geniohyoid, mylohyoid, thyrohyoid, sternohyoid, stylohyoid, and omohyoid manipulate the hyoid bone, moving it anteriorly and caudally, dilating the upper airway. The pharyngeal constrictor muscles assist in swallowing and constrict the airway at normal and elevated lung volumes (Edwards and White 2011).

At the level of the larynx, the muscle in the airway wall transitions to a smooth muscle phenotype. Smooth muscle is found throughout the airways, from the trachea to alveolar ducts.

## Innervation

### *Upper Airways*

The upper airways are innervated by sensory, motor, parasympathetic, and sympathetic neurons (Fig. 2.1a) (Sarin et al. 2006; Yoshida et al. 2000; Undem et al. 1999). Olfaction is carried in cranial nerve I (CN I), and taste is carried in the facial and glossopharyngeal nerves (CN VII and IX). Other sensory modalities are from the mouth, nasal cavity, and nasopharynx are transmitted in the trigeminal nerve (CN V) via the ophthalmic (V1), maxillary (V2), and mandibular (V3) branches. A pharyngeal plexus innervated by the glossopharyngeal (CN IX), vagus (CN X), cranial accessory (CN XI) nerves conveys sensation from the lower aspect of the nasopharynx, the oropharynx, and supralaryngeal pharynx. Sensation from the larynx is carried in the internal, external, and recurrent laryngeal branches of the vagus nerve.

The soft palate and walls of the pharynx contain both constrictor and dilator muscles that move contents of the pharynx to the esophagus, close the nasopharynx and larynx during swallowing, and stabilize the airway during normal breathing. Branchial motor neurons originating in the trigeminal motor nucleus pass through the trigeminal nerve, trigeminal ganglion, and mandibular nerves to innervate the tensor veli palatine, which stiffens the soft palate. The vagus nerve (CN X) innervates the remaining muscles of the soft palate (levator veli palatine, palatoglossus,

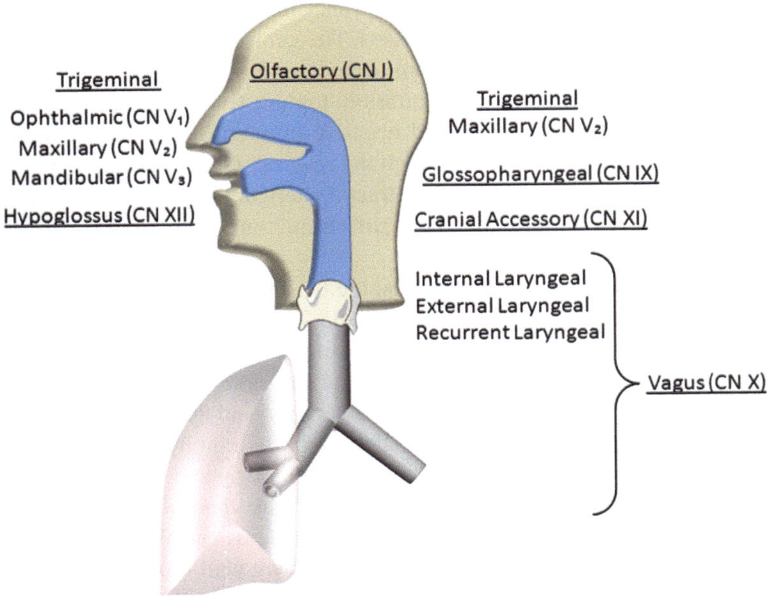


**Fig. 2.1** Cranial nerves innervating the upper and lower airways

palatopharyngeus, musculus uvulae), the major constrictor muscles in the pharyngeal wall (superior, middle, and inferior constrictors), the salpingopharyngeus muscle that draws the larynx upward during swallowing, and the muscle of the larynx. The glossopharyngeal nerve (CN IX) innervates the stylopharyngeus, which also draws the larynx upward, dilating the pharynx. Motor control of the tongue is mainly via the hypoglossal nerve (CN XII), except for the palatoglossus muscle that is innervated from the vagus nerve via the pharyngeal plexus, as mentioned above.

Autonomic innervation of the upper airways is from the deep petrosal, facial, and vagus nerves. Parasympathetic innervation of the nose is via the facial nerve. Preganglionic parasympathetic fibers originate in facial and superior salivatory nuclei, exit the brain stem in the facial nerve (CN VII), and branch into the greater superior petrosal nerve. The greater superior petrosal nerve merges with the deep petrosal nerve to form the Vidian nerve that leads to the pyterygopalatine or sphenopalatine, ganglion. Postganglionic fibers from the spenopalatine ganglion distribute to the surface epithelium, glands, arteries, and veins in the nasal mucosa. Acetylcholine (Ach) is the major preganglionic and postganglionic transmitter, although vasoactive intestinal peptide (VIP), peptide histidine methionine, peptide histidine valine, secretoneurin, and nitric oxide have also been associated with cholinergic neurons (Sarin et al. 2006). Parasympathetic output induces serous and mucous secretions and vasodilation.

Preganglionic sympathetic fibers innervating the nose arise from the thoracic and lumbar regions of the spinal cord and are carried to the superior cervical ganglion via the vagosympathetic trunk. Postganglionic sympathetic fibers from the superior cervical ganglion destined for the nasal cavity and nasopharynx are carried in the deep petrosal nerve, which merges with the greater petrosal nerve to form the Vidian nerve (Sarin et al. 2006). The fibers pass through the sphenopalatine ganglion and are distributed to the mucosa with fibers from the trigeminal nerve. Postganglionic sympathetic fibers innervating the pharyngeal plexus derive from direct gray rami communicans from the superior ganglion. Sympathetic fibers primarily innervate the mucosal vasculature, inducing vasoconstriction. Activation of α1 and α2 adrenoceptors or neuropeptide Y receptors on arterioles and venous sinusoids leads to vasoconstriction, lower mucosal blood flow, and less pooling of blood in the mucosal vasculature (Sarin et al. 2006). Adrenergic stimulation has been associated with secretion by glands, but sympathetic innervation of glands is sparse (Undem et al. 1999).

### *Lower Airways*

The lungs are innervated by parasympathetic cholinergic and parasympathetic noncholinergic neurons carried in the vagus nerve (CN X), and sympathetic adrenergic and sympathetic nonadrenergic neurons carried in spinal nerves between T1 and T6 (Fig. 2.1b) (Lee and Pisarri 2001; Canning 2006). Parasympathetic innervation of the lungs is conserved across species, whereas sympathetic innervation exhibits significant species variation. The majority of sympathetic postganglionic efferent fibers originate in the superior cervical ganglion and thoracic ganglia. Human airway smooth muscle exhibits little sympathetic innervation, whereas other species exhibit significant sympathetic-mediated constriction and relaxation effects based on whether α- or β- adrenoceptors are expressed on the postsynaptic membrane (Canning 2006). Likewise, in humans, a convincing role for sympathetic control of gland and epithelial secretions has not been demonstrated (Rogers 2001).

Parasympathetic innervation of the lungs includes afferent and efferent neurons. Preganglionic parasympathetic efferent neurons emanate from dorsal motor nuclei of the vagus or nucleus ambiguus. Postganglionic fibers originate in plexuses within the airway wall associated with mucosa, submucosa, smooth muscle, peri-tracheal, and peribronchial layers (Wine 2007). Afferent fibers exiting the lungs travel through the vagus nerve to the nodose and intracranial jugular ganglia, which in turn have outputs to the nucleus tractus solitarius. Afferent neurons include myelinated Aδ and nonmyelinated C fibers. Aδ fibers exhibit an organized pattern of terminals with attachments to the mucosal extracellular matrix making them responsive to mechanical deformation of the airway wall (Canning 2011). The Aδ mechanosensitive fibers can be separated into slowly adapting (SAR) and rapidly adapting (RAR) functional phenotypes, with SARs being associated with regulatory inflation and deflation reflexes (e.g., Hering-Breuer); and RARs being polymodal and associated with defensive reflexes such as cough and sneeze (Widdicombe 1982). Lung afferent C-fibers are small, nonmyelinated fibers that terminate in the airway wall, vasculature, and parenchyma. Similar to nociceptors in other tissues, these fibers are polymodal and are typically classified as chemoreceptors (Lee and Pisarri 2001). C fibers in the lungs are classified into two groups, bronchial and pulmonary, based on the circulation that perfuses the tissues they innervate.

In addition to conventional sympathetic adrenergic and parasympathetic cholinergic fibers, the upper and lower airways are replete with neurons that release nonadrenergic noncholinergic transmitters, either in concert with or independent of acetylcholine and norepinephrine. The noncholinergic nonadrenergic (NANC) neurons were originally referred to as a discrete subset (Rogers 2001), but in the last decade there has been increasing reference to these neurons as subtypes of sympathetic and parasympathetic neurons (Canning 2006).

Although less developed than in the gut, the neural network within the airway wall is extensive and exhibits some capacity to control airway functions without efferent input from the central nervous system. One mechanism by which this occurs is antidromic conduction of action potential in branches of afferent nerve fibers. Action potentials generated at sensory nerve terminals in the airway mucosa can be conducted along branches of the afferent neuron leading to the surface epithelium, glands, and blood vessels within the airway wall. Release of neurotransmitters, particularly NANC transmitters, results in intrinsic control of airway functions, initiating responses or modulating centrally mediated responses. Axon reflexes are common in the airways of rats and guinea pigs, but their overall importance in humans is a matter of debate. While direct empirical evidence of the importance of intrinsic control of airway tone and secretory activity is lacking, the fact that airways in transplanted lungs can function relatively normally for years without external innervations argues in favor of some intrinsic mechanism for maintaining airway patency and protecting the airways from environmental insult (Wine 2007) (Fig. 2.2).

## *Mechanical, Thermal, and Chemical Receptors*

Whereas SAR's respond primarily to mechanical deformation, RAR and C-fibers are polymodal, responding to diverse stimuli including temperature, acidity, and osmolarity. Transient receptor potential cation channels (TRP channels) are involved in transduction of environmental stimuli into physiologically relevant cellular responses. TRP channels are express on numerous cell types within the airway wall, including neurons (Fig. 2.3).

TRP channels were first described in relation to phospholipase C (PLC)-dependent phototransduction in *Drosophila* (Hardie and Minke 1995), and later as a family of mammalian proteins involved in capacitative calcium entry induced by diverse stimuli via PLC-dependent and -independent mechanisms (Birnbaumer et al. 1996; Zhu et al. 1996). In 2001, TRPs were implicated in hypoxic vasoconstriction (McDaniel et al. 2001; 2002), bronchoconstriction, and bronchial smooth muscle proliferation (Sweeney et al. 2002); and by 2003 were recognized as potential targets in diverse environmental and inflammatory lung diseases (Li et al. 2003). From a more fundamental standpoint, they constitute a critical interface between the

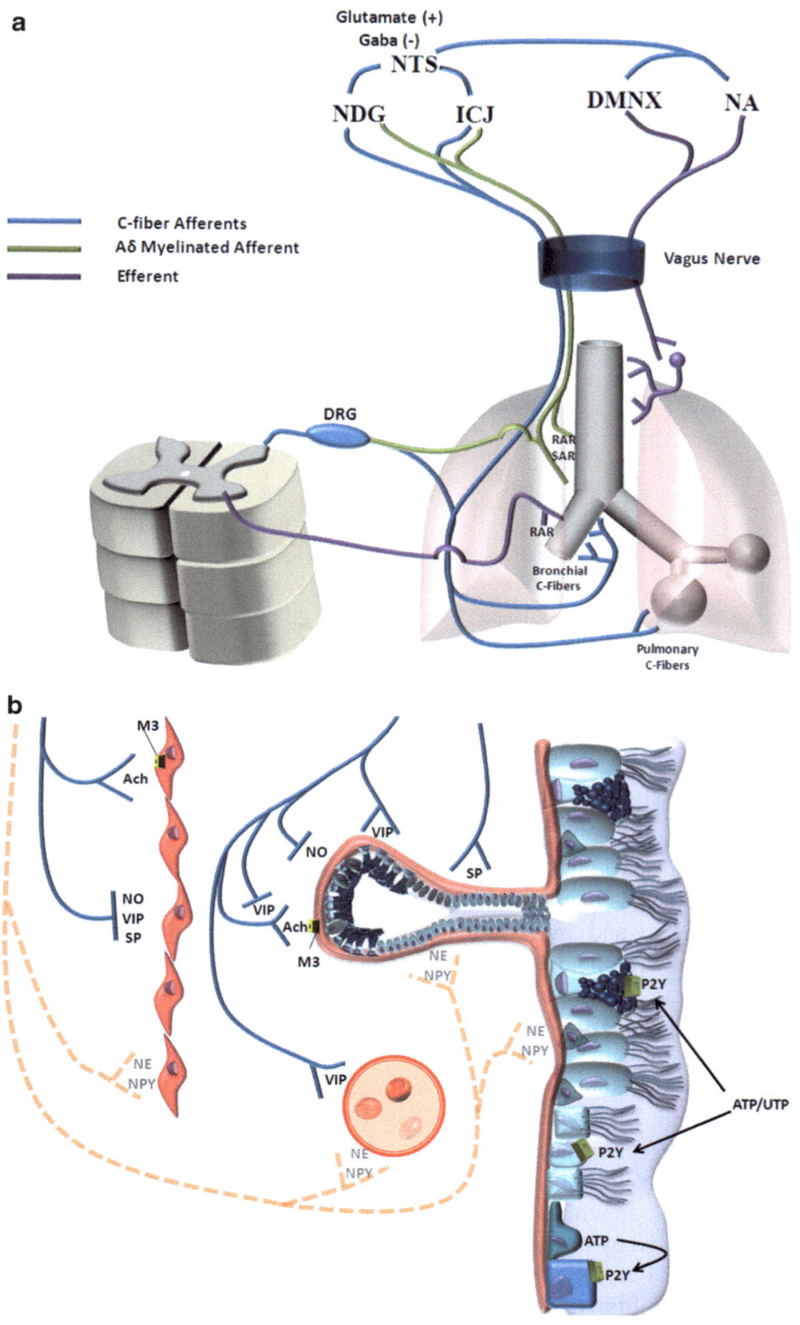


**Fig. 2.2** Innervation of the lower airways. (**a**) Distribution of autonomic fibers. (**b**) End organ innervations within the airway mucosa. *Dashed lines* represent sympathetic fibers, which have minimal activity in humans. *RAR* rapidly adapting receptor, *SAR* slowly adapting receptor, *DRG* dorsal root ganglion, *NDG* nodose ganglion, *ICJ* intracranial jugular ganglion, *NTS* nucleus tractus solitarius, *DMNX* dorsal motor nucleus of cranial nerve X, *NA* nucleus ambiguus, *M3* muscarinic receptor subtype 3, *Ach* acetylcholine, *NO* nitric oxide, *VIP* vasoactive intestinal peptide, *SP* substance P, *NE* norepinephrine, *NPY* neuropeptide Y, *P2Y* purinergic receptor 2Y

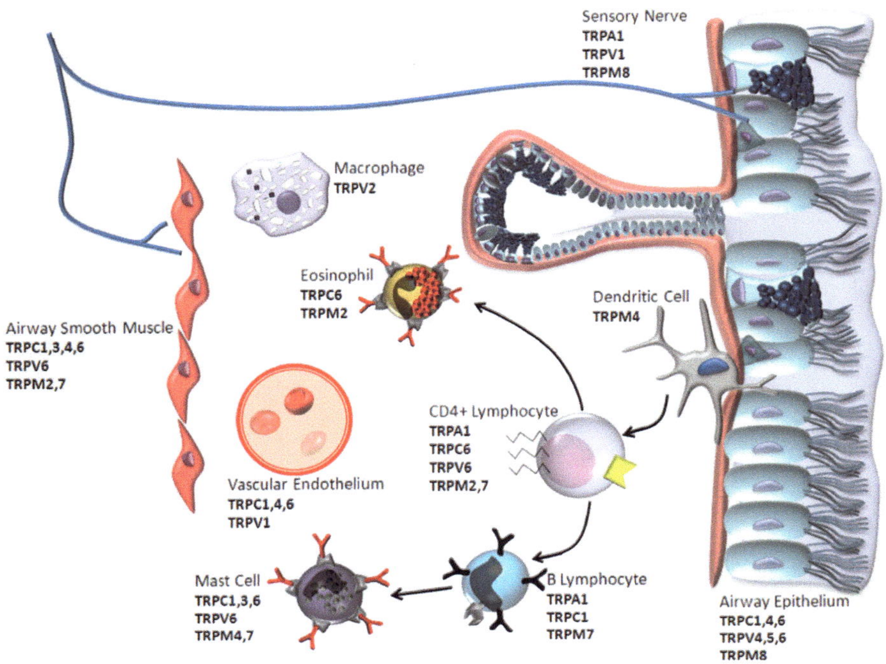


**Fig. 2.3** Expression of transient receptor potential (TRP) cation channel subtypes in the structural and inflammatory cells of the airway mucosa. TRP subtypes are defined in the text

environment and the lungs, transducing changes in temperature, osmolality, pressure, stretch, pH, and chemical stimuli into transmembrane cation fluxes, membrane potential changes, and intracellular second messenger signals. In addition to responding to environmental cues, changes in intracellular second messengers originating from activation of other signaling cascades can modulate TRP function, including their sensitivity to primary stimuli (Moran et al. 2011).

The TRP family has 28 members subdivided into six subfamilies on the basis of sequence homology and chemical activation: TRPC (canonical), TRPV (vanilloid), TRPM (melastatin), TRPA (ankyrin), TRPP (polycystin), and TRPML (mucolipin). Activation of TRP can lead to depolarization due to enhanced cation conductance, elevation of intracellular $Ca^{2+}$ concentration, or hyperpolarization when the channels are co-expressed with BKCa $K^+$ channels (Moran et al. 2011; Kim et al. 2009). TRPs are expressed by many of the major cell types involved in asthma and COPD, and data indicate that TRP channels are involved in osmotic sensing, modulation of vascular permeability, mucociliary clearance, and inflammation (Colsoul et al. 2009). In most cases, in vivo studies confirming physiological and pathophysiological roles for these receptors are lacking, but in the case of TRPA1, TRPC6, TRPV1, TRPV4, and TRPM4 in vivo validation is emerging (Banner et al. 2011). TRPA1 is activated by diverse chemical stimuli, including changes in pH, and cold. TRPV1 is activated by heat, acid, and high chemical stimuli, but at higher concentrations than those known to activate TRPA1. TRPC6 is expressed in vascular smooth muscle and endothelium, and its activity is affected by mechanical stimuli, including stretch. TRPC6 has been linked to hypoxic vasoconstriction in pulmonary vasculature (Weissmann et al. 2006) and plays a role in formation of pulmonary edema following pulmonary ischemia and reperfusion, as well as podocyte formation in kidney cells (Kim et al. 2009). TRPV4 has also been linked to changes in vascular permeability and formation of pulmonary edema induced by high vascular pressure, airway inflation pressures, and tidal volumes (Banner et al. 2011).

TRP channels are expressed on cells involved in innate and adaptive immunity, and have been implicated in inflammatory responses to environmental stimuli. TRPA1 and TRPC6 have been associated with enhanced allergic inflammation (Caceres et al. 2009; Sel et al. 2008). In contrast, TRPV1 has been reported to protect against allergic sensitization to aeroallergens but not sensitization to system allergens (Mori et al. 2011). Differential effects of TRPV1 that are dependent on the route of sensitization is an interesting observation in that neutrophilic inflammation and airway hyperresponsiveness induced by LPS and allergen have also been shown to be affected by the route of sensitization (Wilson et al. 2009), raising the question of whether TRPV plays a role in differentiating between immune responses originating systemically and at a mucosal barrier. TRPM4 has been associated with down-regulation of IgE-mediated mast cell activation in vivo (Banner et al. 2011).

## Reflexes

For this discussion, reflexes in the respiratory system will be separated into two categories, regulatory and defensive. Regulatory reflexes are homeostatic in nature. Physiological parameters are monitored, and ventilation and perfusion are modulated to maintain the composition of arterial blood while maximizing efficiency of breathing and gas exchange. The major physiological parameters monitored in regulatory reflexes are mechanical deformation of airways and blood vessels, $CO_2$ via pH, and arterial partial pressure $O_2$ ( $P_{aO_2}$ ). In contrast, defensive reflexes respond to environmental stimuli to protect cardiopulmonary function. Composition, or quality, of the air is monitored; and ventilation, perfusion, and mucosal functions are modulated to minimize exposure of tissues to injurious, or detrimental factors. The major parameters inducing defensive reflexes are changes in tactile sensation, temperature, acidity, and molecular structures at the mucosal surface.

### *Regulatory Reflexes*

Maintenance of $O_2$, $CO_2$, and pH levels is a primary function of the respiratory system. The basic reflexes linking changes in $O_2$, $CO_2$, and pH to ventilation are described in textbooks of physiology and will not be reiterated here; but changes in sensitivity to $CO_2$ in relation to respiratory drive and sleep apnea and reflex control of the airways by $O_2$ and $CO_2$ deserve consideration. Under normal conditions, hypercapnia and hypoxia are primary stimuli of the respiratory central pattern generator (CPG) in the brainstem. During sleep in normal individuals, the sensitivity to $CO_2$ decreases, resulting in an elevation of $P_{aCO_2}$ by 3–6 mmHg (Dempsey et al. 2010; Skatrud and Dempsey 1983). In parallel, the apnea threshold, or the $P_{aCO_2}$ below which an individual will be apneic, increases in parallel and remains 4–5 mmHg lower than the steady state $P_{aCO_2}$. Normal individuals retain sensitivity to small changes in $CO_2$ during sleep and respond with changes in ventilation that maintain $p_{aCO_2}$ within a narrow range and above the apnea threshold (Naughton 2010). So, $P_{aCO_2}$ remains high but stable. In contrast, patients with sleep apnea do not exhibit elevated $P_{aCO_2}$ during sleep or a reduction in the apnea threshold, resulting in a smaller difference between the steady state $P_{aCO_2}$ during sleep and apnea threshold (Naughton 2010; Xie et al. 2002). Thus, small decreases in $P_{aCO_2}$ lead to apnea and unstable breathing.

During inspiration, negative pressure develops in the airway lumen, acting to collapse the airway and restrict airflow, particularly in the extrathoracic airways that are surrounded by barometric pressure. Reflexes exist to both preempt and respond to collapse of the upper airways. Reflexes that preempt closure of the upper airways originate in the CPG. Many of the muscles of the upper airways receive input from the CPG, which synchronizes their activity with inspiration and expiration and modifies their activity in response to respiratory stimulants and depressants, such as hypoxia, hypercapnia, and opiates. The genioglossus is the upper airway muscle that is best studied in this regard. The genioglossus contracts 50–100 ms before the beginning of inspiration, pulling the tongue forward and down, away from the pharynx, presumably in preparation for the development of negative airway pressure that would act to pull the tongue back into the oropharynx (Edwards and White 2011).

In addition to extrinsic regulation by the CPG, muscles in the pharynx, and the lower airways as well, respond to local deformation of airway and lung tissue leading to reactive regulation of airway diameter, respiratory drive, and cardiac function. The effect of mechanical deformation is observed both within and across regions of the airways. The processes have been defined best in the lower airways, but are also known to be present in the upper airways. Both the active development of compressing transmural pressure during inspiration and passive compression by surrounding tissues tends to collapse the oropharynx. Collapse of the pharyngeal wall is opposed by active and passive forces (Susarla et al. 2010). Negative pressure that develops in the pharynx during inspiration activates mechanoreceptors in the pharyngeal wall, inducing reflex contraction of constrictor muscles that stabilize the wall and oppose collapse. Simultaneously, expansion of the lungs increases traction on the upper airways, stiffening and opposing collapse of the pharynx. Conversely, positive pressure developed during exhalation induces activation of pharyngeal dilator muscles. Simultaneously, loss of traction on the pharynx as the lung deflates leads to progressive loss of tension in the pharyngeal wall during exhalation. The combination of a high level of pharyngeal dilator activity and compression by fat deposits in the wall of the pharynx has been implicated in collapse of the oropharynx late in expiration in obstructive sleep apnea (Susarla et al. 2010).

Pressure changes in the upper airways also affect ventilation (Widdicombe 2011). In adults, negative pressure in the pharynx, particularly in response to nasal obstruction, inhibits respiratory drive and increases expiratory and inspiratory time, and positive pressure has a small stimulatory effect on breathing frequency. Reflex stabilization of the upper airways by positive pressure, and reversing the decrease in respiratory drive associated with negative pressure may underlie the effectiveness of continuous positive airway pressure in alleviating sleep apnea (Widdicombe 2011).

Of the three classes of sensory fibers found in the airways—SAR, RAR, and C-fibers—SAR neurons are most closely associated with regulatory reflexes. Activation leads to tachycardia, relaxation of airway smooth muscle, inhibition of inspiratory drive, and prolongation of expiration (Kubin et al. 2006; Coleridge and Coleridge 1994; Hlastala and Berger 2001). Tachycardia increases cardiac output to accommodate the increase in venous return associated with the lower thoracic pressure and to better match the volumes of blood and air in the lungs. Relaxation of airway smooth muscle allows the airways to expand in concert with the increase in recoil force within the lung tissue. Inhibition of inspiratory drive opposes overinflation, and prolongation of expiration insures that inspiratory and expiratory volumes are matched.

## *Defensive Reflexes*

Defensive reflexes mediate changes in mucociliary clearance, sneezing and coughing to actively clear inhaled agents from the airways. Reflex changes in ventilation and perfusion limit distribution of inspired agents throughout the lungs and to other organs that could be damaged due to exposure to the toxin. Compared to SAR fibers involved in regulatory reflexes, RAR neurons, and C-fibers exhibit greater sensitivity to tactile stimulation, pH, and chemical agents; and play major roles in defensive reflexes. RAR neurons respond to mechanical deformation but also to inhaled irritants (e.g., smoke and ammonia (Kubin et al. 2006)) and low osmolarity solutions (Coleridge and Coleridge 1994). C-fibers are less sensitive to mechanical deformation; but highly sensitive to pH changes, chemicals (e.g., ozone and capsaicin), high osmolarity solutions, and temperature changes (Kubin et al. 2006; Coleridge and Coleridge 1994). Response of the RAR irritant receptors is associated with cough, bronchoconstriction, and mucus secretion (Hlastala and Berger 2001). C-fiber activation is associated with cough, rapid shallow breathing and apnea, bronchoconstriction, mucus secretion, bradycardia, and hypotension (Kubin et al. 2006; Coleridge and Coleridge 1994; Hlastala and Berger 2001).

Under normal conditions, SAR neurons, RAR neurons, and C-fiber neurons are distinct subpopulations physiologically and anatomically. The respond to unique stimuli, exhibit unique temporal responses to stimuli, and terminate in separate regions within the NTS. Yet, outputs from the NTS converge on brainstem and spinal neurons controlling ventilation, cardiac function, airway diameter, salivary and mucus gland secretion, and pain, leading to significant overlap in efferent responses to SAR, RAR, and C-fiber activation (Kubin et al. 2006). Furthermore, physiological differences between the subclasses become blurred in inflammation, which can change the expression patterns of TRP channels in the cells, increasing the diversity of stimuli that activate each neuronal subtype.

Exposure of the nose to diverse environmental stimuli leads to sneezing, mucus secretion, itching, nasal congestion, and nasal obstruction (Tran et al. 2011). Each of these responses can be induced locally, but there is clear evidence of reflex involvement in sneezing, nasal secretion, and congestion (Sarin et al. 2006). Sneezing is induced by irritants or tactile stimulation of the nasal mucosa, but also by exposure of the eyes to bright light or exposure of areas of the skin to sudden changes in temperature will induce sneezing. Rhinorrhea, or excessive nasal secretions, can be induced by local exposure to histamine, allergens, cold air, hypertonic solutions, the TRPV1 activator capsaicin, or bradykinin; but it can also be induced in the contralateral nostril (Sarin et al. 2006). The reflex nature of the response is evident from the fact that the contralateral response is eliminated by cutting the Vidian nerve. Nasal congestion occurs in response to vasodilation of mucosal blood vessels and pooling of blood in the mucosa. Congestion can be induced by exposure of skin at different sites on the body to changes in temperature. The reflex nature of congestion is further indicated by the observation that congestion can cycle from one nostril to the other (Sarin et al. 2006). This nasal cycle can be disrupted by inhibition of either sympathetic or parasympathetic outflow, leading to the idea that the cycling results from oscillating imbalance in parasympathetic-mediated vasodilation and sympathetic-mediated vasoconstriction.

Cough is both a protective mechanism for clearing pathogens, chemicals, and debris from the airways and a chronic, often debilitating, manifestation of infection and inflammation. The role of cough in lung defense is emphasized by the fact that loss of the cough reflex is accompanied by an increase in the incidence of pneumonia (Duarte and Myers 2012). Interestingly, the cough reflex is lost following denervation of the lower airways during lung transplant surgery, but is then partially restored in some cases (Duarte and Myers 2012). The restoration indicates that at least a part of the cough reflex is intrinsic to the lungs and does not require input from the central nervous system.

The cough reflex can be initiated via mechanical or chemical stimuli through parallel vagal afferent pathways. At least two activation pathways exist, one that is activated by capsaicin and inhibited under anesthesia, and another that is not activated by capsaicin and is retained under anesthesia. The former pathway is linked to bronchopulmonary C-fibers (Canning 2011). C-fibers express the transient receptor potential cation channels, TRPV1, which endows them responsiveness to capsaicin, and TRPA1, which is activated by acrolein in cigarette smoke, allyl isothiocyanate, and nicotine (Banner et al. 2011). They terminate in the mucosa, submucosa, parenchyma, and vasculature from the larynx to the peripheral lung. Cough induced by chemical activation of C-fibers is often paroxysmal.

Cough can also be initiated by receptors in the larynx, trachea, and large bronchi that activate Aδ fibers. In contrast to cough initiated by C-fibers, cough associated with Aδ fibers is rarely paroxysmal and is observed under anesthesia. Over 60 years ago, JG Widdicombe described vagal afferent fibers that were insensitive to mechanical stimulation of the airway surface, adapted rapidly to lung inflation, and could induce cough (Widdicombe 1954a, b). This initial description has led to the idea that RAR fibers are cough receptors, but Canning cautions against this interpretation (Canning 2010, 2011). Aδ fibers are not a homogenous population, but rather there are multiple subpopulations that differ in peripheral termination sites, sensitivity to mechanical stimuli, and reflexes they activate. In some cases, activation of RAR fibers and cough can be dissociated, indicating that the cough receptor that activate Aδ fibers are separate entities from RARs. Specifically, stimuli that activate RAR fibers—hyperventilation, breathing against a closed glottis, and bronchoconstriction induced by histamine, neurokinin A, and leukotrienes—do not elicit cough (Canning 2010). The cough receptors do not express the capsaicin receptor, TRPV1, but respond to protons and therefore may express other acid-sensitive ion channels. More definitive identification of cough receptors has been elusive, possibly due to plasticity in the pathway. Undem and colleagues have demonstrated that aeroallergen challenge induces TRPV1 expression in Aδ fibers (Lieu et al. 2012). The aeroallergen-induced change in phenotype increases the range of stimuli that lead to neural activation.

In addition to cough, irritation in the upper airways can induce apnea, bradycardia, and changes in peripheral vascular resistance (Widdicombe 2011). The diving reflex stimulated by exposure of the face and nasal mucosa to cold water is a well-recognized example of a cardiopulmonary reflex originating in the face and upper airways. The apnea and bradycardia induced by immersion in cold water can be so intense as to be fatal. The diving reflex is inhibited by interrupting conduction in the trigeminal nerve and can be mimicked by stimulating the ophthalmic branch ($V_1$) of the trigeminal nerve. The systemic vascular responses to immersion in cold water is species dependent, but in humans exposing the nose to cold water leads to peripheral vasoconstriction and peripheral hypertension, but retention of coronary and cerebral blood flow. The diving reflex also entails closure of the larynx, reducing the risk of aspirating water.

An aspiration reflex is associated with mechanical stimulation of the nose, nasopharynx, and oropharynx. The reflex facilitates clearance of inhaled particles to the esophagus and can be mimicked by stimulation of the glossopharyngeal nerve. The aspiration reflex is closely associated with sniffing induced by some odors, but is unique in the fact that it is elicited by mechanical deformation. The aspiration reflex exhibits species diversity and relatively weak in humans.

Similar to the nose and pharynx, the larynx also exhibits a high density of mechanical, irritant, and chemical receptors. When stimulated, these receptors induce apnea, hypertension, bradycardia, bronchoconstriction, and cough. As would be expected from the diversity of sensory nerve endings, the stimuli affecting the larynx are diverse and include mechanical deformation, ammonia, $SO_2$, smoke,

10–30 % $CO_2$, and osmolarity (Widdicombe 2011). In the case of osmolarity, changes in the concentration of permeant ions, particularly chloride, is a primary stimulus for receptor activation.

## Deposition and Clearance of Airborne Particles

### *Deposition*

Airborne particles are removed from inspired air by the impaction, interception, sedimentation, and diffusion. Impaction is the process by which inertia causes the particle to collide with the wall of the airway where the airstream deviates from a straight path. Particles with diameters greater than 10 μm (e.g., pollens, coarse particulate from mining and grinding activities) are deposit largely in the upper airways due to inertial impaction. Deflection of the inspired air around the turbinates and through the bend in the nasopharynx causes large particles with high inertia to impact with the front edge of the turbinates and posterior wall of the nasopharynx. The degree of impaction is related to the velocity of airflow, and as airflow rates decrease more large particles escape the upper airways and enter the lower airways, depositing in the trachea-bronchial region (Nakorn Tippayawong and Det Damrongsak 2003; Heyder 2004). Large particles escaping the upper airways continue to impact the airway wall at branch points/bifurcations in the lower airways. Interception is a term use to describe deposition resulting from a particle brushing against the wall of the airway and being trapped in the mucus, airway surface liquid, glycocalyx, or cell membranes. Fibers have a particularly high probability of being intercepted by the airways wall. Sedimentation refers to the settling of particles out of the airstream as velocity of airflow decreases. High rates of sedimentation are observed in the distal bronchi and bronchioles, where airflow velocity decreases due to an exponential increase in cross-sectional diameter of the airways. Particles that escape impaction, interception, and sedimentation can come in contact with and deposit on the airway wall via diffusion. Particles with aerodynamic diameters less than 10 μm (e.g., particles from combustion) are carried in the airstream to the lower airways and are considered to be respirable; and particles less than approximately 1 μm are carried into the alveoli; but the composition and surface characteristics of the particles greatly affect their deposition pattern. Hydrophilic particles tend to increase in size as inspired air is humidified, resulting in greater rates of deposition than predicted on their original dimensions (Heyder 2004). Likewise, aggregation of dispersed particles increases deposition within the lungs and consolidation of particles within the airways. Hydrophobic particles exhibit less deposition in the larger airways than expected based on aerodynamic diameter, but greater deposition in distal regions where the hydrophobicity of alveolar surfactant can facilitate their interaction with the airway surface (Heyder 2004).

## *Mucociliary Clearance*

Particles depositing on the airway surface become entrapped in mucus gel layer floating on the airway epithelium. The airway surface is covered by a 7 μm film of electrolyte, the periciliary layer, that supports an overlying layer of mucus that is 7–70 μm thick and composed of electrolyte and gel-forming mucin glycoproteins (Fahy and Dickey 2010; Tarran et al. 2006). Electrolyte and mucins are secreted by both the glands and surface epithelium. Glands are found from the nose through the bronchi, and the density of glands decreases with increasing airway generation. In the large airways, 95 % of the mucus is secreted from submucosal glands, and only 5 % is derived from the surface epithelium, but in airways smaller than 2 mm, non-ciliated cells in the surface epithelium are the only source of mucin glycoproteins (Trout et al. 2001).

The structure of mucus glands was described in 1969 by Meyrick and colleagues from serial thin sectioning of the airway wall (Meyrick et al. 1969), and subsequent studies defined the functional attributes of different regions of the glands (Wine 2007). The prominent portion of the gland observed in histological sections consists of mucous tubules lined by eosinophilic secretory cells. The mucous tubules are flanked by tubules lined with electrolyte secreting epithelial cells. Distally, the serous tubules secrete electrolyte that hydrates the mucus and moves it towards the airway lumen. Proximal to the mucous tubule is the collecting duct, where electrolyte content of the mucus can be adjusted. The gland opens to the airway through a ciliated duct that propels the mucus onto the airway surface.

Mucin glycoproteins impart the gel-like character to mucus. MUCAC and MUC5B are the major polymer-forming mucins in the airways (Fahy and Dickey 2010). MUC5AC is expressed mainly in large proximal airways by the superficial epithelial cells. MUC5B is expressed in glands throughout the proximal airways and by secretory cells in the surface epithelium in both proximal and distal airways. Mucins are stored in secretory cells in a condensed form and hydrated extracellularly following exocytosis (Fahy and Dickey 2010). The mucin glycans provide a substrate which can bind microbial proteins and trap inhaled particles, thereby limit further penetration of the mucosal barrier (Fahy and Dickey 2010). In addition, the gel acts as a sieve with a pore size of approximately 500 nm.

Electrolyte homeostasis in the airways represents a balance in at least three processes: passive transepithelial diffusion of salt and water, transepithelial $Na^+$ absorption mediated by basolateral Na/K ATPase and apical $Na^+$ channels (ENaC), and transepithelial secretion of $Cl^-$ and $HCO_3^-$ via the cystic fibrosis transmembrane regulator (CFTR) and calcium-activated $Cl^-$ channels (CaCC) (Wine 2007; Tarran et al. 2006). CFTR activity is regulated by cAMP, and the importance of this pathway in electrolyte balance is highlighted by the airway dehydration associated with cystic fibrosis. ATP may also play a role in regulating the depth of the periciliary and mucus layers. ATP is released by the epithelium into the airway lumen and acts through P2Y receptors to stimulate airway epithelial $Cl^-$ secretion via CaCC and inhibit airway epithelial $Na^+$ absorption via ENaC (Tarran et al. 2006). Breakdown of ATP to adenosine and subsequent activation of A2b receptors on the apical epithelial surface can regulate CFTR and ENaC secondarily (Tarran et al. 2006). ATP also stimulates surfactant release from Type II pneumocytes and thereby reduces surface tension (Mishra et al. 2011). Surface tension is associated with alveolar edema, and in this context, ATP would reduce the formation of alveolar edema.

The role of purinergic regulation in lung function is well recognized in the context of cystic fibrosis and may also be relevant to asthma. ATP functions in recruitment and activation of dendritic cells, neutrophils, and eosinophils (Mortaz et al. 2010; Willart and Lambrecht 2009; Muller et al. 2010); and can promote allergic responses through the innate immune system by inducing airway epithelial cells to secrete IL-33, which promotes Th2 responses (Kouzaki et al. 2011). Single nucleotide polymorphisms of purinergic receptors are associated with $FEV_1$, $FEV_1/FVC$, airway hyperresponsiveness, and bronchodilator responses; and the associations are affected by house dust mite exposure (Bunyavanich et al. 2012).

## Airway Resistance

The nose accounts for approximately 50 % of the total resistance to airflow in the airways and therefore also accounts for an equivalent proportional decrease in lumenal pressure as air flows between the nares and alveoli. The configuration of the respiratory system leads to region-specific closure of airways during inspiration and expiration. Respiratory muscles act on the chest wall and diaphragm to change the pressure in the pleural space and alveoli, which subsequently drive airflow. The nose accounts for approximately 50 % of the total resistance to airflow through the respiratory system during nasal breathing. The nasal resistance lowers the pressure in the pharynx during inspiration, predisposing the pharynx to collapse during inspiration (Ferris et al. 1964). In contrast, the restriction opposes collapse of the distal airways during exhalation by providing a backpressure in the airway lumen. By comparison, the intrathoracic extrapulmonary airways are surrounded by pleural pressure, which remains negative relative to barometric pressure during quiet breathing. Thus, during normal resting breathing, pleural pressure opposes closure of intrathoracic airways during inspiration. During forced exhalation, pleural pressure can be positive, which tends to compress the intrathoracic extrapulmonary airways. Likewise, intrapulmonary airways are surrounded by alveoli, and development of positive alveolar pressure during exhalation acts as a compressive force. Under normal conditions, the resistance of the distal airways is low, leading to minimal decrease in the luminal pressure, minimizing the pressure differential across the wall of the intrapulmonary airways. Alveolar septa impinge upon the walls of the intrapulmonary airways, and stretch of the septa opposes collapse of the airways, particularly at high lung volumes. Increase in the resistance of the distal airways due to smooth muscle contraction, accumulation of secretions in the airway lumen, or destruction of lung tissue that reduces elastic recoil leads a premature drop in the luminal pressure and dynamic compression of the airways during exhalation (Irvin and Bates 2009).

The collagen and elastin network combined with contractile elements, surface tension, surface-active material, and fluid dynamics result in complex responses of the lungs to applied pressures. The resulting viscoelastic properties of the lungs give rise to tissue resistance that is dependent on breathing frequency, increasing at low frequencies and decreasing at higher frequencies. At respiratory rates of 12–24 bpm, tissue resistance can account for 40 % of the resistance to breathing (Faffe and Zin 2009). The role of tissue resistance in responses to allergen challenge in mice is well established (Irvin and Bates 2009), but less is known about its role in humans. Readers wanting to delve deeper into lung mechanics and models of lung behavior are directed to the excellent review by Faffe and colleagues (Faffe and Zin 2009) as well as the work of Jason Bates (Bates and Lutchen 2005).

## Control of Airway Smooth Muscle

Airway smooth muscle exhibits basal tone; and numerous hormones, neurotransmitters, inflammatory mediators, environmental agents, and therapeutics alter the airway smooth muscle contractile activity. Two primary factors influencing the level of bronchomotor tone under basal conditions is parasympathetic cholinergic stimulation of contraction via M3 receptors on the smooth muscle, and parasympathetic noncholinergic fibers induce bronchodilation via VIP, Substance P, and NO (Canning 2006). While there is abundant expression of VIP in the trachea and bronchi (Groneberg et al. 2006; Kraneveld and Nijkamp 2001; Groneberg et al. 2001), there is a lack of definitive evidence for expression of the known VIP receptors—PAC, VPAC1, and VPAC2—on airway smooth muscle, yet VPAC2 agonists induce bronchodilation both in vivo and in vitro (Tannu et al. 2010). So, the mechanism by which VIP induces smooth muscle relaxation is unclear. Hormonally and therapeutically, bronchodilation via β-adrenergic agonists and elevation of cAMP is well documented.

In humans, SP and NKA contract large airways via activation of NK2 receptors (Kraneveld and Nijkamp 2001). NK1 agonists are without effect. SP and NKA also contract small airways, but the effects are mediated by thromboxane and A2 and NK1 receptors (Kraneveld and Nijkamp 2001).

Mast cell- and basophil-derived mediators, including histamine and cysteinyl leukotrienes, are potent bronchoconstrictors, and bidirectional interaction exists between mast cells and parasympathetic afferents (Kraneveld and Nijkamp 2001). NANC nerve terminals in the airway wall express histamine receptors capable of increasing sensitivity of the neurons to stimuli, lowering the stimulus threshold for release of neuropeptides. In human mast cells, SP can down-regulate FcεRI and the response to IgE (McCary et al. 2010). In vivo, down-regulation of FcεRI would reduce acute bronchoconstriction in response to allergen, which would be in opposition to bronchoconstriction induced by direct effect of SP binding to NK2 receptors airway smooth muscle. Reciprocally, mast cell lines have been shown to express NK1 and NK2 receptors, and SP modulates mast cell activity (Kraneveld and Nijkamp 2001). Similarly, both nerves and mast cells have been shown to secrete and respond to nerve growth factor (NGF) (Kraneveld and Nijkamp 2001). Cholinergic, adrenergic, and nonadrenergic noncholinergic neurotransmitters regulate secretions in the airways. Adrenergic stimulation induces electrolyte secretion onto the airway surface. VIP induces low rates of secretion from glands, and acetylcholine induces high rates of glandular secretion (Wine 2007).

## Control of Mucus Secretion

Control of electrolyte and mucin secretion varies across species and is still not completely understood. In humans, acetylcholine from parasympathetic cholinergic efferent fibers acts on muscarinic $M_3$ receptors to induce both mucin and electrolyte secretion (Rogers 2001; Wine 2007). At least a portion of the Ach-induced electrolyte secretion is secondary to $Ca^{2+}$-induced $Cl^-$ transport that is independent of the cystic CFTR (Wine 2007). Ach-dependent regulation of mucus secretion is thought to be the major pathway controlling reflex stimulation of mucus secretion through the autonomic motor nuclei.

VIP constitutes a second major control pathway in human airways that parallels and modulates Ach-induced mucus secretion. VIP acting on VIP type 1 receptors (VPAC1R) expressed on gland and surface epithelial cells stimulates electrolyte and mucin secretion (Kim et al. 2011; Miotto et al. 2004). Unlike Ach-induced electrolyte secretion, VIP stimulates $HCO_3^-$ secretion that is dependent on CFTR and therefore is impaired in cystic fibrosis (Wine 2007). In addition to the epithelial expression, VIP receptors are also found presynaptically on parasympathetic cholinergic efferent fibers. Activation of these receptors inhibits Ach-induced mucus secretion, and this thought to be the dominant effect of VIP on submucosal glands (Rogers 2001).

Inflammation alters expression of VIP receptors, and it is unclear whether the alteration contributes to, or compensates for increased mucus production. Consistent with this paradigm, in a rat model of airway inflammation, VIP expression in the airway wall was negatively correlated with ozone-induced changes in mucin secretion (Li et al. 2009). In humans, VIP and VIP receptors expression are increased in the nasal mucosa of allergic rhinitis subjects (Kim et al. 2011; Park and Christman 2006) and bronchial mucosa of smokers with chronic bronchitis (Miotto et al. 2004). It is unknown if the increased expression observed in human tissues is related to inhibitory activity at cholinergic synapses, or is associated with NANC stimulation that synergizes with the cholinergic stimulation.

In some species, sensory efferent/axon reflex control of glandular secretion is common and involves CGRP, NKA, and/or SP (Rogers 2001). As stated above, sensory efferent innervation is not common. There is scant evidence of CGRP, NKA, or NKB expression in human airways, but SP is expressed, along with NK1, NK2, and NK3 receptors (Canning 2006). Interestingly, in 2007, Wine and colleagues demonstrated a direct effect of SP on volume secretion by human bronchial glands, the effect was 10 % of what was observed in porcine glands stimulated with

SP and even less and less than 10 % of the secretion rate observed in human glands stimulated with carbachol (Choi et al. 2007). SP was synergized with VIP, but not carbachol, and was shown to involve electrolyte secretion through a CFTR-dependent pathway.

In contrast to glands, secretion of mucins from goblet cells in the surface epithelia is reported to be controlled primarily by ATP and UTP in the airway surface liquid acting on apical P2Y purinoceptors (Davis and Dickey 2008). Bronchioles are normally devoid of goblet cells, and the major nonciliated secretory cell in this region is the Clara cell. Under normal condition, Clara cells secrete mucin glycoproteins in a constitutive fashion, with secretion rates matching production, and no accumulation of glycoproteins in secretory granules. During inflammation, production of mucin glycoproteins increases, and mucin granules appear in the cells, resulting in a goblet cell phenotype.

## Airway Inflammation

The inflammatory response to inhaled pathogens is highly variable and affected by the nature of the agent, its concentration in inspired air, duration and periodicity of exposure, and expression of comorbid conditions. A summary of common inflammatory cells in the lungs and some of their interactions are illustrated in Fig. 2.4. Innate and adaptive responses drive the inflammation, leading to redundancy in the pathways leading to the inflammatory response. Epithelial cells, dendritic cells, macrophages, mast cells, natural killer (NK) cells, and nerves respond to pathogens in the airways and environmental stimuli, altering airway function, mounting defense responses, and initiating inflammation. Interaction with T and B lymphocytes leads to adaptive immune responses, immunologic memory, and efficiency of subsequent responses. There is a tendency in reviews and discussions in this field to focus on pro-inflammatory mechanisms, but it should be noted that counter-regulatory mechanisms are in place that limit the inflammatory response and thereby protect the tissues from intrinsic damage.

*Macrophages* are found in the alveolar, interstitial, and intravascular compartments. The alveolar macrophage exists at the air–tissue interface and acutely responds to environmental stimuli. They stain brightly for nonspecific esterase. Upon activation they secrete reactive oxygen species (ROS) and cytokines, and exhibit Fc-independent phagocytosis (Lohmann-Matthes et al. 1994). Interstitial macrophages exhibit less secretion of ROS and cytokines, but have a greater capacity for antigen presentation. Intravascular macrophages are thought to engulf material then transit from the lung and into the blood. They are distinguished from monocytes by a greater capacity for phagocytosis (Lohmann-Matthes et al. 1994). Dendritic cells are similar to interstitial macrophages, but these cells have even greater capacity for antigen presentation.

Inhaled particles activate macrophages via cell surface receptors (scavenger receptors and pattern recognition receptors (PRRs)) that recognize common

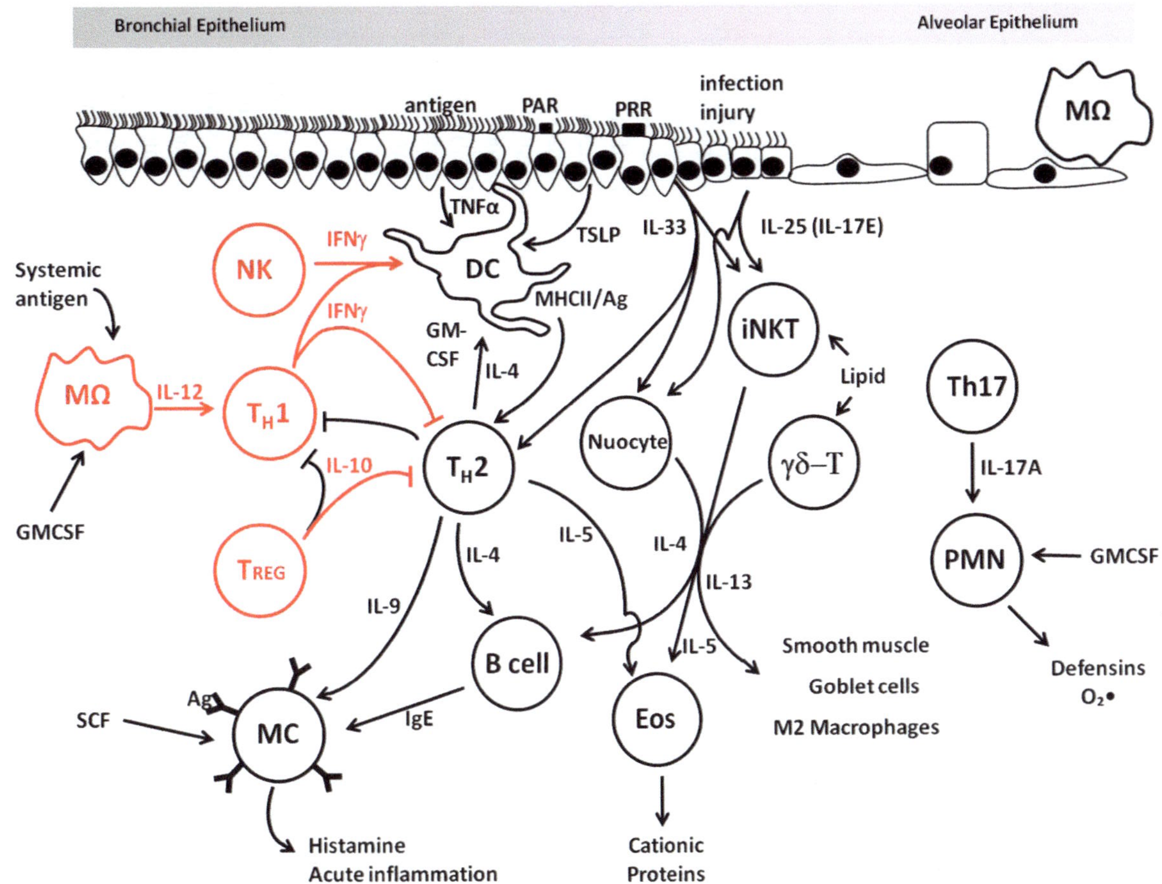


**Fig. 2.4** Overview of cells and cytokines implicated in airway inflammation underlying asthma. *Red* indicates pathways that down-regulate $T_H2$-driven inflammation. *PAR* protease-activated receptor, *PRR* pattern recognition receptor, *MΩ* macrophage, *NK* natural killer cell, *DC* dendritic cell, *Th* T-helper lymphocyte, *iNKT* invariant natural killer T lymphocyte, *γδ-T* γδ-T lymphocyte, *PMN* polymorphonuclear lymphocyte, $T_{reg}$ regulatory T lymphocyte, *B cell* B lymphocyte, *MC* mast cell, *Eos* eosinophil

structures that are shared by broad classes of pathogen (pathogen-associated molecular patterns or PAMPs). Scavenger receptors represent a diverse family of molecules capable of binding inorganic molecules such as silica and titanium, as well as organic molecules such as low density lipoprotein (Murphy et al. 2005). Eight classes of scavenger receptors have been described and are designated A through H. Receptors classes A, B, D, and E, specifically SR-AI/II, MARCO, CD36, CD68, and LOX-1, have been implicated in responses to environmental pathogens (Thakur et al. 2008; Yatera et al. 2011; Lewis et al. 2009). PRRs recognize PAMPs including mannans in the yeast cell wall, bacterial-derived formylated peptides, lipopolysaccharides, and lipoteichoic acids; and PRR–PAMP interaction be direct or may depend on intermediate or adapter molecules. Toll-like receptors (TLRs) bind PAMPs directly. TLR2 and 4 are expressed by alveolar macrophages and mediate many of the responses to pathogens (Xiang et al. 2010; Xiang and Fan. 2010). TLRs also recognize damage-associated molecular patterns (DAMPs), leading macrophages to respond to tissue injury following environmental exposures and inflammatory responses (Xiang et al. 2010). Particles and pathogens may also bind indirectly to macrophages following opsonization with immunoglobulins, complement, or collectins including mannose binding protein and surfactant apoproteins A and D. Opsonized pathogens bind to macrophage via Fc (Fc$\gamma$RI, II, and III; Fc$\varepsilon$RI; and Fc$\alpha$RI), complement receptors (CR1, 3, 4), or collectin receptors (SP-R210, cC1qR, CD14, SRCL) (Selman et al. 2008; Aderem and Underhill 1999; Grubor et al. 2006).

Macrophages play a central role in dust-induced occupational diseases, such as silicosis, asbestosis, and berylliosis. Activation by particles leads to phagocytosis and secretion of ROI (reactive oxygen intermediates such as superoxide, hydrogen peroxide, hydroxyradicals) and RNI (reactive nitrogen intermediates like nitric oxide and peroxynitrite). Activation also alters immune and inflammatory responses via secretion of cytokines (e.g., TNF-$\alpha$, IL-12, TGF-$\beta$) and chemoattractants (e.g., CCL17 and CCL22 act on $T_H2$ cells, and CCL11 attracts eosinophils). The specific stimulus controls the secretory products that are released and the ultimate physiological and pathological responses of the macrophage.

*Dendritic cells* are found throughout the respiratory tract and can be separated into at least five subtypes based on cell surface markers and origin: conventional, plasmacytoid, monocyte-derived inflammatory, innate killer, and alveolar dendritic cells (Hammad and Lambrecht 2011; Lambrecht and Hammad 2009). Dendritic cells play a central role in both initiating immune responses to allergens, microbes, and viruses and maintaining balance within the immune system. Accordingly, different subsets have specialized, and occasionally opposing effects on immune responses. For example, dendritic cells of myeloid origin, including conventional and inflammatory dendritic cells, actively promote $T_H1$ and $T_H2$ immune responses against foreign antigens (Hammad and Lambrecht 2011; Hammad et al. 2010). In contrast, some plasmacytoid dendritic cells have anti-inflammatory activity that leads to apoptosis of eosinophils and lymphocytes through expression of programmed death 1 ligand (PD-1L) (Kool et al. 2009).

In normal lungs, immature dendritic cells express high levels of PRRs, but low levels of accessory molecules necessary for binding and activating naïve

T-lymphocytes (CD40, CD54, CD58, CD80, and CD86). Immature dendritic cells are thereby poised to take up and process antigens, but are inefficient in presenting antigen to lymphocytes. In the presence of inflammatory mediators including GM-CSF, IL-4, CD40L, TNF-α, IL-1β, IL-6, and thymic stromal lymphopoietin (TSLP), DAMPs, PAMPs, or specific ligation with T-helper cells, immature dendritic cells differentiate and express high levels of MHCII and the accessory molecules necessary for efficient antigen presentation. Exposure to antigen and inflammatory mediators, which normally occurs in peripheral tissues, causes the dendritic cell to migrate to the draining lymph nodes where the mature dendritic cell then presents antigens with high efficiency in the T cell zones of the secondary lymphoid tissues. Maturation factors for dendritic cells are prevalent in the mucosa in many diseases, particularly in allergic airways disease, and result in recruitment of monocytes that differentiate into mature dendritic cells (Ganesh et al. 2009; Blanchfield and Mannie 2010; Hamilton and Anderson 2004; Ritz et al. 2002; Soruri and Zwirner 2005).

Dendritic cells process and present both peptide and non-peptide antigens, and the type of antigen affects dendritic cell maturation. Viral- and cell-associated antigens induce maturation to a phenotype characterized by expression of CD70 and Notch Ligand Delta and secretion of IL-12, which promotes development of $T_H1$ cells that are thought to mediate antiviral immunity and promote cell-mediated diseases such as Sarcoidosis (Parisinos 2011). In contrast, soluble peptide allergens induce dendritic cells, particularly myeloid dendritic cells, to mature into a $T_H2$-promoting phenotype thought to play a critical role in allergic respiratory diseases (Tsoumakidou et al. 2008). Interestingly, viral infections are a primary trigger for asthmatic reactions, so the dichotomy between the effects of viral and allergenic antigens is not absolute. Viral exposure has been shown to induce the expression of the high affinity IgE receptor (FcεRI) on murine dendritic cells, and activation of the receptor leads to expression of CCL28, a chemoattractant for T and B lymphocytes (Holtzman et al. 2009; Grayson et al. 2007).

*Lymphocytes* comprise a relatively small percentage of the inflammatory cells in environmental lung diseases compared to macrophages, PMNs, and eosinophils (<10 % of the cells in bronchoalveolar lavage fluid); but are thought to play crucial regulatory roles. All three subtypes (T cells, B cells, and natural killer (NK) cells) are found in the lungs following environmental exposures.

T cells express the CD3 cell surface marker, which is a subunit of the T cell receptor. They are subdivided into CD4+ (T helper ($T_H$), CD4+ T regulatory T ($T_{reg}$), γδ T, and invariant Natural Killer T-lymphocytes (iNKT)) and CD8+ (cytotoxic $T_C$)) cells. $T_H$ cells are further divided into effector and memory $T_H1$, $T_H2$, $T_H9$, and $T_H17$ cells. $T_H1$ cells secrete IFN-γ and promote cellular immunity. $T_H2$ cells secrete IL-4, IL-5, IL-6, IL-9, IL-10, and IL-13 that support humoral immune responses. IL-4 is a key cytokine in needed for differentiation of the $T_H2$ subset and immunoglobulin class switching to the IgE isotype. IL-5 is a primary growth factor for eosinophils, and IL-13 induces smooth muscle and goblet cell growth. IL-6 is a growth factor for T, B, and mast cells. IL-9 also promotes mast cell growth. IL-10 promotes B cell growth, but inhibits $T_H1$ and $T_H2$ responses. $T_H17$ cells secrete IL-17A and F, which promote neutrophilic inflammation. iNKT cells can be activated by glycolipid bound to the MHC-class-I-like cell surface protein, CD1d, leading to secretion of IL-4, IL-5, and IL-13 and $T_H2$-like inflammation (Meyer et al. 2008; Iwamura and Nakayama 2010). iNKT cells are responsive to IL-25 and IL-33, which are expressed by epithelial cells in response to activation of PRRs. iNKT cells may thereby act as effector cells for epithelial cell-initiated responses to diverse environmental stimuli, helping to explain the preponderance of the Th2 response in the allergic lungs. IL-25 is also secreted by mast cells and $T_H2$ lymphocytes. This reciprocal activation of iNKT, mast cells, and $T_H2$ lymphocytes represents a point of synergism between the adaptive and innate immune systems (Iwamura and Nakayama 2010). iNKT cells are relatively resistant to corticosteroids and may contribute to steroid-resistance in asthma. γδ T cells also respond to lipid antigens presented in the context of CD1d on the surface of DCs (Lloyd and Hessel 2010). Some γδ T cells can express cytokines associated with asthma, including IL-5 and IL-13 (Robinson 2010) and IL-17A (Murdoch and Lloyd 2010). However, γδ T cells may not be purely pro-inflammatory and have been associated with resolution of allergic responses in mice (Murdoch and Lloyd 2010).

$T_{reg}$ cells secrete the immunosuppressive cytokines TGF-β and IL-10 and are thought to play an important role in moderating pulmonary allergic sensitivity and immune responsives (Nouri-Aria and Durham 2008; Ray et al. 2010; Wan and Flavell 2007). TGF-β is also implicated in wound healing and tissue remodeling. These cells are therefore capable of down-regulating inflammation and promoting repair of lung tissue. In the lungs, an excessive repair response however may result in fibrosis.

CD8 $T_C$ bind to the non-variable region of MHCI stabilizing the interaction between the $T_C$ cells and cells that express viral antigens in the context of MHCI, positioning the $T_C$ cells to release perforin, granzymes, and granulysin that kill the virus-infected cells. $T_C$ cells differentiate into subsets that are functionally similar to those described for $T_H$ cells, including $T_C1$, $T_C2$, $T_C17$, FOXP3+, γδ+, effector, and memory cells. In a $T_H2$ environment, $T_C$ cells are induced to produce IL-5, augmenting the allergic response and providing a potential mechanism for virus-induced asthma exacerbations (Coyle et al. 1995).

NK cells are CD3 negative cells that lyse cells expressing abnormal levels of MHCI. NK cells play diverse roles in allergic asthma. They can produce large amounts of IFN-γ, and thereby affect DC maturation. They express MHC II, and in the presence of costimulatory molecules present the antigens to $T_H2$ cells (Korsgren et al. 1999), but depletion does not impair antibody responses to antigen (Hanna et al. 2004). Consistent with secretion of IFN-γ, NK cells attenuate ovalbumin-induced airway responses in mice (Wang et al. 1998) and are required for timely resolution of OVA-induced airway inflammation, possibly via Resolvin E1 binding to its receptor, CMKLR1, on NK cells (Matsubara et al. 2007).

Multiple subpopulations of NK cells have been described based on cell surface markers, cytolytic capacity, and cytokine secretion. IL-12 induces a cytolytic phenotype (Haworth et al. 2011). IL-18 also induces differentiation of NK cells towards a phenotype of low cytolytic activity and robust IFN-γ secretion (Moretta et al. 2006).

Exposure to IL-4 inhibits development of a cytolytic phenotype (Agaugue et al. 2008), and a subpopulation of NK cells has been described, NK2 cell, that secrete $T_H2$ cytokines and promote humoral immunity (Moretta et al. 2006). Thus, depending on the environment, NK cells can modulate antigen presentation and development of effector cells.

*Polymorphonuclear leukocytes* (*PMNs*) are prominent in the airways of smokers and are among the first cell types to infiltrate the lung during the airway inflammatory response to allergen. PMNs are also prominent following acute lung injury and in the lungs of subjects who die of status asthmaticus (Deniz et al. 2002). In COPD, PMN numbers correlate with impairment of pulmonary function (Cowburn et al. 2008; Perl et al. 2011). PMNs are activated and recruited to the lungs by diverse signals, including IL-8 acting on the CXCR1 and CXCR2 chemokine receptors and leukotriene-B4 (LTB4), TNF-α, IL-1β, IL-6, and MCP-1 (Bathoorn et al. 2008). Circulating PMN binds to pulmonary capillary endothelial cells via selectins (P-, E-, and L-selectin) and β2-integrins. The majority of transendothelial migration of neutrophils is via active endothelial engulfment triggered by engagement of ICAM1 (Perl et al. 2011; Bathoorn et al. 2008). In the tissues, PMNs migrate to the site of inflammation by phosphoinositide 3-kinase-dependent chemotaxis. Circulating PMNs have a relatively short lifespan (6–12 h), but apoptosis can be inhibited and lifespan extended at sites of inflammation by lipid activators, TNF, IL-1, IL-6, IL-8, GM-CSF, G-CSF, and hypoxia; thereby extending their longevity in the tissues (Cowburn et al. 2008; van Buul et al. 2007). Activated neutrophils secrete elastase, cathepsins, myeloperoxidase, and ROS; all of which can lead to further tissue damage. Macrophages play a role in down-regulating neutrophilic inflammation by phagocytosis of apoptotic neutrophils and secretion IL-10 and TGF-β (Perl et al. 2011). Impairment of macrophages in COPD may contribute to chronic neutrophilic inflammation.

Anti-inflammatory lipid mediators acting on the PMNs, endothelium, and epithelium inhibit PMN migration and promote resolution of neutrophilic inflammation (Cowburn et al. 2008). Five categories of anti-inflammatory mediators have been described: lipoxins, resolvins, protectins, cyclopentenones, and polyisoprenyl phosphates. These mediators reduce PMN migration and inhibit release of pro-inflammatory mediators while increasing apoptosis and clearance by macrophages (Haworth et al. 2011; Campbell et al. 2007; Haworth and Levy 2007). These mediators increase expression of anti-adhesion molecules on epithelium and consequently promote epithelial clearance of PMN (Haworth and Levy 2007).

*Eosinophils* are commonly associated with allergic asthma although their number can vary widely between subtypes of patients (Campbell et al. 2007). Eosinophils are also prevalent in 20–40 % of COPD patients (Welte and Groneberg 2006; Akuthota et al. 2011). Whether eosinophils are bystanders or effectors in these diseases is a matter of debate (Saha and Brightling 2006). IL-5 is a primary eosinophil growth factor, and complement C5a and platelet activating factor are major chemoattractants (Akuthota et al. 2011; Sugita et al. 2003). Other cytokines that are active in eosinophil recruitment include IL-2, IL-3, GM-CSF, eotaxin, and RANTES (Resnick and Weller 1993). Vascular cell adhesion molecule 1 (VCAM-1) is upregulated on endothelial cells by IL-4t does not efficiently interact with neutrophils, which may be why eosinophils accumulate in allergic airways to a greater degree than neutrophils (Resnick and Weller 1993). When activated, eosinophils release cationic proteins, leukotrienes, and ROS (Resnick and Weller 1993). In addition, eosinophils contain over 30 different cytokines that are released in response to specific stimulation (Sugita et al. 2003; Spencer et al. 2009). Eosinophils augment the $T_H2$ response to allergen by production of IL-4 and IL-5 (Spencer et al. 2009). They also inhibit growth of respiratory syncytial virus (Akuthota et al. 2011).

*Mast cells* respond to environmental stimuli through TRPs, PRRs, crosslinking of FcεRI by allergen and allergen-specific IgE. Mast cells originate from a myeloid progenitor that is distinct from the granulocyte and macrophage progenitor. Immature precursor cells are released from the bone marrow and circulate to peripheral tissues where they mature into effector cells. The mechanisms underlying recruitment of mast cell precursors to the lungs have not been fully defined but appear to involve interactions of integrins α4β1 and α4β7 with VCAM-1 in response to LTB4, $PGE_2$, IL-9, and other signals from NKT and $T_{reg}$ cells (Akuthota et al. 2011). In the mucosa, mast cells mature in response to stem cell factor (SCF) produced by the epithelium (Collington et al. 2011; Weller et al. 2011), acting through the c-kit receptor (Wen et al. 1996). When mature, mast cells respond to PAMPs, DAMPs, environmental stimuli, and allergen-specific IgE by immediate release of preformed mediators, including histamine, serotonin, and serine proteases, followed by synthesis and release of cysteinyl leukotrienes (LTC4, D4, E4, and F4), LTB4, thromboxane, and platelet activating factor. Mast cells also release pro-inflammatory cytokines including TNF-α, IL-4, IL-5, IL-6, and IL-13, which augment and prolong mucosal inflammation (Collington et al. 2011).

Mast cell products have widespread effects in the lungs. Histamine induces smooth muscle contraction, increases endothelial permeability, stimulates epithelial secretory activity, and modulates afferent nerve activity. Histamine stimulates or inhibits nerve activity depending on the balance of H1and H3 histamine receptor ligation (Weller et al. 2011). Leukotriene receptors are found on diverse structural and inflammatory cells types and regulate global aspects of airway and vascular function, as well as immunity and inflammation (Weller et al. 2011; Groneberg et al. 2004). LTB4 is a potent chemoattractant and activator of neutrophils, eosinophils, macrophages, T cells, and DCs (Okunishi and Peters-Golden 2011). Mast cells have been implicated in myocardial remodeling and fibrosis (Okunishi and Peters-Golden 2011) and pulmonary responses to silica and nanoparticles (Levick et al. 2011).

*Epithelial cells* have emerged as important participants in inflammatory responses to environmental stimuli. The epithelium expresses a wide array of receptors to monitor inspired air for pathogens and toxins, including protease-activated receptors (PARs), TLRs, nucleotide-binding oligomerization domain [NOD]-like receptors, and TRPs. Activation leads to release of cytotoxic proteins, collectins, and ROS that contribute to killing and clearance of microbes (Brown et al. 2007; Shannahan et al. 2012). Epithelial cells modulate immune responses through release of cytokines that act on dendritic cells and T cells. For example, GM-CSF and TSLP induce dendritic cells to promote $T_H2$ immune responses. IFN-α and -β promote $T_H1$ responses, and IFN-λ (IL-28 and IL-29) promotes $T_{reg}$ growth (Schleimer et al. 2007). IL-33 production by epithelial cells promotes mast cell activation and $T_H2$

cell differentiation, and IL-25 activates iNKT cells to produce $T_H2$ cytokines. Recent studies by McKenzie indicate that IL-25 also induces nuocytes that produce $T_H2$ cytokines (Schleimer et al. 2007). IL-6 production results in the differentiation of antibody-secreting B cells. Ligation of CD40 on epithelial cells can initiate inflammatory cell recruitment via release of RANTES, MCP, CCL28, and IL-8. Epithelial cells can also regulate survival of immune cells via expression of PD-L1, PD-L2, and Fas ligand (Barlow and McKenzie 2011; Neill et al. 2010).

In addition to its roles in immunity and inflammation, the airway epithelium is thought to play an important role in mucosal repair and tissue remodeling through the release of pro-fibrotic mediators and enzymes (Schleimer et al. 2007). The epithelium may play an even more direct role in fibrosis via epithelial–mesenchymal transition (EMT). EMT is a form of epithelial plasticity in which epithelial cells redifferentiate into migratory fibroblastoid cells. It is well recognized that epithelial damage leads to release of TGF-β, epidermal growth factor (EGF), and fibroblast growth factors (FGFs) that facilitate wound healing and promote fibrosis. TGF-β down-regulates E-cadherin and tight junctions between the epithelial cells and upregulates mesenchymal markers (Hackett. 2012). To date, most of the work in this area has been in mice, and definitive evidence of whether EMT plays a role in human airways is lacking.

*Neurons* interact with inflammatory and immune cells in a bidirectional fashion. Afferent nerves express receptors for inflammatory mediators. One prominent example mentioned above is H1 and H3 histamine receptors on afferent parasympathetic neurons (Johnson et al. 2011). Another is LTB4 acting on TRPV1 channels (Groneberg et al. 2004).

Work supporting development of cholinergic antagonists for use in COPD has led to documentation of muscarinic receptors on diverse inflammatory cells that mediate acetylcholine-induced proliferation and chemotaxis (Hwang et al. 2000). At least some of the acetylcholine effects are thought to be due to increased secretion of LTB4. Interestingly, while the clinical use of cholinergic antagonists is increasing, definitive proof of a direct role for acetylcholine in airway inflammation is lacking (Kistemaker et al. 2012).

In contrast to acetylcholine, a strong case is emerging for a role of VIP in immune and inflammatory processes. Two subtypes of VIP receptors with opposing activity have been described, VPAC1 and VPAC2. VPAC1 activation is immunosuppressive, causing down-regulation of both cytotoxic and allergic responses (Kistemaker et al. 2012). VIP induces generation of $T_{reg}$ cells in the spleen of mice (Voice et al. 2002), which may account for some of its immune suppression. VPAC1 is expressed constitutively, and long-acting VIP analogues are being developed as means to suppress inflammation in allergic asthma and COPD (Szema et al. 2011). VPAC1 has also been associated with enhanced Th17 responses, and the impact of VIP-VPAC1 effects in disease has yet to be defined (Onoue et al. 2010, 2011; Misaka et al. 2010).

In contrast to VPAC1, VPAC2 expression is induced following activation of the TCR and is associated with enhanced IgE antibody responses and heightened cutaneous reactions (Yadav et al. 2008). Through VPAC2, VIP augments co-stimulation via B7, inhibits apoptosis of activated $T_H2$ cells, and inhibits IL-12 production, which has the effect of skewing the $T_H1/T_H2$ balance towards $T_H2$ immunity (Voice et al. 2002). The net effect of VPAC2 activation is augmentation of $T_H2$ effector and memory functions in peripheral tissues exposed to allergen.

There is also some evidence that tachykinins modulate inflammatory processes. Alveolar macrophages express NK1 receptors, and exposure to substance P increases metalloproteinase, TNF-α, and IL-1β secretion (Delgado and Ganea 2000; Delgado et al. 2000; Goetzl et al. 2008). Knockout of preprotachykinin A gene attenuates LPS-induced airway hyperreactivity and airway inflammation (Xu et al. 2008, 2011; Xu and Xu 2010). As of 2010, clinical trials with NK receptor antagonists had not validated a role of tachykinins in asthma (Helyes et al. 2010). Expression of NK1 receptors is upregulated by cigarette smoke, which may account for increased susceptibility of smokers to infection, fibrosis, cancer, and emphysema (Ramalho et al. 2011).

## *Counter Regulation*

Numerous negative feedback pathways limit the duration and magnitude of inflammatory responses (Xu et al. 2011; Xu and Xu 2010). Detailed discussion of these mechanisms is beyond the scope of this chapter, but a few examples are noteworthy because they portray a general paradigm. Similar to traditional negative feedback loops in the endocrine system, some mediators released during immune activation act on inhibitory receptors to restrict further cellular activation. Notable examples are nitric oxide, prostaglandins, and catabolites of tryptophan. Prostaglandins produced by the cyclooxygenase pathway interact with heterotrimeric G protein-coupled receptors to stimulate adenylate cyclase formation of cAMP. Nitric oxide produced by nitric oxide synthetase acts through guanylate cyclase to increase cGMP, which in certain cases inhibits immune and inflammatory processes (Bosnjak et al. 2011; Saxon et al. 2008; Cook and Bochner 2010; Bjorgo et al. 2011; Bopp et al. 2009; Baumer et al. 2007; Heijink and Van Oosterhout 2006; Mitkiewicz et al. 2011). Similarly, activation of indoleamine 2,3-dioxygenase and subsequent release of tryptophan metabolites can stimulate aryl hydrocarbon receptors that promote tolerance to aeroallergens (Taher et al. 2008). Inhibitory Fc receptors that bind the Fc domain of IgG, such as FcγRIIB, are expressed on B cells and mast cells, and when activated reduce cellular activation and cytokine production (Taher et al. 2008). Upregulation and activation of decoy cytokine receptors, such as IL-13R α2, can have potent inhibitory and negative feedback consequences, thereby opposing the inflammatory activity of cytokines (Saxon et al. 2008; Karra and Levi-Schaffer 2011; Smith and Clatworthy 2010; Zhu et al. 2010).

In addition to receptors that respond to soluble mediators, there is a plethora of inhibitory receptors that respond to ligands expressed on the surface of activated immune cells. CTLA-4 is expressed on the surface of activated T cells and inhibits CD28 binding to B7 on antigen presenting cells. Expression of CTLA4 limits co-stimulation required for T-cell activation (Mentink-Kane and Wynn 2004). PD-1 acts in a similar fashion. PD-1 is expressed on activated T and B cells, and one of its ligands, PDL-2 is expressed on myeloid dendritic cells and macrophages. Expression of PD-1 provides negative feedback to further activation of T and B cells (Chen and Shi 2006; Bour-Jordan et al. 2011). CD22 and CD72 are co-inhibitory receptors on B cells. Their ligands are expressed on diverse cell types, but when activated simultaneously the B cell is inhibited. Similarly, CD200R is expressed on dendritic cells and macrophages, and CD200 is more widely expressed on epithelium, T cells, and B cells (Chen and Shi 2006; Singh et al. 2011; Okazaki and Honjo 2006). CD200 interaction with CD200R is thought to maintain balance in the lungs between protection and immunopathology (Minas and Liversidge 2006; Gorczynski 2005; Barclay et al. 2002).

TGF-β is a pro-fibrotic growth factor produced by activated monocytes, pulmonary macrophages, eosinophils, neutrophils, airway epithelial cells, smooth muscle cells, mast cells, lung fibroblasts, and T $T_{reg}$ cells (Holt and Strickland 2008). TGF-β is a strong stimulating factor for epithelial cell differentiation and fibroblast secretion of extracellular matrix proteins, contributing to the airway remodeling observed in chronic pulmonary allergic disease pathology. TGF-β can be pro-inflammatory when acting in concert with cytokines such as IL-1, IL-6, IL-23, or IL-4 by augmenting differentiation of $T_H17$ and $T_H2$ cells. TGF-β has pronounced anti-inflammatory activity by inhibiting IgE production, mast cell proliferation, T cell, B cell, NK cell, and cytotoxic lymphocyte function (Commins et al. 2010; Chung and Barnes 1999) or anti-inflammatory role by inhibiting IgE production, mast cell proliferation, T cell, B cell, NK cell, and cytotoxic lymphocyte functions (Chung and Barnes 1999). TGF-β is a primary cytokine responsible for the differentiation of CD4+CD25+T regulatory lymphocytes ($T_{reg}$ cells) that release the anti-inflammatory cytokine IL-10. Reduction in the numbers of $T_{reg}$ cells in hypersensitivity disorders may allow activation of APC and effector cells to promote inflammation. However, the role of $T_{reg}$ cells in pulmonary inflammation may be more complicated because some subsets of $T_{reg}$ cells, particularly the inducible $iT_{reg}$ subset exhibits a high level of plasticity, and can transform into IL-17 and IFN-γ producing effector cells to drive inflammation (Akdis and Akdis 2009). Thus, whether $T_{reg}$ cells act to promote or attenuate inflammation could depend on the local environment.

IL-10, originally named "cytokine synthesis inhibitor factor", is produced by $T_H0$, $T_H1$, $T_H2$, $T_{Reg}$, $T_C$ cells, mast cells, and activated monocytes, macrophages, and dendritic cells. IL-10 decreases $T_H1$ and $T_H2$ cytokine production, suppresses monocyte and macrophage activity, inhibits production of ROI and RNI, and down-regulates secretion of pro-inflammatory cytokines. However, IL-10 is pleiotropic, and while its dominant effect is suppression of adaptive immune responses, it also promotes growth of mast cells, T cells, and induces T cell growth in certain circumstances by induction of the IL-2 receptors (Vock et al. 2010).

Osteopontin (OPN) is a $T_H1$ cytokine with emerging potential for affecting allergic responses. OPN appears to augment primary sensitization, but inhibits responses to secondary antigen exposure (Chung and Barnes 1999; Vock et al. 2010). The complex responses to OPN may be due to different domains on the protein, as ligation of different epitopes with antibodies leads to different effects (Xanthou et al. 2007).

## Remodeling

Repeated exposure of the lungs to irritants and pathogens leads to a constellation of morphological and physiological changes manifested throughout the respiratory tract. The changes manifested in an individual may vary depending on the stimulus, exposure history, genetic and epigenetic background of the individual, and coincident pathogenic conditions or comorbidities.

Irritants and allergens often induce remodeling of the airway wall typically associated with asthma. Smooth muscle hypertrophy, subepithelial collagen deposition, and edema are observed throughout the airways. IL-4, -9, -13, -17, -23, and -25 induce growth of mucin secreting cells in the surface epithelium and submucosal glands (Konno et al. 2011). In mild asthma, the surface epithelium is mainly affected (Turner and Jones 2009; Zuhdi Alimam et al. 2000; Dabbagh et al. 1999), but with increased severity of the disease, submucosal glands enlarge (Ordonez et al. 2001). Small airways that are normally devoid of goblet cells are characterized by Clara cells that differentiate into a mucin-secreting cell phenotype (Dunnill et al. 1969). Corticosteroids are effective in inhibiting mucus hypersecretion in asthma, thereby revealing a major role of inflammatory mediators in mucus hypersecretion (Davis and Dickey 2008).

Deposition of collagens I, III, and V, fibronectin, tenascin, lumican, and biglycan are increased in asthma (Barnes 2002). Increased synthesis is paralleled by an altered balance in metalloproteinase (MMP)-9 and tissue inhibitor of metalloproteinase (TIMP) (Bergeron et al. 2009) resulting in altered ECM turnover and thickening of the lamina reticularis (Suzuki et al. 2001). Degradation of cartilage in the airway wall can also be observed in asthma (Al-Muhsen et al. 2011).

The number and diameter of blood vessels in the airway wall are increased in asthma (Haraguchi et al. 1999; Noble et al. 2002). Epithelial cells, eosinophils, lymphocytes, mast cells, basophils, macrophages, endothelial cells, and smooth muscle cells secrete and angiogenic factors that can drive increase in vascularity, including vascular endothelial growth factor (VEGF), fibroblast growth factor-2 (FGF-2), tryptase, chymase, IL-8, TGF-β, TNF-α, NGF, and angiogenin.

Although not well documented in humans, neural remodeling is likely to occur in asthma. In rhesus macaques, postnatal exposure to house dust mite and ozone reduced neural projections to the epithelium and increased lateral projections to the basal lamina (Dunnill et al. 1969). One year after exposure, nerve density in the airway wall was increased, and projections to the epithelium were abnormal (Larsen et al. 2012; Larson et al. 2004). In rodents, allergic aeroallergens and irritants such as ozone stimulate release of neurotrophins, such as NGF, that promote neural growth within the airway mucosa (Kajekar et al. 2007). Ovalbumin sensitization induces TRPV1 expression in airway Aδ afferent fibers in guinea pigs, which could increase the diversity of stimuli that activate these fibers and lead to cough in allergic asthma (Joos et al. 2000; Ito et al. 2008; Hunter et al. 2011). Another indication of altered neural activity in allergic asthma is that inhibition of TRPA1 inhibits ovalbumin-induced hyperresponsiveness in rats (Lieu et al. 2012).

## Summary

The function of the respiratory system is based on bulk flow of air in response to small pressure gradients developed by respiratory muscle contraction coupled with passive diffusion of gases between inspired air and circulating blood of the alveolar capillaries in response to differential gas pressures. Extensive mechanisms exist to protect the lungs against environmental insults, and many of these processes are adaptive in nature, resulting in memory that increases sensitivity and responsiveness to antigenic stimuli. Adaptations are observed locally and systemically and involve responses by epithelial, nerve, muscle, and immune cells. In over 10 % of the population, the responses to environmental stimuli become pathological and result in excessive sensitivity and aberrant responses to both specific and nonspecific stimuli, and culminate in a progressive and deleterious remodeling of the airways and lungs. Environmental diseases, such as extrinsic asthma, rhinitis, and allergy are increasing and represent major health issues around the world. A better understanding of the mechanisms underlying responses to environmental factors is required for more effective prevention and treatment of these disorders.

## References

Aderem A, Underhill DM. Mechanisms of phagocytosis in macrophages. Annu Rev Immunol. 1999;17:593–623.

Agaugue S, Marcenaro E, Ferranti B, Moretta L, Moretta A. Human natural killer cells exposed to IL-2, IL-12, IL-18, or IL-4 differently modulate priming of naive T cells by monocyte-derived dendritic cells. Blood. 2008;112(5):1776–83.

Akdis CA, Akdis M. Mechanisms and treatment of allergic disease in the big picture of regulatory T cells. J Allergy Clin Immunol. 2009;123(4):735–46. quiz 747–8.

Akuthota P, Xenakis JJ, Weller PF. Eosinophils: offenders or general bystanders in allergic airway disease and pulmonary immunity? J Innate Immun. 2011;3(2):113–9.

Al-Muhsen S, Johnson JR, Hamid Q. Remodeling in asthma. J Allergy Clin Immunol. 2011;128(3):451–62. quiz 463–4.

Banner KH, Igney F, Poll C. TRP channels: emerging targets for respiratory disease. Pharmacol Ther. 2011;130(3):371–84.

Barclay AN, Wright GJ, Brooke G, Brown MH. CD200 and membrane protein interactions in the control of myeloid cells. Trends Immunol. 2002;23(6):285–90.

Barlow JL, McKenzie AN. Nuocytes: expanding the innate cell repertoire in type-2 immunity. J Leukoc Biol. 2011;90(5):867–74.

Barnes PJ. Current and future therapies for airway mucus hypersecretion. Novartis Found Symp. 2002;248:237–49. discussion 249-53, 277-82.

Bates JH, Lutchen KR. The interface between measurement and modeling of peripheral lung mechanics. Respir Physiol Neurobiol. 2005;148(1–2):153–64.

Bathoorn E, Kerstjens H, Postma D, Timens W, MacNee W. Airways inflammation and treatment during acute exacerbations of COPD. Int J Chron Obstruct Pulmon Dis. 2008;3(2):217–29.

Baumer W, Hoppmann J, Rundfeldt C, Kietzmann M. Highly selective phosphodiesterase 4 inhibitors for the treatment of allergic skin diseases and psoriasis. Inflamm Allergy Drug Targets. 2007;6(1):17–26.

Bergeron C, Al-Ramli W, Hamid Q. Remodeling in asthma. Proc Am Thorac Soc. 2009;6(3):301–5.

Birnbaumer L, Zhu X, Jiang M, Boulay G, Peyton M, Vannier B, Brown D, Platano D, Sadeghi H, Stefani E, Birnbaumer M. On the molecular basis and regulation of cellular capacitative calcium entry: roles for Trp proteins. Proc Natl Acad Sci USA. 1996;93(26):15195–202.
Bjorgo E, Moltu K, Tasken K. Phosphodiesterases as targets for modulating T-cell responses. Handb Exp Pharmacol. 2011;204(204):345–63.
Blanchfield JL, Mannie MD. A GMCSF-neuroantigen fusion protein is a potent tolerogen in experimental autoimmune encephalomyelitis (EAE) that is associated with efficient targeting of neuroantigen to APC. J Leukoc Biol. 2010;87(3):509–21.
Bopp T, Dehzad N, Reuter S, Klein M, Ullrich N, Stassen M, Schild H, Buhl R, Schmitt E, Taube C. Inhibition of cAMP degradation improves regulatory T cell-mediated suppression. J Immunol. 2009;182(7):4017–24.
Bosnjak B, Stelzmueller B, Erb KJ, Epstein MM. Treatment of allergic asthma: modulation of Th2 cells and their responses. Respir Res. 2011;12:114.
Bour-Jordan H, Esensten JH, Martinez-Llordella M, Penaranda C, Stumpf M, Bluestone JA. Intrinsic and extrinsic control of peripheral T-cell tolerance by costimulatory molecules of the CD28/B7 family. Immunol Rev. 2011;241(1):180–205.
Brown JM, Swindle EJ, Kushnir-Sukhov NM, Holian A, Metcalfe DD. Silica-directed mast cell activation is enhanced by scavenger receptors. Am J Respir Cell Mol Biol. 2007;36(1):43–52.
Bunyavanich S, Boyce JA, Raby BA, Weiss ST. Gene-by-environment effect of house dust mite on purinergic receptor P2Y12 (P2RY12) and lung function in children with asthma. Clin Exp Allergy. 2012;42(2):229–37.
Caceres AI, Brackmann M, Elia MD, Bessac BF, del Camino D, D'Amours M, Witek JS, Fanger CM, Chong JA, Hayward NJ, Homer RJ, Cohn L, Huang X, Moran MM, Jordt SE. A sensory neuronal ion channel essential for airway inflammation and hyperreactivity in asthma. Proc Natl Acad Sci USA. 2009;106(22):9099–104.
Campbell EL, Louis NA, Tomassetti SE, Canny GO, Arita M, Serhan CN, Colgan SP. Resolvin E1 promotes mucosal surface clearance of neutrophils: a new paradigm for inflammatory resolution. FASEB J. 2007;21(12):3162–70.
Canning BJ. Functional implications of the multiple afferent pathways regulating cough. Pulm Pharmacol Ther. 2011;24(3):295–9.
Canning BJ. Afferent nerves regulating the cough reflex: mechanisms and mediators of cough in disease. Otolaryngol Clin North Am. 2010;43(1):15–25. vii.
Canning BJ. Reflex regulation of airway smooth muscle tone. J Appl Physiol. 2006;101(3): 971–85.
Carati CJ, Gannon BJ. Lymphatic system. In: Anonymous, editor. Encyclopedia of respiratory medicine. New York: Elsevier; 2006. p. 643.
Chen YQ, Shi HZ. CD28/CTLA-4–CD80/CD86 and ICOS–B7RP–1 costimulatory pathway in bronchial asthma. Allergy. 2006;61(1):15–26.
Choi JY, Joo NS, Krouse ME, Wu JV, Robbins RC, Ianowski JP, Hanrahan JW, Wine JJ. Synergistic airway gland mucus secretion in response to vasoactive intestinal peptide and carbachol is lost in cystic fibrosis. J Clin Invest. 2007;117(10):3118–27.
Chung KF, Barnes PJ. Cytokines in asthma. Thorax. 1999;54(9):825–57.
Coleridge HM, Coleridge JC. Pulmonary reflexes: neural mechanisms of pulmonary defense. Annu Rev Physiol. 1994;56:69–91.
Collington SJ, Williams TJ, Weller CL. Mechanisms underlying the localisation of mast cells in tissues. Trends Immunol. 2011;32(10):478–85.
Colsoul B, Nilius B, Vennekens R. On the putative role of transient receptor potential cation channels in asthma. Clin Exp Allergy. 2009;39(10):1456–66.
Commins SP, Borish L, Steinke JW. Immunologic messenger molecules: cytokines, interferons, and chemokines. J Allergy Clin Immunol. 2010;125(2 Suppl 2):S53–72.
Cook ML, Bochner BS. Update on biological therapeutics for asthma. World Allergy Organiz J. 2010;3(6):188–94.
Cowburn AS, Condliffe AM, Farahi N, Summers C, Chilvers ER. Advances in neutrophil biology: clinical implications. Chest. 2008;134(3):606–12.

Coyle AJ, Erard F, Bertrand C, Walti S, Pircher H, Le Gros G. Virus-specific CD8+ cells can switch to interleukin 5 production and induce airway eosinophilia. J Exp Med. 1995;181(3):1229–33.
Dabbagh K, Takeyama K, Lee HM, Ueki IF, Lausier JA, Nadel JA. IL-4 induces mucin gene expression and goblet cell metaplasia in vitro and in vivo. J Immunol. 1999;162(10):6233–7.
Davis CW, Dickey BF. Regulated airway goblet cell mucin secretion. Annu Rev Physiol. 2008;70:487–512.
Delgado M, Ganea D. VIP and PACAP inhibit activation induced apoptosis in T lymphocytes. Ann N Y Acad Sci. 2000;921:55–67.
Delgado M, Leceta J, Sun W, Gomariz RP, Ganea D. VIP and PACAP induce shift to a Th2 response by upregulating B7.2 expression. Ann N Y Acad Sci. 2000;921:68–78.
Dempsey JA, Veasey SC, Morgan BJ, O'Donnell CP. Pathophysiology of sleep apnea. Physiol Rev. 2010;90(1):47–112.
Deniz G, Akdis M, Aktas E, Blaser K, Akdis CA. Human NK1 and NK2 subsets determined by purification of IFN-gamma-secreting and IFN-gamma-nonsecreting NK cells. Eur J Immunol. 2002;32(3):879–84.
Duarte AG, Myers AC. Cough reflex in lung transplant recipients. Lung. 2012;190(1):23–7.
Dunnill MS, Massarella GR, Anderson JA. A comparison of the quantitative anatomy of the bronchi in normal subjects, in status asthmaticus, in chronic bronchitis, and in emphysema. Thorax. 1969;24(2):176–9.
Edwards BA, White DP. Control of the pharyngeal musculature during wakefulness and sleep: implications in normal controls and sleep apnea. Head Neck. 2011;33 Suppl 1:S37–45.
Faffe DS, Zin WA. Lung parenchymal mechanics in health and disease. Physiol Rev. 2009;89(3):759–75.
Fahy JV, Dickey BF. Airway mucus function and dysfunction. N Engl J Med. 2010;363(23):2233–47.
Ferris Jr BG, J M, LH O. Partitioning of respiratory flow resistance in man. J Appl Physiol. 1964;19:653–8.
Forbes LR, Haczku A. SP-D and regulation of the pulmonary innate immune system in allergic airway changes. Clin Exp Allergy. 2010;40(4):547–62.
Ganesh BB, Cheatem DM, Sheng JR, Vasu C, Prabhakar BS. GM-CSF-induced CD11c+CD8a– dendritic cells facilitate Foxp3+ and IL-10+ regulatory T cell expansion resulting in suppression of autoimmune thyroiditis. Int Immunol. 2009;21(3):269–82.
Goetzl EJ, Chan RC, Yadav M. Diverse mechanisms and consequences of immunoadoption of neuromediator systems. Ann N Y Acad Sci. 2008;1144:56–60.
Gorczynski RM. CD200 and its receptors as targets for immunoregulation. Curr Opin Investig Drugs. 2005;6(5):483–8.
Gray H. Anatomy of the human body. New York: Bartelby.com, Inc.; 2000. p. 1396.
Grayson MH, Cheung D, Rohlfing MM, Kitchens R, Spiegel DE, Tucker J, Battaile JT, Alevy Y, Yan L, Agapov E, Kim EY, Holtzman MJ. Induction of high-affinity IgE receptor on lung dendritic cells during viral infection leads to mucous cell metaplasia. J Exp Med. 2007;204(11):2759–69.
Groneberg DA, Hartmann P, Dinh QT, Fischer A. Expression and distribution of vasoactive intestinal polypeptide receptor VPAC(2) mRNA in human airways. Lab Invest. 2001;81(5):749–55.
Groneberg DA, Quarcoo D, Frossard N, Fischer A. Neurogenic mechanisms in bronchial inflammatory diseases. Allergy. 2004;59(11):1139–52.
Groneberg DA, Rabe KF, Fischer A. Novel concepts of neuropeptide-based drug therapy: vasoactive intestinal polypeptide and its receptors. Eur J Pharmacol. 2006;533(1–3):182–94.
Grubor B, Meyerholz DK, Ackermann MR. Collectins and cationic antimicrobial peptides of the respiratory epithelia. Vet Pathol. 2006;43(5):595–612.
Hackett TL. Epithelial-mesenchymal transition in the pathophysiology of airway remodelling in asthma. Curr Opin Allergy Clin Immunol. 2012;12(1):53–9.
Hamilton JA, Anderson GP. GM-CSF biology. Growth Factors. 2004;22(4):225–31.
Hammad H, Lambrecht BN. Dendritic cells and airway epithelial cells at the interface between innate and adaptive immune responses. Allergy. 2011;66(5):579–87.

Hammad H, Plantinga M, Deswarte K, Pouliot P, Willart MA, Kool M, Muskens F, Lambrecht BN. Inflammatory dendritic cells—not basophils—are necessary and sufficient for induction of Th2 immunity to inhaled house dust mite allergen. J Exp Med. 2010;207(10):2097–111.

Hanna J, Gonen-Gross T, Fitchett J, Rowe T, Daniels M, Arnon TI, Gazit R, Joseph A, Schjetne KW, Steinle A, Porgador A, Mevorach D, Goldman-Wohl D, Yagel S, LaBarre MJ, Buckner JH, Mandelboim O. Novel APC-like properties of human NK cells directly regulate T cell activation. J Clin Invest. 2004;114(11):1612–23.

Haraguchi M, Shimura S, Shirato K. Morphometric analysis of bronchial cartilage in chronic obstructive pulmonary disease and bronchial asthma. Am J Respir Crit Care Med. 1999;159(3):1005–13.

Hardie RC, Minke B. Phosphoinositide-mediated phototransduction in Drosophila photoreceptors: the role of Ca2+ and trp. Cell Calcium. 1995;18(4):256–74.

Haworth O, Cernadas M, Levy BD. NK cells are effectors for resolvin E1 in the timely resolution of allergic airway inflammation. J Immunol. 2011;186(11):6129–35.

Haworth O, Levy BD. Endogenous lipid mediators in the resolution of airway inflammation. Eur Respir J. 2007;30(5):980–92.

Heijink IH, Van Oosterhout AJ. Strategies for targeting T-cells in allergic diseases and asthma. Pharmacol Ther. 2006;112(2):489–500.

Helyes Z, Elekes K, Sandor K, Szitter I, Kereskai L, Pinter E, Kemeny A, Szolcsanyi J, McLaughlin L, Vasiliou S, Kipar A, Zimmer A, Hunt SP, Stewart JP, Quinn JP. Involvement of preprotachykinin A gene-encoded peptides and the neurokinin 1 receptor in endotoxin-induced murine airway inflammation. Neuropeptides. 2010;44(5):399–406.

Heyder J. Deposition of inhaled particles in the human respiratory tract and consequences for regional targeting in respiratory drug delivery. Proc Am Thorac Soc. 2004;1(4):315–20.

Hlastala MP, Berger AJ. Physiology of respiration. New York: Oxford University Press; 2001.

Holt PG, Strickland DH. The CD200-CD200R axis in local control of lung inflammation. Nat Immunol. 2008;9(9):1011–3.

Holtzman MJ, Byers DE, Benoit LA, Battaile JT, You Y, Agapov E, Park C, Grayson MH, Kim EY, Patel AC. Immune pathways for translating viral infection into chronic airway disease. Adv Immunol. 2009;102:245–76.

Hunter DD, Carrell-Jacks LA, Batchelor TP, Dey RD. Role of nerve growth factor in ozone-induced neural responses in early postnatal airway development. Am J Respir Cell Mol Biol. 2011;45(2):359–65.

Hwang SW, Cho H, Kwak J, Lee SY, Kang CJ, Jung J, Cho S, Min KH, Suh YG, Kim D, Oh U. Direct activation of capsaicin receptors by products of lipoxygenases: endogenous capsaicin-like substances. Proc Natl Acad Sci USA. 2000;97(11):6155–60.

Irvin CG, Bates JH. Physiologic dysfunction of the asthmatic lung: what's going on down there, anyway? Proc Am Thorac Soc. 2009;6(3):306–11.

Ito W, Tanimoto M, Ono K, Mizuno S, Yoshida A, Koga H, Fuchimoto Y, Kondo N, Tanimoto Y, Kiura K, Matsumoto K, Kataoka M, Nakamura T, Gelfand EW, Kanehiro A. Growth factors temporally associate with airway responsiveness and inflammation in allergen-exposed mice. Int Arch Allergy Immunol. 2008;145(4):324–39.

Iwamura C, Nakayama T. Role of NKT cells in allergic asthma. Curr Opin Immunol. 2010;22(6):807–13.

Johnson JR, Roos A, Berg T, Nord M, Fuxe J. Chronic respiratory aeroallergen exposure in mice induces epithelial-mesenchymal transition in the large airways. PLoS One. 2011;6(1):e16175.

Joos GF, Germonpre PR, Pauwels RA. Role of tachykinins in asthma. Allergy. 2000;55(4): 321–37.

Kajekar R, Pieczarka EM, Smiley-Jewell SM, Schelegle ES, Fanucchi MV, Plopper CG. Early postnatal exposure to allergen and ozone leads to hyperinnervation of the pulmonary epithelium. Respir Physiol Neurobiol. 2007;155(1):55–63.

Karra L, Levi-Schaffer F. Down-regulation of mast cell responses through ITIM containing inhibitory receptors. Adv Exp Med Biol. 2011;716:143–59.

Kelly JT, Prasad AK, Wexler AS. Detailed flow patterns in the nasal cavity. J Appl Physiol. 2000;89(1):323–37.

Kim DH, Park IH, Cho JS, Lee YM, Choi H, Lee HM. Alterations of vasoactive intestinal polypeptide receptors in allergic rhinitis. Am J Rhinol Allergy. 2011;25(1):e44–7.

Kim EY, Alvarez-Baron CP, Dryer SE. Canonical transient receptor potential channel (TRPC)3 and TRPC6 associate with large-conductance Ca2+-activated K+ (BKCa) channels: role in BKCa trafficking to the surface of cultured podocytes. Mol Pharmacol. 2009;75(3):466–77.

Kistemaker LE, Oenema TA, Meurs H, Gosens R. Regulation of airway inflammation and remodeling by muscarinic receptors: Perspectives on anticholinergic therapy in asthma and COPD. Life Sci. 2012;91(21–22):1126–33.

Konno S, Kurokawa M, Uede T, Nishimura M, Huang SK. Role of osteopontin, a multifunctional protein, in allergy and asthma. Clin Exp Allergy. 2011;41(10):1360–6.

Kool M, van Nimwegen M, Willart MA, Muskens F, Boon L, Smit JJ, Coyle A, Clausen BE, Hoogsteden HC, Lambrecht BN, Hammad H. An anti-inflammatory role for plasmacytoid dendritic cells in allergic airway inflammation. J Immunol. 2009;183(2):1074–82.

Korsgren M, Persson CG, Sundler F, Bjerke T, Hansson T, Chambers BJ, Hong S, Van Kaer L, Ljunggren HG, Korsgren O. Natural killer cells determine development of allergen-induced eosinophilic airway inflammation in mice. J Exp Med. 1999;189(3):553–62.

Kouzaki H, Iijima K, Kobayashi T, O'Grady SM, Kita H. The danger signal, extracellular ATP, is a sensor for an airborne allergen and triggers IL-33 release and innate Th2-type responses. J Immunol. 2011;186(7):4375–87.

Kraneveld AD, Nijkamp FP. Tachykinins and neuro-immune interactions in asthma. Int Immunopharmacol. 2001;1(9–10):1629–50.

Kubin L, Alheid GF, Zuperku EJ, McCrimmon DR. Central pathways of pulmonary and lower airway vagal afferents. J Appl Physiol. 2006;101(2):618–27.

Lambrecht BN, Hammad H. Biology of lung dendritic cells at the origin of asthma. Immunity. 2009;31(3):412–24.

Larsen JM, Steen-Jensen DB, Laursen JM, Sondergaard JN, Musavian HS, Butt TM, Brix S. Divergent pro-inflammatory profile of human dendritic cells in response to commensal and pathogenic bacteria associated with the airway microbiota. PLoS One. 2012;7(2):e31976.

Larson SD, Schelegle ES, Walby WF, Gershwin LJ, Fanuccihi MV, Evans MJ, Joad JP, Tarkington BK, Hyde DM, Plopper CG. Postnatal remodeling of the neural components of the epithelial-mesenchymal trophic unit in the proximal airways of infant rhesus monkeys exposed to ozone and allergen. Toxicol Appl Pharmacol. 2004;194(3):211–20.

Lee LY, Pisarri TE. Afferent properties and reflex functions of bronchopulmonary C-fibers. Respir Physiol. 2001;125(1–2):47–65.

Levick SP, Melendez GC, Plante E, McLarty JL, Brower GL, Janicki JS. Cardiac mast cells: the centrepiece in adverse myocardial remodelling. Cardiovasc Res. 2011;89(1):12–9.

Lewis S, Singh D, Evans CE. Cyclic hydrostatic pressure and cotton particles stimulate synthesis by human lung macrophages of cytokines in vitro. Respir Res. 2009;10:44.

Li S, Westwick J, Poll C. Transient receptor potential (TRP) channels as potential drug targets in respiratory disease. Cell Calcium. 2003;33(5–6):551–8.

Li X, Wang XM, Zhang JS. Relevance of vasoactive intestinal peptide and total bronchial mucin in rat lung. Sheng Li Xue Bao. 2009;61(6):539–43.

Lieu TM, Myers AC, Meeker S, Undem BJ. TRPV1 induction in airway vagal low-threshold mechanosensory neurons by allergen challenge and neurotrophic factors. Am J Physiol Lung Cell Mol Physiol. 2012;302(9):L941–8.

Lloyd CM, Hessel EM. Functions of T cells in asthma: more than just T(H)2 cells. Nat Rev Immunol. 2010;10(12):838–48.

Lohmann-Matthes ML, Steinmuller C, Franke-Ullmann G. Pulmonary macrophages. Eur Respir J. 1994;7(9):1678–89.

Matsubara S, Takeda K, Kodama T, Joetham A, Miyahara N, Koya T, Swasey CH, Okamoto M, Dakhama A, Gelfand EW. IL-2 and IL-18 attenuation of airway hyperresponsiveness requires STAT4, IFN-gamma, and natural killer cells. Am J Respir Cell Mol Biol. 2007;36(3):324–32.

McCary C, Tancowny BP, Catalli A, Grammer LC, Harris KE, Schleimer RP, Kulka M. Substance P downregulates expression of the high affinity IgE receptor (FcepsilonRI) by human mast cells. J Neuroimmunol. 2010;220(1–2):17–24.
McDaniel SS, Platoshyn O, Wang J, Yu Y, Sweeney M, Krick S, Rubin LJ, Yuan JX. Capacitative Ca(2+) entry in agonist-induced pulmonary vasoconstriction. Am J Physiol Lung Cell Mol Physiol. 2001;280(5):L870–80.
Mentink-Kane MM, Wynn TA. Opposing roles for IL-13 and IL-13 receptor alpha 2 in health and disease. Immunol Rev. 2004;202:191–202.
Meyer EH, DeKruyff RH, Umetsu DT. T cells and NKT cells in the pathogenesis of asthma. Annu Rev Med. 2008;59:281–92.
Meyrick B, Sturgess JM, Reid L. A reconstruction of the duct system and secretory tubules of the human bronchial submucosal gland. Thorax. 1969;24(6):729–36.
Minas K, Liversidge J. Is the CD200/CD200 receptor interaction more than just a myeloid cell inhibitory signal? Crit Rev Immunol. 2006;26(3):213–30.
Miotto D, Boschetto P, Bononi I, Zeni E, Cavallesco G, Fabbri LM, Mapp CE. Vasoactive intestinal peptide receptors in the airways of smokers with chronic bronchitis. Eur Respir J. 2004;24(6):958–63.
Misaka S, Aoki Y, Karaki S, Kuwahara A, Mizumoto T, Onoue S, Yamada S. Inhalable powder formulation of a stabilized vasoactive intestinal peptide (VIP) derivative: anti-inflammatory effect in experimental asthmatic rats. Peptides. 2010;31(1):72–8.
Mishra A, Chintagari NR, Guo Y, Weng T, Su L, Liu L. Purinergic P2X7 receptor regulates lung surfactant secretion in a paracrine manner. J Cell Sci. 2011;124(Pt 4):657–68.
Mitkiewicz M, Kuropatwa M, Kurowska E, Gorczyca WA. Different effects of soluble and particulate guanylyl cyclases on expression of inflammatory cytokines in rat peripheral blood mononuclear cells. Immunobiology. 2011;216(3):423–30.
Moran MM, McAlexander MA, Biro T, Szallasi A. Transient receptor potential channels as therapeutic targets. Nat Rev Drug Discov. 2011;10(8):601–20.
Moretta L, Ferlazzo G, Bottino C, Vitale M, Pende D, Mingari MC, Moretta A. Effector and regulatory events during natural killer-dendritic cell interactions. Immunol Rev. 2006;214: 219–28.
Mori T, Saito K, Ohki Y, Arakawa H, Tominaga M, Tokuyama K. Lack of transient receptor potential vanilloid-1 enhances Th2-biased immune response of the airways in mice receiving intranasal, but not intraperitoneal, sensitization. Int Arch Allergy Immunol. 2011;156(3):305–12.
Mortaz E, Folkerts G, Nijkamp FP, Henricks PA. ATP and the pathogenesis of COPD. Eur J Pharmacol. 2010;638(1–3):1–4.
Muller T, Robaye B, Vieira RP, Ferrari D, Grimm M, Jakob T, Martin SF, Di Virgilio F, Boeynaems JM, Virchow JC, Idzko M. The purinergic receptor P2Y2 receptor mediates chemotaxis of dendritic cells and eosinophils in allergic lung inflammation. Allergy. 2010;65(12):1545–53.
Murdoch JR, Lloyd CM. Resolution of allergic airway inflammation and airway hyperreactivity is mediated by IL-17-producing {gamma}{delta}T cells. Am J Respir Crit Care Med. 2010;182(4):464–76.
Murphy JE, Tedbury PR, Homer-Vanniasinkam S, Walker JH, Ponnambalam S. Biochemistry and cell biology of mammalian scavenger receptors. Atherosclerosis. 2005;182(1):1–15.
Tippayawong N, Damrongsak D. Prediction of particle deposition in human respiratory system. Thammasat Int J Sci Technol. 2003;8(2):65–71.
Naughton MT. Loop gain in apnea: gaining control or controlling the gain? Am J Respir Crit Care Med. 2010;181(2):103–5.
Neill DR, Wong SH, Bellosi A, Flynn RJ, Daly M, Langford TK, Bucks C, Kane CM, Fallon PG, Pannell R, Jolin HE, McKenzie AN. Nuocytes represent a new innate effector leukocyte that mediates type-2 immunity. Nature. 2010;464(7293):1367–70.
Noble PB, Turner DJ, Mitchell HW. Relationship of airway narrowing, compliance, and cartilage in isolated bronchial segments. J Appl Physiol. 2002;92(3):1119–24.
Nouri-Aria KT, Durham SR. Regulatory T cells and allergic disease. Inflamm Allergy Drug Targets. 2008;7(4):237–52.

Okazaki T, Honjo T. The PD-1-PD-L pathway in immunological tolerance. Trends Immunol. 2006;27(4):195–201.

Okunishi K, Peters-Golden M. Leukotrienes and airway inflammation. Biochim Biophys Acta. 2011;1810(11):1096–102.

Onoue S, Aoki Y, Matsui T, Kojo Y, Misaka S, Mizumoto T, Yamada S. Formulation design and in vivo evaluation of dry powder inhalation system of new vasoactive intestinal peptide derivative ([R(15, 20, 21), L(17), A(24,25), des-N(28)]-VIP-GRR) in experimental asthma/COPD model rats. Int J Pharm. 2011;410(1–2):54–60.

Onoue S, Misaka S, Aoki Y, Karaki S, Kuwahara A, Ohide A, Mizumoto T, Yamada S. Inhalable powder formulation of vasoactive intestinal peptide derivative, [R15,20,21, L17]-VIP-GRR, attenuated neutrophilic airway inflammation in cigarette smoke-exposed rats. Eur J Pharm Sci. 2010;41(3–4):508–14.

Ordonez CL, Khashayar R, Wong HH, Ferrando R, Wu R, Hyde DM, Hotchkiss JA, Zhang Y, Novikov A, Dolganov G, Fahy JV. Mild and moderate asthma is associated with airway goblet cell hyperplasia and abnormalities in mucin gene expression. Am J Respir Crit Care Med. 2001;163(2):517–23.

Orgeig S, Hiemstra PS, Veldhuizen EJ, Casals C, Clark HW, Haczku A, Knudsen L, Possmayer F. Recent advances in alveolar biology: evolution and function of alveolar proteins. Respir Physiol Neurobiol. 2010;173(Suppl):S43–54.

Osborn AG. The nasal arteries. AJR Am J Roentgenol. 1978;130(1):89–97.

Parisinos CA. Sarcoidosis is a Th1/Th17 multisystem disorder: wider implications. Thorax. 2011;66(11):1011–2. author reply 1012.

Park GY, Christman JW. Involvement of cyclooxygenase-2 and prostaglandins in the molecular pathogenesis of inflammatory lung diseases. Am J Physiol Lung Cell Mol Physiol. 2006;290(5):L797–805.

Parungo CP, Colson YL, Kim SW, Kim S, Cohn LH, Bawendi MG, Frangioni JV. Sentinel lymph node mapping of the pleural space. Chest. 2005;127(5):1799–804.

Parungo CP, Ohnishi S, De Grand AM, Laurence RG, Soltesz EG, Colson YL, Kang PM, Mihaljevic T, Cohn LH, Frangioni JV. In vivo optical imaging of pleural space drainage to lymph nodes of prognostic significance. Ann Surg Oncol. 2004;11(12):1085–92.

Perez-Gil J, Weaver TE. Pulmonary surfactant pathophysiology: current models and open questions. Physiology (Bethesda). 2010;25(3):132–41.

Perl M, Lomas-Neira J, Venet F, Chung CS, Ayala A. Pathogenesis of indirect (secondary) acute lung injury. Expert Rev Respir Med. 2011;5(1):115–26.

Raemdonck K, de Alba J, Birrell MA, Grace M, Maher SA, Irvin CG, Fozard JR, O'Byrne PM, Belvisi MG. A role for sensory nerves in the late asthmatic response. Thorax. 2012;67(1):19–25.

Ramalho R, Soares R, Couto N, Moreira A. Tachykinin receptors antagonism for asthma: a systematic review. BMC Pulm Med. 2011;11:41.

Ray A, Khare A, Krishnamoorthy N, Qi Z, Ray P. Regulatory T cells in many flavors control asthma. Mucosal Immunol. 2010;3(3):216–29.

Resnick MB, Weller PF. Mechanisms of eosinophil recruitment. Am J Respir Cell Mol Biol. 1993;8(4):349–55.

Rhee JS, Kimbell JS. The nasal valve dilemma: the narrow straw vs the weak wall. Arch Facial Plast Surg. 2012;14(1):9–10.

Ritz SA, Stampfli MR, Davies DE, Holgate ST, Jordana M. On the generation of allergic airway diseases: from GM-CSF to Kyoto. Trends Immunol. 2002;23(8):396–402.

Robinson DS. The role of the T cell in asthma. J Allergy Clin Immunol. 2010;126(6):1081–91. quiz 1092–3.

Rogers DF. Motor control of airway goblet cells and glands. Respir Physiol. 2001;125(1–2): 129–44.

Saha S, Brightling CE. Eosinophilic airway inflammation in COPD. Int J Chron Obstruct Pulmon Dis. 2006;1(1):39–47.

Salassa JR, Pearson BW, Payne WS. Gross and microscopical blood supply of the trachea. Ann Thorac Surg. 1977;24(2):100–7.

Sarin S, Undem B, Sanico A, Togias A. The role of the nervous system in rhinitis. J Allergy Clin Immunol. 2006;118(5):999–1016.

Saxon A, Kepley C, Zhang K. "Accentuate the negative, eliminate the positive": engineering allergy therapeutics to block allergic reactivity through negative signaling. J Allergy Clin Immunol. 2008;121(2):320–5.

Schleimer RP, Kato A, Kern R, Kuperman D, Avila PC. Epithelium: at the interface of innate and adaptive immune responses. J Allergy Clin Immunol. 2007;120(6):1279–84.

Sel S, Rost BR, Yildirim AO, Sel B, Kalwa H, Fehrenbach H, Renz H, Gudermann T, Dietrich A. Loss of classical transient receptor potential 6 channel reduces allergic airway response. Clin Exp Allergy. 2008;38(9):1548–58.

Selman L, Skjodt K, Nielsen O, Floridon C, Holmskov U, Hansen S. Expression and tissue localization of collectin placenta 1 (CL-P1, SRCL) in human tissues. Mol Immunol. 2008;45(11):3278–88.

Shannahan JH, Kodavanti UP, Brown JM. Manufactured and airborne nanoparticle cardiopulmonary interactions: a review of mechanisms and the possible contribution of mast cells. Inhal Toxicol. 2012;24(5):320–39.

Singh AK, Stock P, Akbari O. Role of PD-L1 and PD-L2 in allergic diseases and asthma. Allergy. 2011;66(2):155–62.

Skatrud JB, Dempsey JA. Interaction of sleep state and chemical stimuli in sustaining rhythmic ventilation. J Appl Physiol. 1983;55(3):813–22.

Smith KG, Clatworthy MR. FcgammaRIIB in autoimmunity and infection: evolutionary and therapeutic implications. Nat Rev Immunol. 2010;10(5):328–43.

Soruri A, Zwirner J. Dendritic cells: limited potential in immunotherapy. Int J Biochem Cell Biol. 2005;37(2):241–5.

Spencer LA, Szela CT, Perez SA, Kirchhoffer CL, Neves JS, Radke AL, Weller PF. Human eosinophils constitutively express multiple Th1, Th2, and immunoregulatory cytokines that are secreted rapidly and differentially. J Leukoc Biol. 2009;85(1):117–23.

Sugita M, Kuribayashi K, Nakagomi T, Miyata S, Matsuyama T, Kitada O. Allergic bronchial asthma: airway inflammation and hyperresponsiveness. Intern Med. 2003;42(8): 636–43.

Susarla SM, Thomas RJ, Abramson ZR, Kaban LB. Biomechanics of the upper airway: changing concepts in the pathogenesis of obstructive sleep apnea. Int J Oral Maxillofac Surg. 2010;39(12):1149–59.

Suzuki R, Kato T, Miyazaki Y, Iwata M, Noda Y, Takagi K, Nakashima N, Torii K. Matrix metalloproteinases and tissue inhibitors of matrix metalloproteinases in sputum from patients with bronchial asthma. J Asthma. 2001;38(6):477–84.

Sweeney M, McDaniel SS, Platoshyn O, Zhang S, Yu Y, Lapp BR, Zhao Y, Thistlethwaite PA, Yuan JX. Role of capacitative Ca2+ entry in bronchial contraction and remodeling. J Appl Physiol. 2002;92(4):1594–602.

Szema AM, Hamidi SA, Golightly MG, Rueb TP, Chen JJ. VIP Regulates the Development & Proliferation of Treg in vivo in spleen. Allergy Asthma Clin Immunol. 2011;7:19.

Taher YA, Piavaux BJ, Gras R, van Esch BC, Hofman GA, Bloksma N, Henricks PA, van Oosterhout AJ. Indoleamine 2,3-dioxygenase-dependent tryptophan metabolites contribute to tolerance induction during allergen immunotherapy in a mouse model. J Allergy Clin Immunol. 2008;121(4):983–91.e2.

Tannu SA, Renzetti LM, Tare N, Ventre JD, Lavelle D, Lin TA, Morschauser A, Paciorek J, Bolin DR, Michel H, Singer L, Hargaden M, Knowles I, Gardiner P, Cazzola M, Calzetta L, Matera MG, Hicks A. Dual bronchodilatory and pulmonary anti-inflammatory activity of RO5024118, a novel agonist at vasoactive intestinal peptide VPAC2 receptors. Br J Pharmacol. 2010;161(6):1329–42.

Tarran R, Button B, Boucher RC. Regulation of normal and cystic fibrosis airway surface liquid volume by phasic shear stress. Annu Rev Physiol. 2006;68:543–61.

Thakur SA, Hamilton Jr RF, Holian A. Role of scavenger receptor a family in lung inflammation from exposure to environmental particles. J Immunotoxicol. 2008;5(2):151–7.

Tran NP, Vickery J, Blaiss MS. Management of rhinitis: allergic and non-allergic. Allergy Asthma Immunol Res. 2011;3(3):148–56.
Trout L, Corboz MR, Ballard ST. Mechanism of substance P-induced liquid secretion across bronchial epithelium. Am J Physiol Lung Cell Mol Physiol. 2001;281(3):L639–45.
Tsoumakidou M, Demedts IK, Brusselle GG, Jeffery PK. Dendritic cells in chronic obstructive pulmonary disease: new players in an old game. Am J Respir Crit Care Med. 2008;177(11):1180–6.
Turner J, Jones CE. Regulation of mucin expression in respiratory diseases. Biochem Soc Trans. 2009;37(Pt 4):877–81.
Undem BJ, McAlexander M, Hunter DD. Neurobiology of the upper and lower airways. Allergy. 1999;54 Suppl 57:81–93.
van Buul JD, Allingham MJ, Samson T, Meller J, Boulter E, Garcia-Mata R, Burridge K. RhoG regulates endothelial apical cup assembly downstream from ICAM1 engagement and is involved in leukocyte trans-endothelial migration. J Cell Biol. 2007;178(7):1279–93.
Vock C, Hauber HP, Wegmann M. The other T helper cells in asthma pathogenesis. J Allergy (Cairo). 2010;2010:519298.
Voice JK, Dorsam G, Chan RC, Grinninger C, Kong Y, Goetzl EJ. Immunoeffector and immunoregulatory activities of vasoactive intestinal peptide. Regul Pept. 2002;109(1–3):199–208.
Wan YY, Flavell RA. Regulatory T cells, transforming growth factor-beta, and immune suppression. Proc Am Thorac Soc. 2007;4(3):271–6.
Wang M, Ellison CA, Gartner JG, HayGlass KT. Natural killer cell depletion fails to influence initial CD4 T cell commitment in vivo in exogenous antigen-stimulated cytokine and antibody responses. J Immunol. 1998;160(3):1098–105.
Weir N. Anatomy of the larynx and tracheobronchial tree. In: Kerr AG, editor. Scott-Brown's otolaryngology. 6th ed. Oxford: Butterworth-Heinemann; 1997. p. 13–4.
Weissmann N, Dietrich A, Fuchs B, Kalwa H, Ay M, Dumitrascu R, Olschewski A, Storch U, Mederos Y, Schnitzler M, Ghofrani HA, Schermuly RT, Pinkenburg O, Seeger W, Grimminger F, Gudermann T. Classical transient receptor potential channel 6 (TRPC6) is essential for hypoxic pulmonary vasoconstriction and alveolar gas exchange. Proc Natl Acad Sci USA. 2006;103(50):19093–8.
Weller CL, Collington SJ, Williams T, Lamb JR. Mast cells in health and disease. Clin Sci (Lond). 2011;120(11):473–84.
Welte T, Groneberg DA. Asthma and COPD. Exp Toxicol Pathol. 2006;57 Suppl 2:35–40.
Wen LP, Fahrni JA, Matsui S, Rosen GD. Airway epithelial cells produce stem cell factor. Biochim Biophys Acta. 1996;1314(3):183–6.
Widdicombe JG. Pulmonary and respiratory tract receptors. J Exp Biol. 1982;100:41–57.
Widdicombe JG. Receptors in the trachea and bronchi of the cat. J Physiol. 1954a;123(1):71–104.
Widdicombe JG. Respiratory reflexes from the trachea and bronchi of the cat. J Physiol. 1954b;123(1):55–70.
Widdicombe JG. Reflexes from the upper respiratory tract. In: Anonymous, editor. Comprehensive physiology. New Jersey: John Wiley & Sons Inc.; 2011.
Willart MA, Lambrecht BN. The danger within: endogenous danger signals, atopy and asthma. Clin Exp Allergy. 2009;39(1):12–9.
Wilson RH, Whitehead GS, Nakano H, Free ME, Kolls JK, Cook DN. Allergic sensitization through the airway primes Th17-dependent neutrophilia and airway hyperresponsiveness. Am J Respir Crit Care Med. 2009;180(8):720–30.
Wine JJ. Parasympathetic control of airway submucosal glands: central reflexes and the airway intrinsic nervous system. Auton Neurosci. 2007;133(1):35–54.
Xanthou G, Alissafi T, Semitekolou M, Simoes DC, Economidou E, Gaga M, Lambrecht BN, Lloyd CM, Panoutsakopoulou V. Osteopontin has a crucial role in allergic airway disease through regulation of dendritic cell subsets. Nat Med. 2007;13(5):570–8.
Xiang M, Fan J. Pattern recognition receptor-dependent mechanisms of acute lung injury. Mol Med. 2010;16(1–2):69–82.

Xiang M, Fan J, Fan J. Association of Toll-like receptor signaling and reactive oxygen species: a potential therapeutic target for posttrauma acute lung injury. Mediators Inflamm. 2010;2010:916425. Epub 2010 Jul 13, 2010.

Xie A, Skatrud JB, Puleo DS, Rahko PS, Dempsey JA. Apnea-hypopnea threshold for CO2 in patients with congestive heart failure. Am J Respir Crit Care Med. 2002;165(9):1245–50.

Xu J, Xu F. Role of neurogenic substance P in overexpression of alveolar macrophages' neurokinin 1 receptor in mice exposed to cigarette smoke. Exp Lung Res. 2010;36(4):243–54.

Xu J, Xu F, Barrett E. Metalloelastase in lungs and alveolar macrophages is modulated by extracellular substance P in mice. Am J Physiol Lung Cell Mol Physiol. 2008;295(1):L162–70.

Xu J, Xu F, Lin Y. Cigarette smoke synergizes lipopolysaccharide-induced interleukin-1beta and tumor necrosis factor-alpha secretion from macrophages via substance P-mediated nuclear factor-kappaB activation. Am J Respir Cell Mol Biol. 2011;44(3):302–8.

Yadav M, Rosenbaum J, Goetzl EJ. Cutting edge: vasoactive intestinal peptide (VIP) induces differentiation of Th17 cells with a distinctive cytokine profile. J Immunol. 2008;180(5):2772–6.

Yatera K, Morimoto Y, Kim HN, Myojo T, Mukae H. Foam cell formation of alveolar macrophages in Clara cell ablated mice inhaling crystalline silica. Inhal Toxicol. 2011;23(12):736–44.

Yoshida Y, Tanaka Y, Hirano M, Nakashima T. Sensory innervation of the pharynx and larynx. Am J Med. 2000;108(Suppl 4a):51S–61.

Zhu X, Jiang M, Peyton M, Boulay G, Hurst R, Stefani E, Birnbaumer L. trp, a novel mammalian gene family essential for agonist-activated capacitative Ca2+ entry. Cell. 1996;85(5):661–71.

Zhu Z, Oh SY, Cho YS, Zhang L, Kim YK, Zheng T. Tyrosine phosphatase SHP-1 in allergic and anaphylactic inflammation. Immunol Res. 2010;47(1–3):3–13.

Zuhdi Alimam M, Piazza FM, Selby DM, Letwin N, Huang L, Rose MC. Muc-5/5ac mucin messenger RNA and protein expression is a marker of goblet cell metaplasia in murine airways. Am J Respir Cell Mol Biol. 2000;22(3):253–60.

# Chapter 3
# Reactive Airways Dysfunction Syndrome (RADS) and Irritant-Induced Asthma

**Stuart M. Brooks**

**Abstract** Irritant-induced asthma signifies nonallergic asthma without latency or immunological sensitization. The acute sudden-onset type that appears within 24-h after a single, massive irritant gas, vapor, or fume exposure is coined Reactive Airways Dysfunction Syndrome (RADS). Almost all cases are accidental and arise without warning such as with an unanticipated explosion, accidental release of irritant(s) held under pressure, activities taking place in a confined space and/or emissions of smoke and irritant gases accompanying a fire. Presumably in some poorly understood manner, the massive irritant exposure leads to persistent airway inflammation, altered airway remodeling, sustained airway hyperresponsiveness and asthmatic symptoms. A second type of irritant-induced asthma emerges not as suddenly as RADS. Individuals are repeatedly exposed to non-massive levels of irritants over a few days, weeks, or months and eventually develop clinical asthma. Ostensibly, this type of asthma is associated with a preexisting susceptibility including asthma in clinical remission or stability. The long-term outcome of subjects with irritant-induced asthma is similar to subjects with allergic occupational asthma. The treatment of irritant-induced asthma is similar to the treatment afforded patients suffering with other types of adult-onset asthma.

**Keywords** Asthma • Reactive airways dysfunction syndrome (RADS) • Irritant-induced asthma • Occupational asthma

---

S.M. Brooks, M.D. (✉)
Department of Environmental & Occupational Health, Health Sciences Center, College of Public Health, University of South Florida, Tampa, FL, USA
e-mail: sbrooks@health.usf.edu

W.J. Meggs (ed.), *The Toxicant Induction of Irritant Asthma, Rhinitis, and Related Conditions*, DOI 10.1007/978-1-4614-9044-9_3,

## Introduction

The link between asthma and workplace exposures are established on four situations/mechanisms: (1) *allergic-type occupational asthma* occurs when an employee is repeatedly exposed to a unique workplace agent (~250 different high- and low-molecular animal, vegetable, and chemical agents) over months or years (latency) that eventuates into immunologic/allergic sensitization to this workplace agent and where subsequent reexposure to the agent, even in low concentrations, initiates new-onset asthma; (2) *single exposure irritant-induced occupational asthma* occurs when an employee inhales a solitary massive concentration of an irritant gas, vapor, or fume and manifests newly developed clinical asthma (asthma symptoms + non-specific airway hyperresponsiveness) within 24-h following the exposure (no latency); (3) *repeated exposure irritant-induced occupational asthma* occurs when a purportedly susceptible employee is repeatedly exposed to non-massive levels of an irritant gas, vapor, or fume (or as a mixture) over a few days, weeks, or months and eventually develops clinical asthma; and (4) *work-aggravated asthma* correspond to preexisting or concurrent asthma that is exacerbated or aggravated by workplace exposures to airborne irritant dusts, gases, vapors, or fumes. Some clinicians differentiate between *work-exacerbated asthma* and *work-aggravated asthma*, based on whether the worker returns to a prior asthma baseline (i.e., work-exacerbated asthma) or not (work-aggravated asthma), but this distinction is not accepted by all. Work-aggravated asthma may be the most common effect of work on asthma (Goe et al. 2004). Up to 20 % of full-time workers with asthma report work-aggravated asthma symptoms on a weekly basis over the preceding month.

Brooks and colleagues declared two archetypical types of irritant-induced asthma (Brooks et al. 1998). Many thousands of workers who yearly seek medical care because of inhalational exposures recover without persistent clinical pulmonary aftermaths and few individuals die (Blanc et al. 1991; Henneberger et al. 2000). The inhalation injury takes longer to resolve in individuals who are left with persistent pulmonary impairment.

## Frequency of Irritant-Induced Asthma

Irritant-induced asthma includes less than one-fifth of workers with the diagnosis of "occupational asthma" (Bernstein et al. 2006; Brooks 2010; Chatkin et al. 1999; Henneberger et al. 2003; Malo et al. 2004; Nemery, 1996, 2006). A retrospective study of 469 asthma claims accepted by the Ontario Workers' Compensation Board between 1984 and 1988 identified 89 subjects (19 %) who developed asthma after an accidental high irritant exposure (i.e., Reactive Airways Dysfunction Syndrome, RADS), 68 people (76 %) reportedly had an exacerbation of preexisting asthma, and 12 subjects (13 %) claimed new-onset irritant-induced asthma (Chatkin et al. 1999). In a specialized chest clinic of Toronto in Canada, a retrospective investigation of 154 patients suspected of work-related asthma seen between 1978 and 1987, showed that 17 % of the cases were considered to represent the diagnoses of "definite" or "possible" RADS/irritant-induced asthma (Tarlo and Broder 1989). The incidence of self-reported asthma and chronic bronchitis in cohorts of Swedish workers were associated with peak concentrations of irritant exposures (Henneberger et al. 2005). According to data published by SWORD (Surveillance of Work-Related and Occupational Respiratory Diseases) and OPRA (Occupational Physicians Reporting Activity) for the span of 10 years, between 1992 and 2001, the incidence of inhalation accidents resulting in occupational asthma and RADS comprised between 13.7 and 29 % of incident work-related respiratory diseases depending on whether cases were reported by chest physicians or occupational physicians (McDonald et al. 2005). In the United States, RADS cases were identified by the four American states (California, Massachusetts, Michigan, and New Jersey) that conducted surveillance for work-related asthma during the period 1993–2003 as part of the Sentinel Event Notification Systems for Occupational Risks (SENSOR). In this sampling period, a total of 445 RADS cases were documented by SENSOR representing 9 % of work-related asthma events including both occupational asthma and RADS (Bernstein et al. 2006).

## RISK Factors for Irritant-Induced Asthma

Risk factors for irritant-induced asthma are not well characterized but likely include the concentration of the offending agent, physical and chemical properties, and host susceptibility factors (Brooks 2011). Other risk factors may relate to the covalent binding properties of the irritant chemical (i.e., halogenated vs. nonhalogenated gas), the chemical's vapor pressure (i.e., high vapor pressure then likelihood of higher levels in air) and physical state (vapor, gas fume, dust), the chemical's water solubility (i.e., may determines upper vs. lower airway involvement) and/or the chemical's ability to react with sulfur or cysteine molecules and thus possess the potential to form double bonds with human proteins. The Quantitative Structure Activity Relationship (QSAR) provides an estimate of the capacity to form chemical cross-linking reactions perhaps an indicator of a chemical's propensity to cause irritancy (Abraham et al. 2003; Alarie 1973, 1981). In an investigation conducted by Kern, RADS cases were confirmed in four individuals and the risk increased in a dose–response manner with exposure intensity (Kern 1991). A massive irritant exposure may lead not only to RADS but could also result in the Adult Respiratory Distress Syndrome, bronchiolitis and perhaps other respiratory outcomes (Brooks 2011; Nemery 1996).

## Clinical Types of Irritant-Induced Asthma

### *Single Exposure Irritant-Induced Occupational Asthma*

*Reactive Airways Dysfunction Syndrome (RADS)* and *Acute Irritant-Induced Asthma* are synonymous with *Single Exposure Irritant-Induced Occupational Asthma.*

This type of irritant-induced asthma emerges as acute new-onset asthma without latency or immunological sensitization beginning within 24-h following a single, massive irritant gas, vapor or fume exposure (Bardana 1999; Brooks et al. 1985; Malo 1998; Tarlo 2010). Generally, it is not possible to accurately gauge the precise concentration of the irritant exposure since almost all cases are accidental and occur without warning such as with an unanticipated explosion, accidental release of irritant(s) held under pressure, when there are activities taking place in a confined space having reduced exchange ventilation rate and/or reduced fresh air make-up and when there are emissions of airborne smoke and irritant gases accompanying a fire. Presumably in some poorly understood manner, a massive irritant exposure leads to persistent airway inflammation, altered airway remodeling, sustained airway hyperresponsiveness, and asthmatic symptoms. It must be stressed that the connotation Reactive Airways Dysfunction Syndrome ("RADS") is not the same as the designation Reactive Airways Disease ("RAD") (Fahy and O' Byrne 2001). The latter is a code word for the general term of "asthma", while RADS refers specifically to acute irritant-induced asthma caused by a high-level irritant exposure. The worker with RADS may initially describe burning of the eyes, nose, and throat in the ensuing minutes after the exposure confirming its irritant nature. Symptoms always begin with coughing appearing almost immediately. Both shortness of breath and chest discomfort are also early complaints but wheezing can take longer to evolve. Workers seek treatment in an emergency facility or a physician's office within a few hours or possibly the next morning and by definition always within 24 h after the accidental exposure. In some cases respiratory symptoms associated with RADS are transient and resolve within 12 weeks or less (Nemery 1996). In other cases of RADS, continuing asthma-type symptoms and nonspecific airway hyperresponsiveness persist for years following the inciting exposure (Malo et al. 2009). The reason for the differences is unknown. One review of RADS cases reported a median duration of symptoms lasting 13 months (Shakeri et al. 2008). The routine chest X-ray is characteristically interpreted as being "negative" without acute infiltrates or pleural changes. When performed, spirometric tests often display "normal" or "mild" airflow limitation with no "significant" response to an inhaled bronchodilator. Among the ten subjects originally described by Brooks and coworkers, four had a reduced Tiffeneau index (Swanney et al. 2008). Persistent airflow limitation occurs only in a small percentage of persons with RADS. Bhérer and coworkers showed airflow obstruction in 31/51 (60 %) subjects assessed 18–24 months after inhalational accidents due to chlorine (Bherer et al. 1994). Some patients demonstrate a mixed spirometric pattern reflecting combined central and peripheral involvement (Charan et al. 1979; Gilbert and Auchincloss 1989). The hallmark of RADS is persistent airway hyperresponsiveness as defined by a "positive" methacholine challenge test (e.g., $PC_{20}$ for methacholine is <8 mg/ml). However, the level of bronchial hyperresponsiveness to methacholine tends to be mild or even borderline in some cases (Lemiere et al. 1997). It is important that other pulmonary conditions, that simulate RADS, are excluded including vocal cord dysfunction. Table 3.1 provides the diagnostic criteria for RADS.

**Table 3.1** Diagnostic criteria for RADS

| | |
|---|---|
| 1. | Absence of preexisting respiratory disorder, asthma symptomatology or a history of asthma in remission and exclusion of conditions that can simulate asthma |
| 2. | Onset of asthma after a single exposure or accident |
| 3. | Exposure is to an irritant vapor, gas, fumes, or smoke in very high concentrations |
| 4. | Onset of asthma occurs within minutes to hours and always less than 24 h after the exposure |
| 5. | Finding of a positive methacholine challenge test (<8 mg/ml) following the exposure |
| 6. | Possible airflow obstruction on pulmonary function testing |
| 7. | Another pulmonary disorder to explain the symptoms and findings is excluded |

## *Repeated Exposure Irritant-Induced Occupational Asthma*

Repeated exposure-type of irritant-induced asthma has been classified under different monikers including: *Repeated Exposure Irritant-Induced Asthma, "Atypical RADS", "Low-Dose RADS", Low-Intensity Chronic Exposure Dysfunction Syndrome (LICEDS), "Not-So-Sudden" Irritant-Induced Asthma, and "Chronic" Irritant-Induced Asthma* (Bernstein et al. 2006; Brooks et al. 1998; Gilbert and Auchincloss 1989; Henneberger et al. 2003; Kipen et al. 1994; Malo et al. 2004; Tabar et al. 1998; Tarlo 2010; Tarlo et al. 2008). In the repeated exposures-type of irritant-induced asthma, the clinical appearance of asthma takes longer to evolve and only after repeated irritant exposures. Table 3.2 suggests the diagnostic criteria needed to establish the diagnosis of repeated exposure irritant-induced occupational asthma (Brooks et al. 2013). Irritant chemicals contribute to the incidence of asthma in children and adults (McConnell et al. 2002; Medina-Ramón et al. 2005; Rumchev et al. 2002; Sherriff et al. 2005; Zock et al. 2010). Numerous epidemiological surveys have been conducted in workers repeatedly exposed to both low and high levels of chlorine, $SO_2$, and/or ozone in pulp and paper mills and other workplaces with high risk of similar exposures (Bherer et al. 1994; Chan-Yeung et al. 1994; Gautrin et al. 1995; Henneberger et al. 2005; Malo et al. 2009; Olin et al. 2002, 2004). Mild increases in bronchial responsiveness and other clinical associations were identified during a 2-year follow-up of Canadian workers experiencing repeated chlorine "puff" exposures (Gautrin et al. 1999). Persistent asthmatic symptoms and presence of nonspecific bronchial hyperresponsiveness and/or variable airflow obstruction was reported among three pulp mill workers experiencing repeated chlorine "gassing" episodes occurring over several years (Chan-Yeung et al. 1994) Among 25 subjects, the onset of asthma symptoms took longer to materialized after repeated irritant exposures transpiring over days, weeks, or months (Brooks et al. 1998). When analyzed, 88 % of subjects were considered "atopic" and 40 % developed new-onset asthma in the setting of underlying preexisting asthma clinically quiescent for at least 1 year before the exposure (Brooks et al. 1998).

Some swimmers, mainly children repeatedly exposed to chlorine chemicals applied for water disinfection, may develop an asthmatic condition (Bougault et al. 2009; Weisel et al. 2009). The water contained in public swimming pools comprises organic precursors from the tap water used to fill the pool as well as precursors from

**Table 3.2** Diagnostic criteria for repeated exposure irritant-induced asthma

1. There is no preceding latency but asthma symptoms commence during repeated intermittent or continuous inhalational exposures to non-massive, moderate, lower intensity but tolerable concentrations of an irritant vapor, gas, fumes, or smoke
2. Asthma symptoms start during the time repeated irritant exposures take place and not after cessation of exposure
3. The duration of the repeated exposures is always more than 24 h and typically does not last longer than 4 months of repeated exposures before asthma symptoms begin. Rarely does the irritant exposure last $\geq$1-year before the initiation of asthma symptoms
4. There is the absence of preexisting asthma symptomatology for the previous 1-year or there may be a past history of childhood asthma that resolved or there was a past history of adult asthma in remission for at least 1-year. There may have also been a diagnosis and/or treatment of bronchial asthma instituted by a previous physician
5. Typical irritant-induced asthma symptoms include episodic coughing, wheezing, and symptoms of "bronchial irritability," (i.e., acute respiratory complaints that follow exposures to various nonspecific irritants, physical factors, and odors). There also may be intermittent chest tightness and nocturnal episodes of coughing, wheezing, and breathlessness
6. Spirometry may be normal, show airflow limitation, and/or demonstrate a positive response ($\geq$12 %) to an inhaled bronchodilator
7. There is a positive methacholine challenge test ($<$8 mg/ml) that confirms the presence of nonspecific airway hyperresponsiveness
8. There must be exclusion of alternative conditions that simulate asthma including vocal cord dysfunction. The possibility of occupational asthma caused by a workplace sensitizer is also eliminated
9. There is no preceding latency but asthma symptoms commence during repeated intermittent or continuous inhalational exposures to non-massive, moderate, lower intensity but tolerable concentrations of an irritant vapor, gas, fumes, or smoke
10. Asthma symptoms start during the time repeated irritant exposures take place and not after cessation of exposure
11. The duration of the repeated exposures is always more than 24 h and typically does not last longer than 4 months of repeated exposures before asthma symptoms begin. Rarely does the irritant exposure last $\geq$1-year before the initiation of asthma symptoms
12. There is the absence of preexisting asthma symptomatology for the previous 1-year or there may be a past history of childhood asthma that resolved or there was a past history of adult asthma in remission for at least 1-year. There may have also been a diagnosis and/or treatment of bronchial asthma instituted by a previous physician
13. Typical irritant-induced asthma symptoms include episodic coughing, wheezing, and symptoms of "bronchial irritability," (i.e., acute respiratory complaints that follow exposures to various nonspecific irritants, physical factors, and odors). There also may be intermittent chest tightness and nocturnal episodes of coughing, wheezing, and breathlessness
14. Spirometry may be normal, show airflow limitation, and/or demonstrate a positive response ($\geq$12 %) to an inhaled bronchodilator
15. There is a positive methacholine challenge test ($<$8 mg/ml) that confirms the presence of nonspecific airway hyperresponsiveness
16. There must be exclusion of alternative conditions that simulate asthma including vocal cord dysfunction. The possibility of occupational asthma caused by a workplace sensitizer is also eliminated

Also, not-so-sudden irritant-induced asthma, "Low-dose RADS" or "low-intensity chronic exposure dysfunction syndrome, 'LICEDS'" swimmers; the latter includes constituents of sweat and urine, skin particles, hair, microorganisms, cosmetics, and other personal care products (Weisel et al. 2009). Disinfection of swimming pools entails generation of "free chlorine" by addition of sodium hypochlorite (liquid bleach), calcium hypochlorite, or chlorine gas (Weisel et al. 2009). The free chlorine reacting with precursor materials form disinfection by-products that include inorganic chloramines, organic chloramines, haloacetonitriles, and other organic compounds (Li and Blatchley 2007). The specific types and levels of disinfection by-products formed depend on numerous factors, including the type and amount of disinfectant used, characteristics of the swimming pool and pool water, and swimmer hygiene. For lifeguards at swimming pools, an exposure–response relationship has been identified between trichloramine, measured as total chloramines, and irritant eye, nasal, and throat symptoms, although not chronic respiratory symptoms or bronchial hyperresponsiveness (Massin et al. 1998).

## Etiological Agents for Irritant-Induced Asthma

The originally reported causative agents of RADS include: uranium hexafluoride gas, floor sealant, spray paint containing significant concentrations of ammonia, heated acid, 35 % hydrazine, fumigating fog, metal coating remover, and smoke (Brooks et al. 1985). Cases of inhalation accidents were reported to Surveillance Of Work-Related and Occupational Respiratory Disease (SWORD) and the Open Public Records Act (OPRA) between 1992 and 2001. The offending agents were classified into five categories with different physical properties: the most frequently reported were irritant gases (42 %) followed by solvent vapors (18 %), metallic fumes (11 %), acid mists (9 %), and other (18 %) (McDonald et al. 2005). When comparing subjects with inhalation injuries to those with immunological occupational asthma, there is a predominance of men (McDonald et al. 2005; Tarlo and Broder 1989) and smoking whereas atopy is less frequent. Table 3.3 lists reported causes of irritant-induced asthma and RADS.

**Table 3.3** Causes of irritant-induced asthma and RADS

| Exposure | Agent or process |
|---|---|
| Acids | Glacial acetic, sulfuric, hydrochloric, hydrofluoric acid |
| Alkali | Ammonia, bleach, calcium oxide, sodium hydroxide, World Trade Center dust, air bag emissions |
| Gases | Chlorine, sulfur dioxide, mustard, ozone, hydrogen sulfide, phosgene, nitrogen dioxide; dinitrogen tetroxide |
| Spraying | Spraying of paints and coatings |
| Explosion | Irritant gases, vapors, and fume releases under pressure; uranium hexafluoride; World Trade Center disaster |
| Fire/pyrolysis | Combustion and pyrolysis products of fires, burning paint fumes, pyrolysis products of polyvinylchloride (PVC) meat wrapping film; smoke inhalation, chlorofluorocarbons degradation, urea fumes |

(continued)

**Table 3.3** (continued)

| Exposure | Agent or process |
|---|---|
| Confined spaces | Epichlorohydrin, acrolein, floor sealant, metal coating remover, biocides, fumigating aerosol, cleaning aerosol sprays, mixture of drain cleaning agents |
| Environment and workplace | $SO_2$ gas in a pyrite dust explosion; locomotive and diesel exhaust; dunsmuir metam sodium spill; aerosols of metalworking fluids including aldehyde and formaldehyde; aluminum smelter workers exposed to pot-room fumes; metal processing plant and c chlorine gas exposures; bleachery workers with ozone and chlorine dioxide/$SO_2$ gassings; chlorine gas "puffs" among pulp mill workers and chlorine gassing incidents; sodium persulfate; inorganic salts used as oxidizing agents in hair bleaches and hair-coloring preparation; shoe and leather workers exposed to the organic solvents; workers exposed to $SO_2$ from apricot sulfurization tunnel construction workers, cleaning and disinfecting workers in the food industry, chili pepper pickers, dust exposure in Norwegian smelters; 2-hydroxyethyl methacrylate and methyl methacrylate in dentists; synthetic leather workers exposed to organic solvents toluene, xylene, and methylethyl ketone; eucalyptus; fragranced aerosol products; gases from liquid manure; steam system additive 2-diethylaminoethanolamine; irritant gas containing chromate at a chrome pellet manufacturing plant; bromochlorodifluoromethane and bromotrifluoromethane |

## Pathology of RADS and Irritant-Induced Asthma

The pathological features of RADS showing mononuclear cell inflammation, denuded epithelium, and edematous mucosa, first communicated in a sentinel publication, were similar to findings described in later publications (Bernstein and Bernstein 1989; Brooks et al. 1985; Deschamps et al. 1992, 1994; Lemiere et al. 2000). Additional pathological findings included mucosal squamous cell metaplasia, thickening of the basement membrane and reticular and collagen-associated bronchial wall fibrosis (Deschamps et al. 1992; Deschamps et al. 1994; Gautrin et al. 2006). A subject suffering from RADS following a single exposure to a mixture containing an isocyanate disclosed mostly T-lymphocytes inflammatory response (Lemiere et al. 1996). Purportedly, a case of RADS in a worker exposed to chlorine gas revealed sequences of changing pathological changes (Lemiere et al. 1997). Serial bronchial biopsies were acquired at 3 and 15 days and then 3 and 5 months after the inhalational accident. Initially, there was bronchial mucosal denudation with sloughing of epithelial cells and infiltration of a submucosal fibrinohemorrhagic exudate. Subsequent changes exhibited subepithelial edema and cellular regeneration of the basal and parabasal cells; even later, there was deposition of collagen. In another human investigation, the chronic pathological changes of irritant-induced asthma studied on average of 11 years after an inhalational accident suggested the important cellular role for the eosinophil (Takeda et al. 2009). A rat model reported maximum epithelial flattening and necrosis occurring between

1 and 3 days after a single high-level exposure to chlorine gas; bronchoalveolar lavage revealed associated neutrophilic inflammation (Demnati et al. 1998). With time, there was the decline in the amount of epithelial flattening and cellular necrosis as more goblet cells and smooth muscle cells appeared; some rats were left with persisting epithelial aberrations (Demnati et al. 1998).

## Mechanisms to Explain Irritant-Induced Asthma

The mechanism(s) to explain the two types of irritant-induced asthma is/are still poorly understood but there are potential reasons.

### *Genetic Factors*

Molecular alteration in a gene sequence might impose greater host susceptibility for lung injury (Adcock et al. 1994; Bird 2007; Duffy et al. 1998; Glavan et al. 2011; Holroyd et al. 1997; Leikauf et al. 2002; Levitt and Matthay 2010; Piirla et al. 2001; Puthothu et al. 2006; Samet et al. 2001; Wesselkamper et al. 2000; Wikman et al. 2002; Wilk et al. 2012). For example, the changes in gene structure that result in the inability to efficiently detoxify reactive oxygen species (ROS) can serve as subcellular messengers for numerous genetic pathways (Allen and Tresini 2000; Wesselkamper et al. 2000). The cellular damage caused by persistent oxidant stress might lead to an overwhelming of the pulmonary antioxidant defenses resulting in perpetuation of airway inflammation, airway hyperresponsiveness, and other characteristics of irritant-induced asthma (Kelly 2003). A mouse model of chlorine-induced pulmonary injury supports the hypothesis that some of the functional and pathological airways changes in asthma relate to induction of oxidative stress (Martin et al. 2003). Among lung antioxidants, glutathione is considered a susceptibility factor for asthma (Aynacioglu et al. 2004; Lee et al. 2004; Mapp et al. 2002; Piirla et al. 2001; Tamer et al. 2004). It is hypothesized that glutathione-S-transferase pi (GSTP1) influences how an individual handles an inflammatory-derived ROS burden. Possibly, the intermediate electrophilic metabolites, arising in the first phase of detoxification, are not metabolized by GST enzymes in asthmatic patients and are not excreted. These intermediate metabolites can damage cells and generate oxidative stress, and therefore contribute to the pathogenesis of asthma. In the occupational setting, inadequate antioxidant defense and genetic factors are implicated in the pathogenesis of isocyanate-induced asthma (Wikman et al. 2002; Wisnewski and Redlich 2001; Yucesoy et al. 2012). Polymorphic variant in the class $\pi$ glutathione-S-transferase locus (GSTP1) confers susceptibility to developing toluene di-isocyanate (TDI) asthma, and the homozygosity for the Val105-encoding alleles confers protection (Aynacioglu et al. 2004).

## *Ionic Channels*

Irritant exposures may alter pulmonary ionic channels such as the transient receptor potential vanilloid-1 ($TRPV_1$) and $TRPA_1$ (Adcock, 2009; Bautista et al. 2005; Brooks 2010; Huang 2004; Macpherson et al. 2007; McNamara et al. 2007; Medvedeva et al. 2008). Normally, these channels are primed to recognize irritant chemical and to counter with appropriate neurogenic and biochemical rejoinders (Brooks 2008 #2677; Nilius et al. 2005; Takemura et al. 2008; Taylor-Clark et al. 2008; Trevisani et al. 2007; Zhang et al. 2008). When there is significant cellular damage from a high-level irritant exposure, cells release inflammatory products such as bradykinin, ATP, prostaglandin $E_2$, nerve growth factor (NGF), proteases, and serotonin that sustain and potentiate the responsiveness of $TRPV_1$ and $TRPA_1$ receptors/channels (Bengtson et al. 2008; Gatti et al. 2006; Nakatsuka and Gu 2006; Vaughan et al. 2006). $TRPV_1$ and $TRPA_1$ channels manifest much higher neuronal $Ca^{2+}$ responsiveness to irritant chemicals, in such a sustained and potentiated state, and introduce changes leading to irritant-induced asthma. Previously unresponsive neuronal tissues can gain higher sensitivity and display more prolonged neuronal signaling (Woolf and Ma 2007). Neuropeptides released from activated nerve endings lead to localized neurogenic inflammation (see below). The finality of the various alterations leads to sustained airway inflammation, neural plasticity, airway remodeling, persistent airway hyperresponsiveness, and clinical asthma symptoms.

## *Tachykinins and Neurotrophins*

Tachykinins and neurotrophins release and actions propound an alternative explanation for airway inflammation and hyperresponsiveness following irritant-induced airway epithelial injury (e.g., RADS) (Groneberg et al. 2004a, b; Piedimonte 1995). Neuropeptides that are released from nerve endings evoke neurogenic inflammation (Amadesi et al. 2004; Groneberg et al. 2004a, b; Meggs 1993, 1994; Shusterman 1994; Trevisani et al. 2007; Watanabea et al. 2006; Widdicombe 2003). NGF, accumulating in inflamed tissue, induces different cells to discharge pro-inflammatory mediators. Neurogenic inflammation is sustained, in part, by the release of these cytokines and pro-inflammatory molecules, which function in both an autocrine and paracrine manner to create a feedback mechanism to induce more NGF release (Olgart and Frossard 2002). Under the influence of inflammation, nerves undergo remodeling (i.e., neural plasticity) (Jacoby 2003). Neural plasticity in an inflamed airway may both increase synthesis of tachykinins and facilitates their release (Jacoby 2003; Quarcoo et al. 2004). Neural plasticity manifests nervous hyperactivity, which may translate as bronchial hyperresponsiveness (Jacoby 2003).

## *Airway Smooth Muscle*

Airway smooth muscle (ASM) cells regulate airway tone in asthma through the release and response to various cytokines, growth factors, and mediators of airway inflammation (Joubert and Hamid 2005; Lazaar et al. 2005). Increases in ASM mass, epithelial goblet cell hyperplasia, bronchial epithelial abnormalities, lamina reticularis thickening, proliferation of airway blood vessels and nerves are key structural changes in the airways of asthmatics. Borger et al. proposed that the pathogenesis of asthma may relate to an abnormal phenotype of airway smooth muscle where there is faster proliferation of ASM cells, which could contribute to the increase in ASM mass found in patients with asthma (Borger et al. 2006). $PGE_2$ is the major prostanoid produced by ASM cells and can lead to the inhibition of ASM cellular proliferation. Cultured ASM cells of patients with asthma produce less prostaglandin $E_2$ but show greater number of E-prostanoid receptors on the cell membrane (Borger et al. 2006). Both $PGE_2$ and $PGF_2\alpha$ directly activate lung C-fibers.

## *Abnormal Airway Remodeling*

The initiation of an abnormal epithelial–mesenchymal trophic unit (EMTU) in response to an irritant may be because the bronchial epithelial cells of asthmatics are more responsive to environmental irritants (Holgate et al. 2004).

## *Subclinical Asthma*

Severe early-onset asthma, appearing first during childhood, is associated with a strong allergic component, eosinophilic inflammation, and diminished anti-inflammatory response to corticosteroid resistance. Adult-onset asthma without airway eosinophilia may signify a distinct clinical type of asthma (Wenzel 2005). Feasibly, the asymptomatic individual with roots of childhood asthma may have their asthma exacerbated or aggravated by accidental single or repeated irritant exposures (Bradding and Green 2010; Brooks et al. 1998; Sessions 2009). The reason for this conclusion is because the type of asthma originating in infancy or childhood was believed to have an encouraging future prognosis. Presumably, many cases went into "remission" or displayed a reduction in asthma symptoms between the ages of 10 and 20 years (Panhuysen et al. 1997). It is now recognized that this assumption is not always correct. While the severity of asthma symptoms fluctuates with time, the inherited tendency towards respiratory symptoms never disappears; and, a majority of young adults who seem to be free of asthmatic symptoms do, in fact, have persistent asthma symptoms (Barr and Logan 1964; Riiser et al. 2012;

Roorda 1996; Sears 2012). Even in the absence of current asthma symptoms, asymptomatic asthmatic subjects can still demonstrate substantial air flow limitation and show increases in bronchial hyperresponsiveness (Boulet 2003; Cooper et al. 1977; Ferguson 1988; Friberg et al. 1988).

### *Asthma Clinical Phenotype*

Perhaps, repeated exposure-type irritant-induced asthma exemplifies a distinct asthma phenotype dependent on the type of airway cellular inflammation and the airway's unique response to environmental stimuli (Haldar et al. 2008; O'Donnell and Frew 2002; Wenzel 2006). Bronchoscopic evaluation of the types of airways' cells has been utilized to investigate difficult-to-treat asthma and define asthma phenotypes (Good et al. 2012; Wenzel 2006; Wenzel et al. 1999).

## Prognosis of Irritant-Induced Asthma

The long-term outcome of irritant-induced asthma was examined in a follow-up study of 35 subjects reassessed nearly 14 years after their inhalational accident (Malo et al. 2009). The type of causal agent, the interval since the accident, and a visit to an emergency room or a hospitalization were not predictors of prognosis. In this investigation, asthma symptoms persisted in all subjects and more than two-thirds required inhaled corticosteroids. Nearly 50 % revealed bronchial obstruction and 75 % showed bronchial hyperresponsiveness. One quarter of the sample of subjects manifested bronchial eosinophilic inflammation. Workers often reported impaired smell after the inhalational accidents. It seems that the long-term outcome of subjects with irritant-induced asthma is similar to subjects with allergic occupational asthma. As for allergic-type occupational asthma, approximately 25 % of subjects show a disappearance of bronchial hyperresponsiveness 2 years after the inhalational accident with a plateau afterwards (Malo et al. 1994).

## Treatment of Irritant-Induced Asthma

The treatment of RADS is similar to the treatment afforded patients suffering from an acute inhalational injury. Aerosolized bronchodilators are essential for treating bronchoconstriction (as measured by spirometry) or bronchospasm (as determined by auscultation finding of wheezing). The beneficial effect of parenteral steroids has been shown in an animal model of RADS in which dexamethasone was administered immediately before chlorine inhalation (Demnati et al. 1998). There are no human study showing efficacy of oral corticosteroids in the treatment of RADS cases; and possibly oral steroids may not be effective. Inhaled steroids have been found effective in reducing airway hyperresponsiveness in a case considered to be RADS (Lemiere et al. 1997). A substantial number of patients with RADS show biopsy findings of eosinophilic inflammation many years after the acute inhalational accident (Malo et al. 2009). These findings are used as a justification for employing inhaled steroids to treat RADS.

## Other Diagnoses to Consider

### *Vocal Cord Dysfunction*

Psychogenic factors are believed to contribute to cases of Vocal Cord Dysfunction (VCD). Unlike asthmatics, VCD patients (often women) rarely awaken from sleep by attacks. About 10 % of patients referred for refractory asthma have a diagnosis of VCD. An additional 33 % have VCD accompanying asthma. Perkner et al. reported on 11 cases of VCD in which there was a temporal association between VCD onset and occupational or environmental irritant exposure (Perkner et al. 1998). A definitive VCD diagnosis requires visualization of the vocal cords via laryngoscopy (Poonai et al. 2000). Speech therapy is the first line of treatment for VCD and may be sufficient to correct the disorder. Therapy involves techniques emphasizing decreasing laryngeal muscle tone, largely by helping patients focus on expiration, rather than inspiration. Bronchodilator inhalers and corticosteroids used to treat asthma are not effective.

### *Airway Sensory Hyperreactivity*

Some individuals report upper and lower airway symptoms induced by scents and inhaled chemicals such as perfumes, flowers, colored paints, cigarette smoke, and automobile exhaust fumes (Shusterman 2002; Ternesten-Hasseus et al. 2002). There is increased cough sensitivity by capsaicin challenge testing but no greater sensitivity to methacholine; there are also poorer quality of life scores (Millqvist et al. 2000; Ternesten-Hasseus et al. 2007).

### *Odor-Triggered Panic Attacks*

There are cases of episodic dyspnea associated with central and autonomic nervous system symptomatology following odor recognition (Shusterman and Dager 1991). Dager et al. reported that three patients with "panic disorder precipitated by exposure to organic solvents" responded with typical panic symptoms after intravenous sodium lactate challenges (Dager et al. 1987). Similar type "chemically sensitive" patients can also react to $CO_2$ provocation with panic-like symptoms (Poonai et al. 2000). Possibly, the process evolves as a Pavlovian'-type conditioning to an odorant (Shusterman et al. 1988).

## *World Trade Center Entities*

Respiratory disorders among rescue workers that developed after the World Trade Center collapse on September 11, 2001, several respiratory illnesses were described among rescue workers include persistent airway hyperreactivity, chronic cough, and acute eosinophilic pneumonia (Banauch et al. 2003; Prezant et al. 2002; Rom et al. 2002). The designation of RADS for rescue workers involved in the collapse of the World Trade Center has been called into question, and it is important to emphasize that high-level dust exposures are rarely etiologic in causing RADS (Truncale and Brooks 2004).

## References

Abraham MH, Hassanisadi M, Jalali-Heravi M, Ghafourian T, Cain WS, C.-M. JE. Draize rabbit eye test compatibility with eye irritation thresholds in humans: a quantitative structure-activity relationship analysis. Toxicol Sci. 2003;76:384–91.

Adcock IM, Brown CR, Kwon O, Barnes PJ. Oxidative stress induces NF kappa B DNA binding and inducible NOS mRNA in the human epithelial cell line A549. Biochem Soc Trans. 1994;22(2):186S.

Adcock J. TRPV1 receptors in sensitization of cough and pain reflexes. Pulm Pharmacol Ther. 2009;22:65–70.

Alarie Y. Sensory irritation by airborne chemicals. CRC Crit Rev Toxicol. 1973;3:299–363.

Alarie Y. Dose-response analysis of animal studies: prediction of human responses. Environ Health Perspect. 1981;9:9–13.

Allen RG, Tresini M. Oxidative stress and gene regulation. Free Radic Biol Med. 2000;28:463–99.

Amadesi S, Nie J, Vergnolle N, Cottrell GS, Grady EF, Trevisano M, Bunnet NW. Protease-acivated receptor-2 sensitizes the capsaicin receptor transient receptor potential vanilloid receptor 1 to induce hyperalgesia. J Neurosci. 2004;24:4300–12.

Aynacioglu AS, Nacak M, Filiz A, Ekinci E, Roots I. Protective role of glutathione S-transferase P1 (GSTP1) Val105Val genotype in patients with bronchial asthma. Br J Clin Pharmacol. 2004;57(2):213–7.

Banauch GI, Alleyne D, Sanchez R, Olender K, Cohen HW, Weiden M, Prezant DJ. Persistent hyperreactivity and reactive airway dysfunction in firefighters at the World Trade Center. Am J Respir Crit Care Med. 2003;168(1):54–62.

Bardana EJ. Reactive airways dysfunction syndrome (RADS): guidelines for diagnosis and treatment and insight into likely prognosis. Ann Allergy Asthma Immunol. 1999;83(6 Pt 2):583–6.

Barr LW, Logan GB. Prognosis of children having asthma. Pediatrics. 1964;34:856–60.

Bautista DM, Movahead P, Hinman A, Axelsson HE, Sterner O, Hogestatt ED, Zygmunt PM. Pungent products from garlic activate the sensory ion channel TRPA1. Proc Natl Acad Sci USA. 2005;102:12248–52.

Bengtson SH, Eddleston J, Morgelin M, Zuraw BL, Herwald H. Regulation of Kinin B2 receptors by bradykinin in human lung cells. Biol Chem. 2008;380:1435–40.
Bernstein IL, Chan-Yeung M, Luc-Malo J, Bernstein DI. Definition and classification of asthma in the workplace. In: Bernstein IL, Chan-Yeung M, Malo J-L, Bernstein DI, editors. Asthma in the workplace and related conditions. 3rd ed. New York, NY: Taylor & Francis; 2006. p. 1–8.
Bernstein IL, Bernstein DI. Reactive airways dysfunction syndrome (RADS) after exposure to toxic ammonia fumes. J Allergy Clin Immunol. 1989;83:173–9.
Bherer L, Cushman R, Jp C, Quevillon M, Cote G, Bourbeau J, Jl M. Survey of construction workers repeatedly exposed to chlorine over a three to six month period in a pulpmill: II. Follow up of affected workers by questionnaire, spirometry, and assessment of bronchial responsiveness 18 to 24 months after exposure ended. Occup Environ Med. 1994;51(4):225–8.
Bird A. Perceptions of epigenetics. Nature. 2007;447:396–8.
Blanc PD, Galbo M, Hiatt P, Olson KR. Morbidity following acute irritant inhalation in a population based study. JAMA. 1991;266:664–9.
Borger P, Tamm M, Black JL, Roth M. Asthma: is it due to an abnormal airway smooth muscle cell? Am J Respir Crit Care Med. 2006;174:367–72.
Bougault V, Turmel J, St-Laurent J, Bertrand M, Boulet L-P. Asthma, airway inflammation and epithelial damage in swimmers and cold-air athletes. Eur Respir J. 2009;33:740–6.
Boulet L-P. Asymptomatic airway hyperresponsiveness. Am J Respir Crit Care Med. 2003;167:371–8.
Bradding P, Green RH. Subclinical phenotypes of asthma. Curr Opin Allergy Clin Immunol. 2010;10(1):54–9.
Brooks SM. Occupational, environmental, and irritant induced cough. In: Ken GE, Altman W, Irwin RS editors. Cough: an interdisciplinary problem. Otolaryngol Clin North Am. 2010;43:85–96.
Brooks SM. Irritant induced airways disorders. In: David Bernstein D, Rafeul Alam R editors. Occupational asthma. Immunol Allergy Clin North Am. 2011;31:747–68.
Brooks SM, Gautrin D, Malo J-L. Reactive airways dysfunction syndrome and irritant induced asthma. In: Bernstein IL, Chan Yeung M, Malo J-L, Di B, editors. Asthma in the workplace. New York: Marcel Dekker; Taylor & Francis Group partners; 2013.
Brooks SM, Hammad Y, Richards I, Giovinco-Barbas J, Jenkins K. The spectrum of irritant-induced asthma: sudden and not-so-sudden onset and the role of allergy. Chest. 1998;113(1): 42–9.
Brooks SM, Weiss MA, Bernstein IL. Reactive airways dysfunction syndrome (RADS). Persistent asthma syndrome after high level irritant exposures. Chest. 1985;88(3):376–84.
Chan-Yeung M, Lam S, Kennedy SM, Frew AJ. Persistent asthma after repeated exposure to high concentrations of gases in pulpmills. Am J Respir Crit Care Med. 1994;149:1676–80.
Charan N, Meyer C, Lakshminarayan S, Spencer T. Pulmonary injuries associated with acute sulfur dioxide inhalation. Am Rev Respir Dis. 1979;119(4):555–60.
Chatkin JM, Tarlo SM, Liss G, Banks D, Broder I. The outcome of asthma related to workplace irritant exposures: a comparison of irritant-induced asthma and irritant aggravation of asthma. Chest. 1999;116(6):1780–5.
Cooper DM, Cutz E, Levison H. Occult pulmonary abnormalities in asymptomatic asthmatic children. Chest. 1977;71(3):361–5.
Dager SR, Holland JP, Cowley DS, Dunner DL. Panic disorder precipitated by exposure to organic solvents in the work place. Am J Psychiatry. 1987;144:1056–8.
Demnati R, Fraser R, Ghezzo H, Martin JG, Plaa G, Malo JI. Time-course of functional and pathological changes after a single high acute inhalation of chlorine in rats. Eur Respir J. 1998;11(4):922–8.
Deschamps D, Rosenberg N, Soler P, Maillard G, Fournier E, Salson D, Gervais P. Persistent asthma after accidental exposure to ethylene oxide. Br J Ind Med. 1992;49(7):523–5.
Deschamps D, Soler P, Rosenberg N, Baud F, Gervais P. Persistent asthma after inhalation of a mixture of sodium hypochlorite and hydrochloric acid. Chest. 1994;105:1895–6.
Duffy DI, Mitchell CA, Martin NG. Genetic and environmental risk factors for asthma: a cotwin-control study. Am J Respir Crit Care Med. 1998;157(3 Pt 1):840–5.

Fahy JV, O' Byrne P. "Reactive airways disease". A lazy term of uncertain meaning that should be abandoned. Am J Respir Crit Care Med. 2001;163:822–3.

Ferguson AC. Persisting airway obstruction in asymptomatic children with asthma with normal peak expiratory flow rates. J Allergy Clin Immunol. 1988;82(1):19–22.

Friberg S, Bevegard S, Graff-Lonnevig V. Asthma from childhood to adult age: a prospective study of twenty subjects with special reference to the clinical course and pulmonary function. Acta Paediatr Scand. 1988;77:424–31.

Gatti R, Andre E, Amadesi S, Dinh TQ, Fischer A, Bunnett NW, Trevisano M. Protease-activated receptor-2 exaggerates TRPV1-mediated cough in guinea pigs. J Appl Physiol. 2006;101: 506–11.

Gautrin D, Bernstein IL, Brooks SM, Henneberger PK. Reactive airways dysfunction syndrome, or irritant-induced asthma. In: Bernstein IL, Chan Yeung M, Luc-Malo J ,Bernstein DI, editors. Asthma in the Workplace. 2006.

Gautrin D, Leroyer C, L'Archeveque J, Jg D, Girard D, Jl M. Cross-sectional assessment of workers with repeated exposure to chlorine over a three year period. Eur Respir J. 1995;8(12): 2046–54.

Gautrin D, Leroyer C, Infante-Rivard C, Ghezzo H, Dufour JG, Girard D, Malo JL. Longitudinal assessment of airway caliber and responsivenesss in workers exposed to chlorine. Am J Respir Crit Care Med. 1999;160:1232–7.

Gilbert R, Auchincloss J. Reactive airways dysfunction syndrome presenting as a reversible restrictive defect. Lung. 1989;167(1):55–61.

Glavan BJ, Holden TD, Goss CH, Black RA, Neff MJ, Nathens AB, ARDSnet Investigators. Genetic variation in the FAS gene and associations with acute lung injury. Am J Respir Crit Care Med. 2011;183(3):356–63.

Goe S, Henneberger P, Reilly M, Rosenman K, Schill D, Valiante D, Filios MS. A descriptive study of work aggravated asthma. Occup Environ Med. 2004;61:512–7.

Good Jr JT, Kolakowski CA, Groshong SD, Murphy JR, Martin RJ. Refractory asthma: importance of bronchoscopy to identify phenotypes and direct therapy. Chest. 2012;141(3): 599–606.

Groneberg DA, Niimi A, Dinh QT, Cosio B, Hew M, Fischer A, Chung KF. Increased expression of transient receptor potential vanilloid-1 in airway nerves of chronic cough. Am J Respir Crit Care Med. 2004a;170:1276–80.

Groneberg DA, Quarcoo D, Frossard N, Fischer A. Neurogenic mechanisms in bronchial inflammatory diseases. Allergy. 2004b;59(11):1139–52.

Haldar P, Pavord ID, Shaw DE, Berry MA, Thomas M, Brightling CE, Green RH. Cluster analysis and clinical asthma phenotypes. Am J Respir Crit Care Med. 2008;178:218–24.

Henneberger PK, Derk SJ, Davis L, Tumpowsky C, Reilly MJ, Rosenman KD, . . . Tift B. Work-related reactive airways dysfunction syndrome cases from surveillance in selected US states. J Occup Environ Med. 2003;45(4):360-8.

Henneberger PK, Metayer C, Layne LA, Althouse R. Nonfatal work-related inhalations: surveillance data from hospital emergency departments, 1995–1996. Am J Ind Med. 2000;38:140–8.

Henneberger PK, Olin A-C, Andersson E, Hagberg S, Torén K. The incidence of respiratory symptoms and diseases among pulp mill workers with peak exposures to ozone and other irritant gases. Chest. 2005;128:3028–37.

Holgate ST, Holloway J, Wilson S, Bucchieri F, Puddicombe S, Davies DE. Epithelial-mesenchymal communication in the pathogenesis of chronic asthma. Proc Am Thorac Soc. 2004;1:93–8.

Holroyd KJ, Eleff SM, Zhang L-Y, Jakab GJ, Kleeberger SR. Genetic modeling of susceptibility to nitrogen dioxide-induced lung injury in mice. Am J Physiol. 1997;273:L595–L602.

Huang C-L. The transient receptor potential superfamily of ion channels. J Am Soc Nephrol. 2004;15:1690–9.

Jacoby DB. Airway neural plasticity. The nerves they are a-changin'. Am J Respir Cell Mol Biol. 2003;28:138–41.

Joubert P, Hamid Q. Role of airway smooth muscle in airway remodeling. J Allergy Clin Immunol. 2005;116(3):713–6.

Kelly FJ. Oxidative stress: its role in air pollution and adverse health effects. Occup Environ Med. 2003;60:612–6.

Kern DG. Outbreak of the reactive airways dysfunction syndrome after a spill of glacial acetic. Am Rev Respir Dis. 1991;144:1058–64.

Kipen HM, Blume R, Hutt D. Asthma experience in an occupational and environmental medicine clinic. Low-dose reactive airways dysfunction syndrome [see comments]. J Occup Med. 1994;36(10):1133–7.

Lazaar AL, Panettieri J, Reynold A. Airway smooth muscle: a modulator of airway remodeling in asthma. J Allergy Clin Immunol. 2005;116(3):488–95.

Lee Y-L, Lin Y-C, Wang J-Y, Hsiue T-R, Guo YL. Glutathione S-transferase P1 gene polymorphism and air pollution as interactive risk factors for childhood asthma. Clin Exp Allergy. 2004;34:1707–13.

Leikauf GD, McDowell SA, Wesselkamper SC, Hardie WD, Leikauf JE, Korfhagen TR, Prows DR. Acute lung injury: functional genomics and genetic susceptibility. Chest. 2002;121:70S–5.

Lemiere C, Malo J-L, Boulet LP, Boutet M. Reactive airways dysfunction syndrome induced by exposure to a mixture containing isocyanate: functional and histopathologic behaviour. Allergy. 1996;51(4):262–5.

Lemiere C, Jl M, Boutet M. Reactive airways dysfunction syndrome due to chlorine: sequential bronchial biopsies and functional assessment. Eur Respir J. 1997;10:241–4.

Lemiere C, Chaboilliez S, Trudeau C, Taha R, Maghni K, Martin JG, Hamid Q. Characterization of airway inflammation after repeated exposures to occupational agents. J Allergy Clin Immunol. 2000;106(6):1163–70.

Levitt J, Matthay MA. The utility of clinical predictors of acute lung injury: towards prevention and earlier recognition. Expert Rev Respir Med. 2010;4(6):785–97.

Li J, Blatchley III ER. Volatile disinfection byproduct formation resulting from chlorination of organic-nitrogen precursors in swimming pools. Environ Sci Technol. 2007;41:6732–9.

Macpherson LJ, Dubin AE, Evans MJ, Marr F, Schultz PG, Cravatt BF, Patapoutian A. Noxious compounds activate TRPA1 ion channels through covalent modification of cysteines. Nature. 2007;445:541–5.

Malo J-L. Irritant-induced asthma and reactive airways dysfunction syndrome. Can Respir J. 1998;5(1):66–7.

Malo J-L, Lemiere C, Gautrin D, Labrecque M. Occupational asthma. Curr Opin Pulm Med. 2004;10(1):57–61.

Malo JL, Cartier A, Boulet LP, L'Archeveque J, Saint-Denis F, Bherer L, Courteau JP. Bronchial hyperresponsiveness can improve while spirometry plateaus two to three years after repeated exposure to chlorine causing respiratory symptoms. Am J Respir Crit Care Med. 1994;150(4):1142–5.

Malo JL, L'Archeveque J, Castellanos L, Lavoie K, Ghezzo H, Maghni K. Long-term outcomes of acute irritant-induced asthma. Am J Respir Crit Care Med. 2009;179:923–8.

Mapp CE, Fryer AA, De Marzo N, Pozzato V, Padoan M, Boschetto P, Spiteri MA. Glutathione S-transferase GSTP1 is a susceptibility gene for occupational asthma induced by isocyanates. J Allergy Clin Immunol. 2002;109:867–72.

Martin JG, Campbell HR, Iijima H, Gautrin D, Malo J-L, Eidelman DH, Maghni K. Chlorine-induced injury to the airways in mice. Am J Respir Crit Care Med. 2003;168(5):568–74.

Massin N, Bohadana AB, Wild P, Hery M, Toamain JP, Hubert G. Respiratory symptoms and bronchial responsiveness in lifeguards exposed to nitrogen trichloride in indoor swimming pools. Occup Environ Med. 1998;55(4):258–63.

McConnell R, Berhane K, Gilliland F, London SJ, Islam T, Gauderman WJ, . . . Peters JM. Asthma in exercising children exposed to ozone: a cohort study. Lancet. 2002; 359:386–91.

McDonald JC, Chen Y, Zekveld C, Cherry NM. Incidence by occupation and industry of acute work related respiratory diseases in the UK, 1992–2001. Occup Environ Med. 2005;62(12): 836–42.

McNamara CR, Mandel-Brehm J, Bautista DM, Siemens J, Deranian KL, Zhao M, . . . Fanger CM. TRPA1 mediates formalin-induced pain. Proc Natl Acad Sci USA. 2007;104:13525–30.

Medina-Ramón M, Zock JP, Kogevinas M, Sunyer J, Torralba Y, Borrell A, . . . JM., A. Asthma, chronic bronchitis, and exposure to irritant agents in occupational domestic cleaning: a nested case-control study. Occup Environ Med. 2005;*62*:598–606.

Medvedeva YV, Kim M-S, Usachev YM. Mechanisms of prolonged presynaptic $Ca2^{+}$ signaling and glutamate release induced by TRPV1 activation in rat sensory neurons. J Neurosci. 2008;28:5295–311.

Meggs WJ. Neurogenic inflammation and sensitivity to environmental chemicals. Environ Health Perspect. 1993;101(3):234–8.

Meggs WJ. RADS and RUDS–the toxic induction of asthma and rhinitis. J Toxicol Clin Toxicol. 1994;32(5):487–501.

Millqvist E, Lowhagen O, Bende M. Quality of life and capsaicin sensitivity in patients with sensory airway hyperreactivity. Allergy. 2000;55:540–5.

Nakatsuka T, Gu JG. P2X purinoceptors and sensory transmission. Pflugers Arch. 2006;452:598–607.

Nemery B. Late consequences of accidental exposure to inhaled irritants: RADS and the Bhopal disaster. Eur Respir J. 1996;8:1973–6.

Nemery B. Inhalation injury, chemical. In: Nemery B, editor. Occupational diseases. London: Elsevier; 2006. p. 208–16.

Nilius B, Voets T, Peters I. TRP channels in disease. Sci STKE. 2005;295:1–9.

O'Donnell RA, Frew AJ. Is there more than one inflammatory phenotype in asthma? Thorax. 2002;57(7):566–8.

Olgart C, Frossard N. Nerve growth factor and asthma. Pulm Pharmacol Ther. 2002;15(1): 51–60.

Olin AC, Andersson E, Andersson M, Granung G, Hagberg S, Toren K. Prevalence of asthma and exhaled nitric oxide are increased in bleachery workers exposed to ozone. Eur Respir J. 2004;23(1):87–92.

Olin AC, Granung G, Hagberg S, Adriansson M, Brisman J, Dalander O, Toren K. Respiratory health among bleachery workers exposed to ozone and chlorine dioxide. Scand J Work Environ Health. 2002;28(2):117–23.

Panhuysen CIM, Vonk JM, Koeter GH, Schouten JP, Van Altena R, Bleecker ER, Postma DS. Adult patients may outgrow their asthma. A 25-year follow-up study. Am J Respir Crit Care Med. 1997;155:1267–72.

Perkner JJ, Fennelly KP, Balkissoon R, Bartelson BB, Ruttenber AJ, Wood 2nd RP, Newman LS. Irritant-associated vocal cord dysfunction. J Occup Environ Med. 1998;40(2):136–43.

Piedimonte G. Tachykinin peptides, receptors, and peptidases in airway disease. Exp Lung Res. 1995;21:809–34.

Piirla P, Wikman H, Luukkonen R, Kaaria K, Rosenberg C, Nordman H, Hirvonen A. Glutathione S-transferase genotype and allergic responses to diisocyanate exposure. Pharmacogenetics. 2001;11:437–45.

Poonai N, Antony MM, Binkley KE, Stenn P, Swinson RP, Corey P, Tarlo SM. Carbon dioxide inhalation challenges in idiopathic environmental intolerance. J Allergy Clin Immunol. 2000;105:358–63.

Prezant DJ, Weiden M, Banauch GI, McGuinness G, Rom WN, Aldrich TK, Kelly JJ. Cough and bronchial responsiveness in firefighters at the World Trade Center site. N Engl J Med. 2002;347:806–15.

Puthothu B, Krueger M, Heinze J, Forster J, Heinzmann A. Impact of IL8 and IL8-Receptor alpha polymorphisms on the genetics of bronchial asthma and severe RSV infections. Clin Mol Allergy. 2006. Retrieved from http://www.pubmedcentral.nih.gov/picrender.fcgi?artid=1388233&blobtype=pdf.

Quarcoo D, Schulte-Herbruggen O, Lommatzsch M, Schierhorn K, Hoyle GW, Renz H, Braun A. Nerve growth factor induces increased airway inflammation via a neuropeptide-dependent mechanism in a transgenic animal model of allergic airway inflammation. Clin Exp Allergy. 2004;34:1146–51.

Riiser A, Hovland V, Carlsen K-H, Mowinckel P, Carlsen KCL. Does bronchial hyperresponsiveness in childhood predict active asthma in adolescence? Am J Respir Crit Care Med. 2012;86(6):493–500.

Rom WN, Weiden M, Garcia R, Yie TA, Vathesatogkit P, Tse DB, McGuinniess G,. . . P. Acute eosinophilic pneumonia in a New York city firefighter exposed to World Trade Center dust. Am J Respir Crit Care Med 2002;166:797–800.

Roorda RJ. Prognostic factors for the outcome of childhood asthma in adolescence. Thorax. 1996;51 Suppl 1:S7–12.

Rumchev KB, Spickett JT, Bulsara MK, Phillips MR, Stick SM. Domestic exposure to formaldehyde significantly increases the risk of asthma in young children. Eur Respir J. 2002;20(2):403–8.

Samet JM, Hatch GE, Horstman D, Steck-Scott S, Arab L, Bromberg PA, Devlin RB. Effect of antioxidant supplementation on ozone-induced lung injury in human subjects. Am J Respir Crit Care Med. 2001;164:819–25.

Sears MR. Predicting new and persistent asthma. Am J Respir Crit Care Med. 2012;186(6): 469–79.

Sessions CK. Asthma, active component, U.S. Armed Forces, 1999–2008. Silver Spring, MD: Armed Forces Health Surveillance Center (AFHSC). 2009. Retrieved from http://afhsc.army.mil/viewMSMR?file=2009/v16_n07.pdf.

Shakeri MS, Dick FD, Ayres JG. Which agents cause reactive airways dysfunction syndrome (RADS)? A systematic review. Occup Med (Lond). 2008;58:205–11.

Sherriff A, Farrow A, Golding J, Henderson J. Frequent use of chemical household products is associated with persistent wheezing in pre-school age children. Thorax. 2005;60:45–9.

Shusterman D. Neurogenic inflammation: additional points. Environ Health Perspect. 1994;102(1):12–3.

Shusterman D. Review of the upper airway, including olfaction, as mediator of symptoms. Environ Health Perspect. 2002;4:649–53.

Shusterman D, Balmes J, Cone J. Behavioral sensitization to irritants/odorants after acute overexposures. J Occup Med. 1988;30:565–7.

Shusterman DJ, Dager SR. Prevention of psychological disability after occupational respiratory exposures. Occup Med. 1991;6:11–27.

Swanney MP, Ruppel G, Enright PL, Pedersen OF, Crapo RO, Miller MR, Quanjer PH. Using the lower limit of normal for the FEV1/FVC ratio reduces the misclassification of airway obstruction. Thorax. 2008;63:1046–105.

Tabar AI, Alvarez MJ, Acero S, Olaguibel JM, Garcia BE, Quirce S. Reactive airways dysfunction syndrome: two case reports. J Investig Allergol Clin Immunol. 1998;8(2):119–22.

Takeda N, Maghni K, Daigle S, L'Archevêque J, Castellanos L, Al-Ramli W, Hamid Q. Long-term pathologic consequences of acute irritant-induced asthma. J Allergy Clin Immunol. 2009;124(5):975–81.

Takemura M, Quarcooa D, Niimib A, Dinhc Q, Geppettid P, Fischera A, . . . DA, G. Is TRPV1 a useful target in respiratory diseases? Pulm Pharmacol Ther. 2008;21:833–9.

Tamer L, Çalikoğlu M, Ates NA, Yildirim H, Ercan B, Saritas E, Atik U. Glutathione-S-transferase gene polymorphisms (GSTT1, GSTM1, GSTP1) as increased risk factors for asthma. Respirology. 2004;9(4):493–8.

Tarlo SM. Irritant-induced asthma. PCCSU. 2010;24:1–6 (Lesson 22).

Tarlo SM, Balmes J, Balkissoon R, Beach J, Beckett W, Bernstein D, Heitzer J. Diagnosis and management of work-related asthma. American College of Chest Physicians Consensus Statement. Chest. 2008;134(3 (suppl)):1S–41.

Tarlo SM, Broder I. Irritant-induced occupational asthma. Chest. 1989;96(2):297–300.

Taylor-Clark TE, McAlexander MA, Nassenstein C, Sheardown SA, Wilson S, Thornton J, Undem BJ. Relative contributions of TRPA1 and TRPV1 channels in the activation of vagal bronchopulmonary C-fibres by the endogenous autacoid 4-oxononenal. J Physiol. 2008;586:3447–59.

Ternesten-Hasseus E, Farbrot A, Lowhagen O, Millqvist E. Sensitivity to methacholine and capsaicin in patients with unclear respiratory symptoms. Allergy. 2002;57:501–7.

Ternesten-Hasseus E, Lowhagen O, Millqvist E. Quality of life and capsaicin sensitivity in patients with airway symptoms induced by chemicals and scents: a longitudinal study. Environ Health Perspect. 2007;115:425–9.

Trevisani M, Siemens J, Matwrazzi S, Bautista DM, Nassini R, Campi B, … P., G.. 4-Hydroxynonenal, an endogenous aldehyde, causes pain and neurogenic inflammation through activation of the irritant receptor TRPA1. Proc Natl Acad Sci USA. 2007;104: 13519–24.

Truncale T, Brooks SM. World Trade Center dust and airway reactivity (letter to the editor). Am J Respir Crit Care Med. 2004;169:883–5.

Vaughan R, Szewczyk JM, Lanos M, DeSesa CR, Gianutsos G, Morris JB. Adenosine sensory transduction pathways contribute to activation of the sensory irritation response to inspired irritant vapors. Toxicol Sci. 2006;93:411–21.

Watanabea N, Horie S, Michaelb GJ, Keira S, Spinaa D, Pagea CP, Priestley JV. Immunohistochemical co-localization of transient receptor potential vanilloid (TRPV)1 and sensory neuropeptides in the guinea-pig respiratory system. Neuroscience. 2006;141:1533–54.

Weisel CP, Richardson SD, Nemery B, Aggazzotti G, Baraldi E, Blatchley ER, . . . Sattar SA. Childhood asthma and environmental exposures at swimming pools: state of the science and research recommendations. Environ Health Perspect. 2009;117(4):500–7.

Wenzel S. Severe asthma in adults. Am J Respir Crit Care Med. 2005;172(2):149–60.

Wenzel SE. Asthma: defining of the persistent adult phenotypes. Lancet. 2006;368:804–13.

Wenzel SE, Schwartz LB, Langmack EL, Halliday JL, Trudeau JB, Gibbs RL, Chu HW. Evidence that severe asthma can be divided pathologically into two inflammatory subtypes with distinct physiologic and clinical characteristics. Am J Respir Crit Care Med. 1999;160:1001–8.

Wesselkamper SC, Prows DR, Biswas P, Willeke K, Bingham E, Leikauf GD. Genetic susceptibility to irritant-induced acute lung injury in mice. Am J Physiol Lung Cell Mol Physiol. 2000;279:L575–82.

Widdicombe JG. Overview of neural pathways in allergy and asthma. Pulm Pharmacol Ther. 2003;16(1):23–30.

Wikman H, Piirla P, Rosenberg C, Luukkonen R, Kaaria K, Nordman H, Hirvonen A. N-Acetyltransferase genotype as modifiers of diisocyanate exposure-associated asthma risk. Pharmacogenetics. 2002;12:227–33.

Wilk JB, Shrine NRG, Loehr LR, Zhao JH, Manihaikul A, Lopez LM, Stricker BH. Genome-wide association studies identify chrna5/3 and htr4 in the development of airflow obstruction. Am J Respir Crit Care Med. 2012;186(7):622–32.

Wisnewski AV, Redlich CA. Recent advances in diisocyanate asthma. Curr Opin Pulm Med. 2001;1:169–75.

Woolf CJ, Ma Q. Nociceptors – noxious stimulus detectors. Neuron. 2007;55:353–64.

Yucesoy BB, Johnson VJ, Lummus ZL, Kissling GE, Fluharty KK, Gautrin DD, . . . DI, B.. Genetic variants in antioxidant genes are associated with diisocyanate-induced asthma. Toxicol Sci. 2012;129(1):166–73.

Zhang G, Lin R-LL, Wiggers M, Snow DMM, Lee L-YL. Altered expression of TRPV1 and sensitivity to capsaicin in pulmonary myelinated afferents following chronic airway inflammation in the rat. J Physiol. 2008;586:5771–86.

Zock JP, Vizcaya D, Le Moual N. Update on asthma and cleaners. Curr Opin Allergy Clin Immunol. 2010;10:114–20.

# Chapter 4
# Acute Toxicity of Respiratory Irritant Exposures

**Susan Ney Miller**

**Abstract** Acute toxicity of respiratory irritant exposure is a heterogeneous group of gases with similar clinical symptomatology. Symptoms are largely based on water solubility with more water-soluble irritants causing symptoms in the upper respiratory system and less water-soluble irritants causing symptoms in the lower respiratory system. Ammonia, more water soluble, and phosgene, less water soluble, are hallmark examples of exposures. Large concentration of exposure or long time of exposure may cause any symptoms along the respiratory tract. Hypoxia can occur with any exposure that limits the amount of inspired oxygen to less than 21 %. Acute lung injury and acute respiratory distress syndrome are the most severe forms of toxicity. While most of the toxicity is limited to the respiratory system, some exposures can also cause systemic effects with hydrogen fluoride, hydrogen sulfide, and cyanide being classic examples of this. Chronic symptoms can occur after a one-time acute exposure. Treatment is largely supportive, focusing on maintaining the airway and oxygenation/ventilation.

**Keywords** Acute toxicity • Respiratory irritant • Ammonia • Phosgene • Chloride • Cyanide • Hydrogen fluoride • Hydrogen sulfide • Bhopal • Smoke • Smog • Treatment

## Introduction

While the acute clinical symptoms are similar, acute toxicity of respiratory irritant exposures is caused by a heterogeneous group of gases. Some exposures have associated chronic toxicity and will be touched on briefly in this chapter.

S.N. Miller, M.D. (✉)
Division of Toxicology, Department of Emergency Medicine, Brody School of Medicine at East Carolina University, Greenville, NC 27858, USA
e-mail: millersu@ecu.edu

W.J. Meggs (ed.), *The Toxicant Induction of Irritant Asthma, Rhinitis, and Related Conditions*, DOI 10.1007/978-1-4614-9044-9_4,

## *Pathophysiology*

While respiratory irritants are a large group of xenobiotics, their end-effects of mucosal lining damage are the same. There are two basic mechanisms that lead to mucosal lining damage: (1) destruction via acid or base formation, which often requires dissolution of the xenobiotic in the water found in the epithelial lining of the lungs, and (2) destruction by free radical formation or oxidation. There is considerable overlap in mechanism of action for many irritants (Sciuto 1998).

## *Clinical Manifestations*

Acute toxicity of a respiratory irritant exposure is defined by symptom onset within seconds to up 24 hours after a gas exposure. Symptoms, as well as symptom onset, are largely based on the water solubility of the gas, if that gas forms an acid or base when dissolved in the water of the respiratory tract (Kimbell et al. 1993). Generally, more water-soluble gases produce immediate symptoms confined to the upper airways. Ammonia is the hallmark example of a more water-soluble gas. Symptoms of upper airway irritation include nasopharyngeal or oropharyngeal pain, drooling, cough, mucosal edema, and stridor. Conversely, less water-soluble gases produced delayed symptoms in the lower airways. Phosgene is the hallmark example of a less water-soluble gas. Symptoms of lower airway irritation include tracheobronchitis, bronchitis, bronchospasm, and acute lung injury (ALI). Respiratory irritants with a moderate or intermediate water solubility can produce both upper and lower airway symptoms; an example of this is chlorine (Nelson et al. 2011). Exceptions can occur to this water solubility rule (Nelson et al. 2011; Medical Management 2007; Borak and Diller 2001). With exposure to large concentrations, less water-soluble gases can produce more immediate and/or upper airway symptoms. With prolonged exposure times, more water-soluble gases can produce more delayed and/or lower airway symptoms. Any gaseous exposure in high enough concentration can produce effects similar to a simple asphyxiant such as there is simply not enough oxygen in the breathable air and hypoxemia results (Nelson et al. 2011). Some respiratory irritants form free radicals, rather than acids or bases, which then cause local tissue destruction; examples include oxides of nitrogen, oxygen, and ozone. Signs of severe exposure of any respiratory irritant include altered mental status, respiratory insufficiency, cardiovascular instability, loss of consciousness, or seizures (Kales and Christiani 2004) (Table 4.1).

ALI and its most severe form, acute respiratory distress syndrome (ARDS) are the most characteristic and serious clinical manifestations of respiratory irritant exposure (Nelson et al. 2011). ALI and ARDS are nonspecific syndromes seen in a variety of severe physiologic insults, including but not limited to toxic exposures, trauma, and sepsis (Avecillas et al. 2006; Bernard et al. 1994; Rubenfeld and Herridge 2007). Acute onset, pulmonary inflammation, and alveolar filling are the definition of ALI with a clinical, radiographic, and physiologic pattern. Clinically,

**Table 4.1** Hypoxia level verses symptoms (Nelson et al. 2011)

| Inspired oxygen concentration | Signs and symptoms |
|---|---|
| 21 % (normal air) | None |
| 12–16 % | Tachypnea, hyperpnea, hypocapnia, tachycardia, reduced attention/alertness, euphoria, headache, mild incoordination |
| 10–14 % | Altered judgement, incoordination, muscle fatigue, cyanosis |
| 6–10 % | Nausea, vomiting, lethargy, air hunger, sever incoordination, coma |
| Less than 6 % | Gasping respiration, seizure, coma, death |

patients may present with dyspnea, chest tightness/pain, cough, frothy sputum, wheezing, rales, and hypoxemia. Radiographically, bilateral pulmonary infiltrates and a normal cardiac silhouette are typical. Physiologically, ALI is different from congestive heart failure in that the alveolar leakage is not solely due to pulmonary capillary hypertension. ARDS is defined as ALI plus the ratio of partial pressure of dissolved oxygen to inspired oxygen ($PaO_2/FiO_2$) below 200 mmHg (Avecillas et al. 2006; Bernard et al. 1994; Rubenfeld and Herridge 2007).

A potential long-term consequence of single acute exposure to a respiratory irritant is development of Reactive Airways Dysfunction Syndrome (RADS). This syndrome occurs in the absence of primary asthma before the exposure and is otherwise similar to asthma clinically. RADS has been demonstrated after numerous different exposures. Symptoms may last for weeks to years after exposure and are treated the same as asthma with bronchodilators and corticosteroids. Smoking may play an additive role, prolonging symptomatology (Nelson et al. 2011; Brooks and Bernstein 2011; Meggs 1994).

# Major Irritants

## *Ammonia*

Ammonia ($NH_3$) is the prototypical example of a more water-soluble gas and it dissolves easily in water to form a base, ammonium hydroxide ($NH_4OH$). It is a common industrial and household chemical used in a variety of ways: as a fertilizer, in the manufacturing of plastics and explosives, in refrigeration, and as a cleaner. Ammonia has a characteristic smell, which can serve as a warning to exposure. Sinusitis, acute and chronic, can develop after exposure (Brautbar 1998). Bronchiectasis, airway hyper-reactivity, bronchiolitis obliterans, and chronic obstructive pulmonary dysfunction (COPD) may all develop after an acute exposure to ammonia and acute effects have worn off (Tonelli and Pham 2009). Chronic, low-level exposures and repetitive, high-level exposures have both lead to pulmonary fibrosis (Brautbar et al. 2003). Outside of the respiratory tract, corneal ulceration/perforation, glaucoma, and cataracts can occur and may develop up to weeks after exposure (Warden 2005).

## Chloramines

Chloramines are a series of chlorinated nitrogenous compounds that are typically generated when sodium hypochlorite (NaOCl) bleach and ammonia come into contact (Krenzelok and Mrvos 1995). This contact frequently occurs when bleach and ammonia are mixed to combine their cleaning powers (Gapany-Gapanavicius et al. 1982), but they are also known to form in places where sodium hypochlorite and nitrogen mix (examples: swimming pools (Thickett et al. 2002), chicken processing plants (King et al. 2006), and septic systems (Minami et al. 1992)). Upon dissolving chloramines in water, ammonia, hypochlorous acid (HOCl), and oxygen radicals are formed. Less water soluble than ammonia, chloramines still produce immediate symptoms, although the symptoms may be mild and result in prolonged or recurrent exposures (Krenzelok and Mrvos 1995).

## Hydrogen Fluoride

While inhalational injury is thought to be unlikely at concentrations less than 60 %, there are a few reported cases of pulmonic injury occurring at much lower concentrations. Most inhalational exposures occur in the occupational setting; however, they have also occurred outside the workplace (Franzblau and Sahakian 2003; Bennion and Franzblau 1997). Inhalational exposures to hydrogen fluoride are often accompanied by dermal/topical exposures to the face, head, and neck (Takase et al. 2004; Blodgett et al. 2001; Kono et al. 2000).

Presenting symptoms of acute inhalation injury from hydrofluoric acid have a wide range from without symptoms (Braun et al. 1984), to mild symptoms (eye irritation, cough, hemoptysis, oropharyngeal burning, mild wheezing) (Kono et al. 2000; Braun et al. 1984; Lund et al. 1997), to major symptoms (severe wheezing, pulmonary edema, cyanosis, acute respiratory failure) (Blodgett et al. 2001; Kono et al. 2000; Chela et al. 1989), and systemic toxicity (Blodgett et al. 2001). This is related to the concentration of hydrofluoric acid and time exposed. Death by inhalation of hydrofluoric acid can occur from systemic symptoms (Blodgett et al. 2001), immediate respiratory effects of pulmonary edema with or without hemorrhage (Tepperman 1980; Watson et al. 1973), chemical pneumonitis (Dieffenbacher and Thompson 1962), or long-term complications (Braun et al. 1984) of repeated pneumonias, respiratory insufficiency, and tracheobronchial hemorrhage. Patients have survived potentially fatal inhalational exposures after prolonged ventilatory support and hospital stays (Skolnik 2010; Shin et al. 2007; Tsonis et al. 2008). After a one-time acute inhalation exposure, chronic upper respiratory symptoms of hoarseness, thickened/scarred vocal cords, recurrent coughing spells, and nasal pain have been reported (Braun et al. 1984). Reactive airway dysfunction has also been reported after a single acute exposure to hydrofluoric acid (Franzblau and Sahakian 2003).

In addition to the generalized treatments described later for any respiratory irritant exposure, hydrofluoric acid inhalation patients can be given nebulized calcium to bind the fluoride and try to prevent local and systemic toxicity. A 2.5 % solution for nebulization can be made with either 1.5 mL of 10 % calcium gluconate with 4.5 mL of sterile water/saline or 0.15 g calcium gluconate in 6 mL sterile water/saline (Mathieu et al. 2001).

## *Hydrogen Chloride/Chlorine*

Hydrogen chloride (HCl) gas dissolves in water to form hydrochloric acid, which is how hydrochloric acid is manufactured. During fires, firefighters, and victims can be exposed to hydrogen chloride through the burning of polyvinyl chloride (PVC) (Orzel 1993). Symptoms are usually immediate due to high water solubility of HCl.

Chlorine gas is used throughout industry as an oxidizing agent and occupational exposure is common. It was also used in World War I by both the French and German armies. Household exposure is common and is usually the byproduct of mixing almost any acid with hypochlorite bleach, which is typically done to combine cleaning powers (Krenzelok and Mrvos 1995). Chlorine gas can also form in degrading swimming pool tablets (Wood et al. 1987). Chlorine gas has a characteristic smell but distinguishing permissible air levels by smell is difficult. Chlorine gas dissolves at a moderate in water and forms hydrochloric and hypochlorous (HClO) acids. Hypochlorus acid then further decomposes and forms additional hydrochloric acid and liberates an oxygen free radical. Because these reactions are dependent on the rate chlorine gas dissolves in water, initial symptoms may be absent or very mild and even in moderate exposures, it may take hours for symptoms to develop (Fleta et al. 1986; Winder 2001). Fatalities have been reported after large acute exposures (Winder 2001). After low-to-moderate level recurring exposures, increased bronchial responsiveness, and asthma-like symptoms are possible (Gautrin et al. 1999).

## *Hydrogen Sulfide*

Hydrogen sulfide is a byproduct found in sewage and manure pits. It also occurs naturally in volcanoes, caves, and sulfur springs. In industry, exposure can occur in water treatment plants, nylon/synthetic rubber production, and petroleum/natural gas production. The admixture of acid to clean up Plaster of Paris (used in casting of fractures) can liberate hydrogen sulfide and expose health-care workers (Peters 1981). Hydrogen sulfide has also gained internet fame as a method of self-harm, known as "detergent suicides" which started in Japan. Lay-rescuers and first responders, as well as innocent bystanders, are at risk without proper protection (Goode 2011). It has a characteristic rotten egg smell but rapid olfactory fatigue allows for continued exposure. Hydrogen sulfide can also turn silver greenish-black, giving additional clues to exposure (Nelson et al. 2011). At low-moderate levels, hydrogen sulfide has rapid onset of upper airways symptoms (Tanaka et al. 1999). At higher concentrations, asphyxiation, leading to its reputation as a "knock-down gas," and systemic toxicity predominate (Burnett et al. 1977; Reiffenstein et al. 1992).

## *Sulfur Dioxide and Sulfuric Acid*

Sulfur dioxide ($SO_2$) is used widely in industry and is a byproduct of smelting and oil refinery (Nelson et al. 2011). It is highly water soluble and has a characteristic smell as a potential warning of its presence. Sulfur dioxide can easily be converted into sulfuric acid ($H_2SO_3$) within water droplets, "acid rain," in the presences of catalytic metals such as iron and manganese (Nelson et al. 2011). These irritants are a major environmental concern due to these severe health consequences. There is a dose-related bronchospasm that occurs with exposure to sulfur dioxide and sulfuric acid and can make bronchospasm particularly difficult to treat in known asthmatics. The most famous example is the London Fog of 1952 during which about 4,000 deaths occurred due to respiratory causes (Nelson et al. 2011). A large acute exposure to sulfur dioxide or sulfuric acid can upper and lower airway symptoms (Charan et al. 1979) and can produce RADS or asthma-like symptoms for years after exposure (Piirila et al. 1996).

## *Phosgene*

Perhaps the most studied of the respiratory irritants due to its development and use during World War I, phosgene (carbonyl chloride, $COCl_2$) is also used in the synthesis of many organic compounds and is a byproduct of combustion of chlorinated organic compounds. It has a characteristic odor of fresh hay. Because of the low water solubility, symptoms of exposure generally are in the lower respiratory tract, especially ALI, and may take up to 24 h after exposure to develop (Borak and Diller 2001). Phosgene, once dissolved in water, forms hydrochloric acid and reactive oxygen species (Sciuto 1998).

## *Oxides of Nitrogen*

Oxides of nitrogen are a group of oxidized nitrogenous compounds ($NO_x$) that when dissolved in water form reactive nitrogen species, such as peroxynitrite ($ONOO^-$), plus nitric acid ($HNO_3$) and nitric oxide (NO) (Gaston et al. 1994). Silo Filler's Disease is the hallmark occupational exposure of this irritant. Nitrogen dioxide ($NO_2$) is produced during the decomposition of silage and in a poorly ventilated silo, it can accumulate (Zwemer et al. 1992; Douglas et al. 1989). Exposure to oxides of nitrogen can also occur during pyrolysis, especially in confined spaces of chemicals, or with the use of propane-powered Zamboni machines (Nelson et al. 2011). Immediate asphyxiation or delayed lower pulmonary toxicity can occur (Zwemer et al. 1992; Douglas et al. 1989). Oxides of nitrogen may also cause systemic toxicity in the form of methemoglobinemia (Heal and Spencer 1995). From one acute exposure, bronchiolitis obiliterans, a chronic lung disease characterized by inflammation of small airways, can develop (Zwemer et al. 1992).

## *Ozone*

Formed by the reaction of UV light on oxygen, ozone is mainly found in the stratospheric part of the Earth's atmosphere. Its concentration may increase on aircraft. It is a potent oxider and is used commercially as a bleaching agent, as an alternative to chlorine. It can also be found occupationally, in welding, in photocopying and laser printing, and near high-voltage electrical equipment. Because it is a potent oxider, its mechanism of action is through generation of free radicals and generally produces lower pulmonary toxicity symptoms (Nelson et al. 2011).

## *Riot Control Agents*

Riot control agents are a group of respiratory irritants that are used to try to control large crowds. Chloroacetophenone and chlorobenxylidenmalononitrile (often referred to by their military designations of CN and CS, respectively, or its common name of Mace) are commonly referred to as "tear gases" because the ocular symptoms predominate at low-level exposures. CN and CS are the most commonly used (Blain 2003). At higher concentrations of exposure, laryngospasm, ALI, and deaths have occurred (Thomas et al. 2002). CN/CS are alkylates agent similar to mustard agents, which may account for their toxicity (Cucinell et al. 1971). Pepper spray, oleoresin capsicum, has replaced Mace in civilian use and its active ingredient is capsaicin. Capsaicin stimulates the receptor transient receptor potential vanilloid-1 (TRPV1) and releases substance P (Xu et al. 2012). It is through substance P that capsaicin produces pain sensation and inflammation of lung tissue, resulting in bronchoconstriction and ALI (Billmire et al. 1996). Capsaicin is consider less toxic that CN and CS but has been responsible for severe outcomes (Billmire et al. 1996; Steffee et al. 1995).

## *Metals and Polymers*

Metal fume fever (Antonini et al. 2003) and polymer fume fever (Shusterman 1993) are two clinically similar scenarios of self-limiting flu-like illness after exposure to volatized metals or fluorinated polymers. Symptoms generally develop within

12 hours of exposure, consist of fevers, cough, chest pain, and dyspnea, and resolve within 48 hours of exposure. Radiographic imaging is usually normal. Tolerance can develop but also can quickly wane, giving rise to the nickname "Monday Morning Fever," since most of these exposures are occupationally based. In the case of metals, zinc is the most commonly implicated (Nelson et al. 2011). Symptom etiology appears to be a mix of activation of pro-inflammatory cytokines and direct toxicity (Blanc et al. 1991). Metal pneumonitis is the most severe form in which ALI has developed and may also be associated with systemic toxicity of the metal (Huang et al. 2008). Patient experiencing metal fume fever are treated with supportive care (antipyretics, analgesics) and generally discharged (Antonini et al. 2003), whereas patients with metal pneumonitis are drastically sicker, require admission, and should receive corticosteroids (Huang et al. 2008). Chelation is reserved for patients with systemic metal toxicity.

### *Oxygen*

Seemingly paradoxically, at high levels, oxygen is an irritant gas. Oxygen toxicity causes more pulmonary toxicity than CNS or retinal toxicity. Oxygen is the ultimate acceptor in the electron transport chain; it is this oxidizing capability that allows oxygen to remove electrons from other molecules and form reactive oxygen species (Sanders et al. 1999). About 5 % of all patients undergoing hyperbaric oxygen therapy will develop ALI (Smerz 2004). Delayed pulmonary fibrosis may develop at atmospheric sea level with lower concentrations of oxygen. While studies have demonstrated that humans can tolerate 100 % oxygen at sea level for 48 hours without acute pulmonary toxicity (Smerz 2004), it is the goal to reduce the amount of supplemental oxygen to as low as possible as soon as possible in patient's requiring oxygen. Currently, positive end-expiratory pressure (PEEP) ventilation is only mechanism for reducing oxygen requirement and this may not work as well as hoped (Babu et al. 2005). Reducing the amount of inspired oxygen may also be more important in patients exposed to any respiratory irritant, as these patients appear more susceptible to oxygen toxicity (Sinclair et al. 2004).

## Irritants that Can Cause Systemic Toxicity

### *Cyanide*

Cyanide rapid diffuses across alveolar membranes when inhaled and rapidly distributes to organs where toxicity develops (Nelson et al. 2011). While mild corrosive injury of the lungs may be seen, systemic toxicity symptoms overwhelmingly predominate. Cyanide is an inhibitor of multiple enzymes, the most important being, cytochrome oxidase at cytochrome $a_3$, a key enzyme in oxidative phosphorylation in the electron transport chain (Way et al. 1988). Hydrogen ions, despite adequate

**Table 4.2** Dosing antidotes for cyanide and hydrogen sulfide toxicity

| Drug | Dose | Notes |
|---|---|---|
| Amyl nitrite | Break ampule, inhale 50 % of time | CN, $H_2S$; only use if no IV access |
| Sodium nitrite | 300 mg IV (adult);<br>0.2 mL/kg IV of 3 % solution (pediatric);<br>given at 2.5–5 mL/min;<br>half-dose may be repeated in 2 h | CN, $H_2S$ |
| Sodium thiosulfate | 12.5 g IV (adult);<br>2 m/kg IV of 25 % solution (pediatric);<br>given over 15 min;<br>may be repeated 2 h later | CN only |
| Hydroxocobalamin | 5 g IV (adult);<br>70 mg/kg IV (pediatric); given over 15 min;<br>may be repeated 2 h later | CN only |

oxygen, are no longer combine with oxygen, ATP is not formed, and acidemia results. Because of the failure of aerobic metabolism to form ATP, anaerobic metabolism kicks in and lactate is formed in abundance (Singh et al. 1989). Cyanide also has effects on NMDA (Patel et al. 1994) and voltage-gated calcium channels (Jensen et al. 2002) which downstream effects cause the formation of reactive oxygen species. Cyanide is detoxified by the body through the enzyme rhodanese, which adds a sulfur moiety to the cyanide converting it to thiocyanate, which is then excreted by the kidneys.

Acute systemic toxicity by inhalation of cyanide includes progressive hypoxia symptoms and cardiovascular collapse (Gill et al. 2004). ALI may be from direct toxicity or from the progressive hypoxia. Cherry-red skin coloring is a result of increased amount of oxygen in venous blood (Singh et al. 1989).

Treatment for cyanide toxicity starts with good supportive care, oxygenation, ventilation, and sodium bicarbonate (Burrows and Way 1977) for acidemia. Historically, cyanide was treated with a 3-part kit of amyl nitrite, sodium nitrite, and sodium thiosulfate (Chen and Rose 1952). The nitrites cause a methemoglobinemia, which provides a temporary place for the body to put cyanide, since cyanide has a greater affinity for methemoglobin that cytochrome $a_3$. Sodium thiosulfate donates a sulfur to cyanide, converting it to thiocyanate. Hydroxocobalamin is an alternative antidote to cyanide toxicity (Bismuth et al. 1988). The central cobalt moiety of hydroxocobalamin complexes with cyanide and forms cyanocobalamin, also known as vitamin B12. Cynaocobalamin is excreted by the kidneys or releases the cyanide slowly enough to allow the body to detoxify itself via rhodanese. Hydroxocobalamin and sodium thiosulfate can be used together (Reade et al. 2012). See Table 4.2 for dosing for these antidotes.

## *Hydrogen Sulfide*

Hydrogen sulfide, at high-level exposures, is at risk for systemic toxicity (Reiffenstein et al. 1992). The toxicity is similar to cyanide, inhibiting the same cytochrome a3 enzyme involved in oxidative phosphorylation. The major mechanism of detoxification is nonenzymatic oxidation to thiosulfate and polysufides. Hydrogen sulfide does not cause significant levels of sulfhemoglobin (Policastro and Otten 2007) (76). Acute systemic toxicity includes rapid loss of consciousness and hypoxia (45, 46). Cardiac toxicity (ischemia, infarction, dysrhythmia) (Gregorakos et al. 1995) and trauma from the knockdown of sudden loss of consciousness (Gabbay et al. 2001) are possible. Treatment is supportive; there is no known antidote. The formation of methemoglobinemia by nitrites and hyperbaric oxygen therapy can be considered (Reiffenstein et al. 1992).

## *Oxides of Nitrogen*

Methemoglobinemia may result from an exposure to oxides of nitrogen, in particular nitric oxide (Heal and Spencer 1995; Hunter et al. 2011); however, at typical doses used for nitric oxide therapy in hospital, systemic toxicity is rare (Hamon et al. 2010). Methemoglobin occurs when the hemoglobin's iron molecule is oxidized from its ferrous state ($Fe2+$) to its ferric state ($Fe3+$). Since normal body function has an element of oxidative stress produced, normal methemoglobin levels are approximately 1 % (Nelson et al. 2011). Cyanosis is the hallmark presenting sign with methemoglobin levels between 10 and 20 %. As the level of methemoglobin increases so do the severity of symptoms: headache, dyspnea, syncope, metabolic acidosis, dysrhythmias, seizures, coma, and death. Patient may exhibit an oxygen saturation mismatch when comparing their pulse oximetry saturation to one on an arterial blood gas. Initial treatment is increasing inspired oxygen and methylene blue. Methylene blue is dosed at 1 mg/kg and given intravenously and may need to be re-dosed. Methylene blue is typically reserved for symptomatic patients or methemoglobin levels greater than 25 %. If methylene blue fails, exchange transfusions and hyperbaric oxygen theoretically may be beneficial. Methylene blue, a mild oxidizer itself, can be used with caution in patients with G6PD deficiency and may be a cause of methylene blue treatment failure; patients with G6PD deficiency should be monitored for hemolysis after treatment (Nelson et al. 2011; Coleman and Coleman 1996).

## *Hydrogen Fluoride*

Patients appear to be most at risk for developing systemic toxicity after inhalational exposure to hydrofluoric acid of greater than 60 % concentration (Greco et al. 1988) but can occur at concentrations as low as 5 % (Dunser et al. 2004). Electrolyte disturbances and cardiac dysrhythmias appear to be the most common systemic symptoms. Hypocalcemia, hypomagnesemia, and hyperkalemia all can occur in HF inhalational exposure (Blodgett et al. 2001). Prolonged QTc interval on EKG is often the first clue to systemic toxicity (Greco et al. 1988). These three electrolyte disturbances can contribute to cardiac dysrhythmias, particularly ventricular tachycardia and fibrillation. Ventricular tachycardia and fibrillation can occur independent of the electrolyte disturbances due to direct toxicity of fluoride ion to cardiac tissue (Vohra et al. 2008).

Empiric calcium and magnesium should be given if the clinician suspects the inhalation exposure was high enough to cause systemic symptoms. Calcium, magnesium, and potassium levels should be monitored frequently and any abnormal levels should be corrected immediately. Standard ACLS protocols for ventricular tachycardia and fibrillation should be followed but correcting electrolyte disturbances should occur concurrently. Urinary alkalization with sodium bicarbonate may increase fluoride excretion by the kidneys (Ekstrand et al. 1980). Fluoride is dialyzable and has been used as treatment for systemic toxicity (Bjornhagen et al. 2003).

## Treatment

Some respiratory irritants, especially those with systemic toxicity concerns, have specific decontamination considerations and treatments. Please see the discussions under the individual irritants in the preceding sections for further details/ management.

Treatment of a respiratory irritant begins with the ending of exposure (Kales and Christiani 2004). If indoors and the source is indoors, exposed persons should be moved outside or to a well-ventilated, unexposed room. If indoors and the source is outside, windows and doors should be closed and ventilation systems turned off. If outdoors, exposed persons should be moved upwind and as far away from the source as possible. Contaminated clothing should be removed which can eliminate up to 90 % of trapped chemicals (Kales and Christiani 2004; Henretig et al. 2002). Irrigation first with water and then washed with soap and water is a simple and effective method of further decontamination, in most exposure situations (Kales and Christiani 2004; Borak and Diller 2001; Henretig et al. 2002). Ideally, decontamination occurs prior to patients arriving to health-care facilities. However, even in mass causality situations, many exposed persons will self-transport (Kales and Christiani 2004). If exposed persons arrive still contaminated, they should be decontaminated either outside or in a separate, closed-off area of the hospital to contain the exposure and prevent secondary exposure within the hospital.

Treatment should next focus on the ABCs of emergency management of any patient and providing supplemental oxygen. Early endotracheal intubation should be considered in patients with hoarseness, stridor, upper airway burns, or altered mental status, as these are signs of severe upper airway involvement with impending loss of airway or inability of the patient to maintain his own airway (Kales and Christiani 2004). Bronchospasm and wheezing due to respiratory irritant exposure are treated with bronchodilators (typically inhaled beta-agonists), similar to asthma (Medical Management 2007). Albuterol is the most commonly used bronchodilator.

If the exposure is severe enough and ALI or ARDS have developed, these are treated in respiratory irritant exposure the same as from any other cause (Nelson et al. 2011). Using low tidal volumes (6 mL/kg) during mechanical ventilation and keeping plateau pressures less than 30 mmHg reduce the inflammatory response, need for prolonged mechanical ventilation, and mortality (Rubenfeld and Herridge 2007; Artigas et al. 1998). The use of prone positions, PEEP, and inversed inspiratory-to-expiratory ratios improve oxygenation but not overall outcomes (Avecillas et al. 2006; Rubenfeld and Herridge 2007; Artigas et al. 1998). The amount of inspired oxygen ($FiO_2$) should be reduced as much as possible, as soon as possible, to help reduce oxygen toxicity, which respiratory irritant exposure patients may be more susceptible (Sinclair et al. 2004).

Patient should be placed on bed rest and limit their physical activity. Increasing physical exertion actually increases inflammation and severity of symptoms (Medical Management 2007; Borak and Diller 2001).

Corticosteroids are frequently used in the treatment of asthma to reduce the inflammatory response. In a respiratory irritant exposure, the medical literature is limited on this topic to case reports and animal studies. In ARDS caused by trauma or sepsis, corticosteroids improved some lung function but not overall mortality (88). In a case report of two sisters exposed to chlorine, the sister who received corticosteroids had a better outcome (Chester et al. 1977). In rats, with chlorine exposure reduced inflammatory markers on bronchial lavage and increase lungs function have been demonstrated after dexamethasone (Demnati et al. 1998). Other animal models have shown similar results with budesonide (Wang et al. 2004, 2005). Short-term corticosteroids should be considered given the low risk and potential benefit (Borak and Diller 2001; Prevention 2002).

Neutralization of acid or alkaline exposure has always been attractive. In gastrointestinal exposures, this is contraindicated but with the larger surface area to allow heat dissipation and smaller amount of acid present in respiratory exposure, nebulized neutralization therapy becomes an option. For acids and acid-forming irritants, nebulized bicarbonate may be given. Chlorine and chloramine exposures make up most of the reported use of nebulized bicarbonate (Sexton and Pronchik 1998). Dosage of nebulized bicarbonate is typically 1 mL of 7.5 % or 8.4 % sodium bicarbonate diluted in 3 mL of sterile water to give an approximate 2 % solution (Nelson et al. 2011; Sexton and Pronchik 1998). For bases and alkaline-forming irritants, there have been no reported attempts and there are no recommendations for neutralization.

Most other treatments are experimental at best. Antioxidants seem beneficial on theoretical basis, by preventing free radical formation or scavenging free radicals after they have formed. Only *N*-acetylcysteine has demonstrated benefit in mild to moderate ALI after phosgene exposure; however *N*-acetylesteine did not alter progression to respiratory failure (Suter et al. 1994). Antibiotics are not indicated unless the patient has clinical signs of super-infection (Borak and Diller 2001). Diuretics, commonly used to treat cardiogenic causes of pulmonary edema, have no role in ALI treatment (Medical Management 2007). Perfluorocarbon partial liquid ventilation is attractive because in animal models, it improves oxygenation (without increasing supplemental oxygen given) and may have an anti-inflammatory effect

(Sinclair et al. 2004). Exogenous surfactant has demonstrated improvement of oxygen exchange in ARDS but not benefitted overall survival. Most of the patients enrolled in the exogenous surfactant studies, however, are patients with ARDS from sepsis and not respiratory irritant exposure (Spragg et al. 2004).

## Special Topics

### *Smoke Inhalation*

This unique exposure is a combination of simple asphyxiants, irritant toxins, and chemical asphyxiants (Orzel 1993). The composition of smoke varies dependent on the materials, oxygen availability, and temperature of the combustion and may vary by location within the same fire. Treating physicians should be ready for any degree of respiratory compromise and systemic toxicity (Table 4.3).

### *Air Pollution and Smog*

Air pollution and smog is a variable mixture of respiratory irritants, asphyxiants, and particulate matter, usually as a result of incomplete combustion. Respiratory

**Table 4.3** Major components of smoke (Nelson et al. 2011)

| Thermal degradation xenobiotic | Source material | Toxicity |
|---|---|---|
| Ammonia | Nylon, silk, plastics, melamine resins | Pulmonary irritant |
| Carbon dioxide | Complete combustion carbon-containing materials | Simple asphyxiant |
| Carbon monoxide | Incomplete combustion of carbon-containing materials | Chemical asphyxiant |
| Chlorine | Plastics | Pulmonary irritant |
| Cyanide | Wool, nylon, plastics, nitrogen-containing materials, melamine resins | Chemical asphyxiant |
| Hydrogen chloride | Wool, acrylic, plastics, PVC, fire-retardant materials | Pulmonary irritant |
| Hydrogen fluoride | Fluorated resins | Pulmonary irritant, other systemic toxicity |
| Hydrogen sulfide | Rubber | Pulmonary irritant, chemical asphyxiant |
| Isocyanates | Nitrogen-containing materials | Pulmonary irritant |
| Oxides of nitrogen | Nitrogen-containing materials, plastics | Pulmonary irritant, chemical asphyxiant |
| Phosgene | Wool, plastics | Pulmonary irritant |
| Sulfur dioxide | Sulfur-containing materials, rubber | Pulmonary irritant |

irritants involved include but are not limited to oxides of nitrogen, sulfur dioxide/sulfuric acid, and ozone. This generally is a low-level constant exposure; however, asthma and other pulmonary diseases are effected by daily variations. Repeated studies have demonstrated that on days when as air pollution increases, visits to emergency departments and admissions to the hospital increase in patients with asthma, chronic obstruction pulmonary disease, and congestive heart failure (Delfino et al. 2009; Lavigne et al. 2012; Meng et al. 2010; Rappold et al. 2011; Searing and Rabinovitch 2011; Stieb et al. 2009).

## *Isocyanates/Bhopal*

In 1984, methyl isocyanate was released from a factory in Bhopal, India, causing one of the largest civilian toxic disasters. At least 2,500 deaths and 200,000 injuries resulted. Some victims demonstrated ALI and at 10-year follow-up, survivors demonstrated continued small-airway obstruction (Misra et al. 1987; Bucher 1987; Mehta et al. 1990; Naik et al. 1986; Varma and Guest 1993). Methyl isocyanate is the most potent respiratory irritant of the isocyanates. Isocyanates are used in industry in the formation of polymers.

## Summary

Despite being a heterogeneous group of xenobiotics, respiratory irritants have common symptomatology and basic supportive treatment after acute exposure. ALI and ARDS are the most severe and feared forms of pulmonary toxicity. A few xenobiotics also have systemic toxicity concerns. Chronic toxicity may also be a concern, even after a one-time acute exposure.

## References

Antonini JM, Lewis AB, Roberts JR, Whaley DA. Pulmonary effects of welding fumes: review of worker and experimental animal studies. Am J Ind Med. 2003;43(4):350–60.

Artigas A, Bernard GR, Carlet J, Dreyfuss D, Gattinoni L, Hudson L, et al. The American-European Consensus Conference on ARDS, part 2: ventilatory, pharmacologic, supportive therapy, study design strategies, and issues related to recovery and remodeling. Acute respiratory distress syndrome. Am J Respir Crit Care Med. 1998;157(4 Pt 1):1332–47. Epub 1998/05/01.

Avecillas JF, Freire AX, Arroliga AC. Clinical epidemiology of acute lung injury and acute respiratory distress syndrome: incidence, diagnosis, and outcomes. Clin Chest Med. 2006;27(4):549–57. abstract vii.

Babu PBR, Chidekel A, Shaffer TH. Hyperoxia-induced changes in human airway epithelial cells: the protective effect of perflubron. Pediatr Crit Care Med. 2005;6(2):188–94.

Bennion JR, Franzblau A. Chemical pneumonitis following household exposure to hydrofluoric acid. Am J Ind Med. 1997;31(4):474–8.
Bernard GR, Artigas A, Brigham KL, Carlet J, Falke K, Hudson L, et al. The American-European Consensus Conference on ARDS. Definitions, mechanisms, relevant outcomes, and clinical trial coordination. Am J Respir Crit Care Med. 1994;149(3 Pt 1):818–24. Epub 1994/03/01.
Billmire DF, Vinocur C, Ginda M, Robinson NB, Panitch H, Friss H, et al. Pepper-spray-induced respiratory failure treated with extracorporeal membrane oxygenation. Pediatrics. 1996;98(5):961–3.
Bismuth C, Baud FJ, Pontal PG. Hydroxocobalamin in chronic cyanide poisoning. J Toxicol Clin Exp. 1988;8(1):35–8.
Bjornhagen V, Hojer J, Karlson-Stiber C, Selden AI, Sundbom M. Hydrofluoric acid-induced burns and life-threatening systemic poisoning–favorable outcome after hemodialysis. J Toxicol Clin Toxicol. 2003;41(6):855–60.
Blain PG. Tear gases and irritant incapacitants. 1-chloroacetophenone, 2-chlorobenzylidene malononitrile and dibenz[b, f]-1,4-oxazepine. Toxicol Rev. 2003;22(2):103–10.
Blanc P, Wong H, Bernstein MS, Boushey HA. An experimental human model of metal fume fever. Ann Intern Med. 1991;114(11):930–6.
Blodgett DW, Suruda AJ, Crouch BI. Fatal unintentional occupational poisonings by hydrofluoric acid in the U.S. Am J Ind Med. 2001;40(2):215–20.
Borak J, Diller W. Phosgene exposure: mechanisms of injury and treatment strategies. J Occup Environ Med. 2001;43:110–9.
Braun J, Stoss H, Zober A. Intoxication following the inhalation of hydrogen fluoride. Arch Toxicol. 1984;56(1):50–4.
Brautbar N. Ammonia exposure: a common cause for sinusitis. A case report and review of the literature. Toxicol Ind Health. 1998;14(6):891–5.
Brautbar N, Wu MP, Richter ED. Chronic ammonia inhalation and interstitial pulmonary fibrosis: a case report and review of the literature. Arch Environ Health. 2003;58(9):592–6.
Brooks SM, Bernstein IL. Irritant-induced airway disorders. Immunol Allergy Clin North Am. 2011;31(4):747–68. vi.
Bucher JR. Methyl isocyanate: a review of health effects research since Bhopal. Fundam Appl Toxicol. 1987;9(3):367–79.
Burnett WW, King EG, Grace M, Hall WF. Hydrogen sulfide poisoning: review of 5 years' experience. Can Med Assoc J. 1977;117(11):1277–80.
Burrows GE, Way JL. Cyanide intoxication in sheep: therapeutic value of oxygen or cobalt. Am J Vet Res. 1977;38(2):223–7.
Charan NB, Myers CG, Lakshminarayan S, Spencer TM. Pulmonary injuries associated with acute sulfur dioxide inhalation. Am Rev Respir Dis. 1979;119(4):555–60. Epub 1979/04/01.
Chela A, Reig R, Sanz P, Huguet E, Corbella J. Death due to hydrofluoric acid. Am J Forensic Med Pathol. 1989;10(1):47–8.
Chen KK, Rose CL. Nitrite and thiosulfate therapy in cyanide poisoning. JAMA. 1952;149(2): 113–9.
Chester EH, Kaimal J, Payne Jr CB, Kohn PM. Pulmonary injury following exposure to chlorine gas. Possible beneficial effects of steroid treatment. Chest. 1977;72(2):247–50.
Coleman MD, Coleman NA. Drug-induced methaemoglobinaemia. Treatment issues. Drug Saf. 1996;14(6):394–405.
Cucinell SA, Swentzel KC, Biskup R, Snodgrass H, Lovre S, Stark W, et al. Biochemical interactions and metabolic fate of riot control agents. Fed Proc. 1971;30(1):86–91.
Delfino RJ, Chang J, Wu J, Ren C, Tjoa T, Nickerson B, et al. Repeated hospital encounters for asthma in children and exposure to traffic-related air pollution near the home. Ann Allergy Asthma Immunol. 2009;102(2):138–44.
Demnati R, Fraser R, Martin JG, Plaa G, Malo JL. Effects of dexamethasone on functional and pathological changes in rat bronchi caused by high acute exposure to chlorine. Toxicol Sci. 1998;45(2):242–6.

Dieffenbacher PF, Thompson JH. Burns from exposure to anhydrous hydrofluoric acid. J Occup Med. 1962;4:325–6.
Dote T, Kono K, Usuda K, Shimizu H, Kawasaki T, Dote E. Lethal inhalation exposure during maintenance operation of a hydrogen fluoride liquefying tank. Toxicol Ind Health. 2003;19: 51–4.
Douglas WW, Hepper NG, Colby TV. Silo-filler's disease. Mayo Clin Proc. 1989;64(3): 291–304.
Dunser MW, Ohlbauer M, Rieder J, Zimmermann I, Ruatti H, Schwabegger AH, et al. Critical care management of major hydrofluoric acid burns: a case report, review of the literature, and recommendations for therapy. Burns. 2004;30(4):391–8.
Ekstrand J, Ehrnebo M, Whitford G, Jarnberg P. Fluoride pharmacokinetics during acid-base balance changes in man. Eur J Clin Pharmacol. 1980;18(2):189–94.
Fleta J, Calvo C, Zuniga J, Castellano M, Bueno M. Intoxication of 76 children by chlorine gas. Hum Toxicol. 1986;5(2):99–100.
Franzblau A, Sahakian N. Asthma following household exposure to hydrofluoric acid. Am J Ind Med. 2003;44(3):321–4.
Gabbay DS, De Roos F, Perrone J. Twenty-foot fall averts fatality from massive hydrogen sulfide exposure. J Emerg Med. 2001;20(2):141–4.
Gapany-Gapanavicius M, Molho M, Tirosh M. Chloramine-induced pneumonitis from mixing household cleaning agents. Br Med J (Clin Res Ed). 1982;285(6348):1086.
Gaston B, Drazen JM, Loscalzo J, Stamler JS. The biology of nitrogen oxides in the airways. Am J Respir Crit Care Med. 1994;149(2 Pt 1):538–51.
Gautrin D, Leroyer C, Infante-Rivard C, Ghezzo H, Dufour JG, Girard D, et al. Longitudinal assessment of airway caliber and responsiveness in workers exposed to chlorine. Am J Respir Crit Care Med. 1999;160(4):1232–7.
Gill JR, Marker E, Stajic M. Suicide by cyanide: 17 deaths. J Forensic Sci. 2004;49(4):826–8.
Goode E. Chemical suicides, popular in Japan, are increasing in the US. The New York Times. 2011. http://www.nytimes.com/2011/06/19/us/19chemical.html. Accessed 14 Jan 2012.
Greco RJ, Hartford CE, Haith Jr LR, Patton ML. Hydrofluoric acid-induced hypocalcemia. J Trauma. 1988;28(11):1593–6.
Gregorakos L, Dimopoulos G, Liberi S, Antipas G. Hydrogen sulfide poisoning: management and complications. Angiology. 1995;46(12):1123–31.
Hamon I, Gauthier-Moulinier H, Grelet-Dessioux E, Storme L, Fresson J, Hascoet JM. Methaemoglobinaemia risk factors with inhaled nitric oxide therapy in newborn infants. Acta Paediatr. 2010;99(10):1467–73.
Heal CA, Spencer SA. Methaemoglobinaemia with high-dose nitric oxide administration. Acta Paediatr. 1995;84(11):1318–9.
Henretig FM, Cieslak TJ, Eitzen Jr EM. Biological and chemical terrorism. J Pediatr. 2002;141(3): 311–26.
Huang K-L, Chen C-W, Chu S-J, Perng W-C, Wu C-P. Systemic inflammation caused by white smoke inhalation in a combat exercise. Chest. 2008;133(3):722–8.
Hunter L, Gordge L, Dargan PI, Wood DM. Methaemoglobinaemia associated with the use of cocaine and volatile nitrites as recreational drugs: a review. Br J Clin Pharmacol. 2011;72(1):18–26.
Jensen MS, Ahlemeyer B, Ravati A, Thakur P, Mennel HD, Krieglstein J. Preconditioning-induced protection against cyanide-induced neurotoxicity is mediated by preserving mitochondrial function. Neurochem Int. 2002;40(4):285–93.
Kales SN, Christiani DC. Acute chemical emergencies. N Engl J Med. 2004;350(8):800–8.
Kimbell JS, Gross EA, Joyner DR, Godo MN, Morgan KT. Application of computational fluid dynamics to regional dosimetry of inhaled chemicals in the upper respiratory tract of the rat. Toxicol Appl Pharmacol. 1993;121(2):253–63.
King BS, Page EH, Mueller CA, Dollberg DD, Gomez KE, Warren AM. Eye and respiratory symptoms in poultry processing workers exposed to chlorine by-products. Am J Ind Med. 2006;49(2):119–26.

Kono K, Watanabe T, Dote T, Usuda K, Nishiura H, Tagawa T, et al. Successful treatments of lung injury and skin burn due to hydrofluoric acid exposure. Int Arch Occup Environ Health. 2000;73 Suppl:S93–7.

Krenzelok E, Mrvos R. Chlorine/chloramine. J Toxicol Clin Toxicol. 1995;33(4):355–7.

Lavigne E, Villeneuve PJ, Cakmak S. Air pollution and emergency department visits for asthma in Windsor, Canada. Can J Public Health. 2012;103(1):4–8.

Lund K, Ekstrand J, Boe J, Sostrand P, Kongerud J. Exposure to hydrogen fluoride: an experimental study in humans of concentrations of fluoride in plasma, symptoms, and lung function. Occup Environ Med. 1997;54(1):32–7.

Mathieu L, Nehles J, Blomet J, Hall AH. Efficacy of hexafluorine for emergent decontamination of hydrofluoric acid eye and skin splashes. Vet Hum Toxicol. 2001;43(5):263–5.

Medical management of chemical casualties handbook. 4th ed. Aberdeen Proving Ground, MD: U.S Army Medical Research Institus of Chemical Defense, Chemical Caualty Division; 2007.

Meggs WJ. RADS and RUDS—The toxic induction of asthma and rhinitis. J Toxicol Clin Toxicol. 1994;32(5):487–501.

Mehta PS, Mehta AS, Mehta SJ, Makhijani AB. Bhopal tragedy's health effects. A review of methyl isocyanate toxicity. JAMA. 1990;264(21):2781–7.

Meng Y-Y, Rull RP, Wilhelm M, Lombardi C, Balmes J, Ritz B. Outdoor air pollution and uncontrolled asthma in the San Joaquin Valley, California. J Epidemiol Community Health. 2010;64(2):142–7.

Minami M, Katsumata M, Miyake K, Inagaki H, Fan XH, Kubota H, et al. Dangerous mixture of household detergents in an old-style toilet: a case report with simulation experiments of the working environment and warning of potential hazard relevant to the general environment. Hum Exp Toxicol. 1992;11(1):27–34.

Misra NP, Pathak R, Gaur KJ, Jain SC, Yesikar SS, Manoria PC, et al. Clinical profile of gas leak victims in acute phase after Bhopal episode. Indian J Med Res. 1987;86 Suppl:11–9.

Naik SR, Acharya VN, Bhalerao RA, Kowli SS, Nazareth H, Mahashur AA, et al. Medical survey of methyl isocyanate gas affected population of Bhopal. Part I. General medical observations 15 weeks following exposure. J Postgrad Med. 1986;32(4):175–84.

Nelson L, Lewin N, Howland M, Hoffman R, Goldfrank L, Flomenbaum N, editors. Goldfranks's toxicologic emergencies. 9th ed. New York: The McGraw-Hill Compaines; 2011.

Orzel RA. Toxicological aspects of firesmoke: polymer pyrolysis and combustion. Occup Med. 1993;8(3):414–29.

Patel MN, Peoples RW, Yim GK, Isom GE. Enhancement of NMDA-mediated responses by cyanide. Neurochem Res. 1994;19(10):1319–23.

Peters JW. Hydrogen sulfide poisoning in a hospital setting. JAMA. 1981;246(14):1588–9.

Piirila PL, Nordman H, Korhonen OS, Winblad I. A thirteen-year follow-up of respiratory effects of acute exposure to sulfur dioxide. Scand J Work Environ Health. 1996;22(3):191–6. Epub 1996/06/01.

Policastro MA, Otten EJ. Case files of the University of Cincinnati fellowship in medical toxicology: two patients with acute lethal occupational exposure to hydrogen sulfide. J Med Toxicol. 2007;3(2):73–81.

Prevention and treatment of injury from chemical warfare agents. Med Lett Drugs Ther. 2002;44(1121):1–4. Epub 2002/02/22.

Rappold AG, Stone SL, Cascio WE, Neas LM, Kilaru VJ, Carraway MS, et al. Peat bog wildfire smoke exposure in rural North Carolina is associated with cardiopulmonary emergency department visits assessed through syndromic surveillance. Environ Health Perspect. 2011;119(10):1415–20. Epub 2011/06/28.

Reade MC, Davies SR, Morley PT, Dennett J, Jacobs IC, Australian RC. Review article: management of cyanide poisoning. Emerg Med Australas. 2012;24(3):225–38.

Reiffenstein RJ, Hulbert WC, Roth SH. Toxicology of hydrogen sulfide. Annu Rev Pharmacol Toxicol. 1992;32:109–34.

Rubenfeld GD, Herridge MS. Epidemiology and outcomes of acute lung injury. Chest. 2007;131(2):554–62.

Sanders KA, Huecksteadt T, Xu P, Sturrock AB, Hoidal JR. Regulation of oxidant production in acute lung injury. Chest. 1999;116(1 Suppl):56S–61.

Sciuto AM. Assessment of early acute lung injury in rodents exposed to phosgene. Arch Toxicol. 1998;72(5):283–8. Epub 1998/06/18.

Searing DA, Rabinovitch N. Environmental pollution and lung effects in children. Curr Opin Pediatr. 2011;23(3):314–8. Epub 2011/04/07.

Sexton JD, Pronchik DJ. Chlorine inhalation: the big picture. J Toxicol Clin Toxicol. 1998;36(1–2):87–93.

Shin JS, Lee S-W, Kim N-H, Park J-S, Kim KJ, Choi S-H, et al. Successful extracorporeal life support after potentially fatal pulmonary oedema caused by inhalation of nitric and hydrofluoric acid fumes. Resuscitation. 2007;75(1):184–8.

Shusterman DJ. Polymer fume fever and other fluorocarbon pyrolysis-related syndromes. Occup Med. 1993;8(3):519–31.

Sinclair SE, Altemeier WA, Matute-Bello G, Chi EY. Augmented lung injury due to interaction between hyperoxia and mechanical ventilation. Crit Care Med. 2004;32(12):2496–501.

Singh BM, Coles N, Lewis P, Braithwaite RA, Nattrass M, FitzGerald MG. The metabolic effects of fatal cyanide poisoning. Postgrad Med J. 1989;65(770):923–5.

Skolnik S. Acute inhalation exposure to hydrogen fluoride. J Occup Environ Hyg. 2010;7(6):D31–3.

Smerz RW. Incidence of oxygen toxicity during the treatment of dysbarism. Undersea Hyperb Med. 2004;31(2):199–202.

Spragg RG, Lewis JF, Walmrath H-D, Johannigman J, Bellingan G, Laterre P-F, et al. Effect of recombinant surfactant protein C-based surfactant on the acute respiratory distress syndrome. N Engl J Med. 2004;351(9):884–92.

Steffee CH, Lantz PE, Flannagan LM, Thompson RL, Jason DR. Oleoresin capsicum (pepper) spray and "in-custody deaths". Am J Forensic Med Pathol. 1995;16(3):185–92.

Stieb DM, Szyszkowicz M, Rowe BH, Leech JA. Air pollution and emergency department visits for cardiac and respiratory conditions: a multi-city time-series analysis. Environ Health. 2009;8:25. Epub 2009/06/12.

Suter PM, Domenighetti G, Schaller MD, Laverriere MC, Ritz R, Perret C. N-acetylcysteine enhances recovery from acute lung injury in man. A randomized, double-blind, placebo-controlled clinical study. Chest. 1994;105(1):190–4.

Takase I, Kono K, Tamura A, Nishio H, Dote T, Suzuki K. Fatality due to acute fluoride poisoning in the workplace. Leg Med (Tokyo). 2004;6(3):197–200.

Tanaka S, Fujimoto S, Tamagaki Y, Wakayama K, Shimada K, Yoshikawa J. Bronchial injury and pulmonary edema caused by hydrogen sulfide poisoning. Am J Emerg Med. 1999;17(4):427–9.

Tepperman PB. Fatality due to acute systemic fluoride poisoning following a hydrofluoric acid skin burn. J Occup Med. 1980;22(10):691–2.

Thickett KM, McCoach JS, Gerber JM, Sadhra S, Burge PS. Occupational asthma caused by chloramines in indoor swimming-pool air. Eur Respir J. 2002;19(5):827–32.

Thomas RJ, Smith PA, Rascona DA, Louthan JD, Gumpert B. Acute pulmonary effects from o-chlorobenzylidenemalonitrile "tear gas": a unique exposure outcome unmasked by strenuous exercise after a military training event. Mil Med. 2002;167(2):136–9.

Tonelli AR, Pham A. Bronchiectasis, a long-term sequela of ammonia inhalation: a case report and review of the literature. Burns. 2009;35(3):451–3.

Tsonis L, Hantsch-Bardsley C, Gamelli RL. Hydrofluoric acid inhalation injury. J Burn Care Res. 2008;29(5):852–5.

Varma DR, Guest I. The Bhopal accident and methyl isocyanate toxicity. J Toxicol Environ Health. 1993;40(4):513–29.

Vohra R, Velez LI, Rivera W, Benitez FL, Delaney KA. Recurrent life-threatening ventricular dysrhythmias associated with acute hydrofluoric acid ingestion: observations in one case and implications for mechanism of toxicity. Clin Toxicol (Phila). 2008;46(1):79–84.

Wang J, Zhang L, Walther SM. Administration of aerosolized terbutaline and budesonide reduces chlorine gas-induced acute lung injury. J Trauma. 2004;56(4):850–62. Epub 2004/06/10.
Wang J, Winskog C, Edston E, Walther SM. Inhaled and intravenous corticosteroids both attenuate chlorine gas-induced lung injury in pigs. Acta Anaesthesiol Scand. 2005;49(2):183–90. Epub 2005/02/18.
Warden CR. Respiratory agents: irritant gases, riot control agents, incapacitants, and caustics. Crit Care Clin. 2005;21(4):719–37. vi.
Watson AA, Oliver JS, Thorpe JW. Accidental death due to inhalation of hydrofluoric acid. Med Sci Law. 1973;13(4):277–9.
Way JL, Leung P, Cannon E, Morgan R, Tamulinas C, Leong-Way J, et al. The mechanism of cyanide intoxication and its antagonism. Ciba Found Symp. 1988;140:232–43.
Winder C. The toxicology of chlorine. Environ Res. 2001;85(2):105–14.
Wood BR, Colombo JL, Benson BE. Chlorine inhalation toxicity from vapors generated by swimming pool chlorinator tablets. Pediatrics. 1987;79(3):427–30.
Xu YP, Zhang JW, Li L, Ye ZY, Zhang Y, Gao X, et al. Complex regulation of capsaicin on intracellular second messengers by calcium dependent and independent mechanisms in primary sensory neurons. Neurosci Lett. 2012;517(1):30–5.
Zwemer Jr FL, Pratt DS, May JJ. Silo filler's disease in New York State. Am Rev Respir Dis. 1992;146(3):650–3.

# Chapter 5
# Particulate Exposure and Cardiovascular Inflammation

**Christopher J. Wingard, Emily Cozzi, Michael R. Van Scott, and Robert M. Lust**

**Abstract** The cardiovascular complications following pulmonary exposure to a variety of unrelated materials can manifest as adverse outcome events. While the specific underlying mechanisms are yet to be fully elucidated the cardiovascular system response to exposures is manifested as a more robust response. In this chapter we describe cardiovascular responses to ambient particulate matter (PM) $CeO_2$, Printex 90 (P90), and multi-walled carbon nanotube (MWCNT) nanoparticles. The inherent complexity of ambient sources of PM and the growing diversity of specifically engineered PM reinforce a need to understand the broader impact of exposures. Mice were exposed to 100 μg of PM or vehicle by intratracheal instillation. MWCNT, P90, and ambient PM all increased the ischemic-reperfusion injury compared to vehicle. Ambient PM and P90 decreased total blood leukocyte counts, while MWCNT induced a larger increase in plasma fibrinogen than ambient PM. Only ambient PM affected blood palette numbers and endothelial mediated relaxations. MWCNT exposure augmented the constrictor response but had no effect on endothelial dependent responses. These results illustrate our increasing yet limited understanding of the integrative nature of the cardiovascular system with neural, humeral, and immune systems and only begins to hint at the importance of a hypersensitive state on physiological and pathophysiological processes.

**Keywords** Myocardial infarction • Vascular dysfunction • Pulmonary instillation • Multi-walled carbon nanotube • Ambient ultrafine particles • Cerium oxide

---

C.J. Wingard, Ph.D. (✉) • E. Cozzi, Ph.D. • M.R. Van Scott, Ph.D. • R.M. Lust, Ph.D.
Department of Physiology, Brody School of Medicine at East Carolina University,
600 Moye Boulevard, 6N98, Greenville, NC 27834, USA
e-mail: wingardc@ecu.edu

W.J. Meggs (ed.), *The Toxicant Induction of Irritant Asthma, Rhinitis, and Related Conditions*, DOI 10.1007/978-1-4614-9044-9_5,

## Introduction

Inflammation is a common feature of hypersensitivity disorders as well as other environmental diseases. In this chapter, we discuss the phenomenon that immune activation or suppression underlying inflammation in one organ system can change the responsiveness of other organ systems to imposed stress. A notable example of this phenomenon is the impact of asthma on cardiovascular disease. Cardiovascular complications are common in asthma and, in many cases, are due to asthma therapeutics with cardiovascular side effects. However, there is direct evidence from animal studies demonstrating an intrinsic link between aeroallergen exposure and sensitivity of the cardiovascular system to imposed stresses. Furthermore, there is a growing body of literature demonstrating that pulmonary exposure to particles not associated with asthma has similar effects on the cardiovascular system.

In 2004, Hazarika and colleagues proposed that aeroallergen challenge directly affects the response of the myocardium to stress. The hypothesis was tested by comparing the myocardial response to ischemia and reperfusion in rabbit and mouse models of allergic asthma. Allergen sensitization and challenge increased the size of myocardial infarction following ischemia and reperfusion of coronary vasculature, and the difference in the response to the imposed cardiovascular stress could not be attributed to asthma therapeutics (Hazarika et al. 2004, 2007). Hazarika et al. went on to demonstrate that aeroallergen challenge reduced endothelial dependent and independent relaxation of aortic smooth muscle, providing a potential mechanism by which aeroallergen challenge affected the outcome of ischemia and reperfusion of the myocardium (Hazarika et al. 2010). The observations by Hazarika could not be explained by an adjuvant effect of the ambient particles, since exposure to the allergens and ambient particles occurred at different times. The transduction mechanism by which aeroallergen challenge induced a systemic response remains unknown, but the findings provide proof that environmental agents associated with airway hypersensitivity and responsiveness can alter the sensitivity of the cardiovascular system to intrinsic factors controlling its function.

Links between environmental exposure of the lungs and cardiovascular sensitivity to stress have been suspected for years, and the environmental agents are not limited to allergens and adjuvants. Data linking particulate air pollution to morbidity and mortality in humans has been accumulating in earnest for the last 80 years. The most notable air pollution events occurred as "killer fogs" in the Meuse Valley, Belgium (1930); Donora, Pennsylvania (1948); and London (1952 and 1956). In Donora and the Meuse Valley, smog was associated with a relatively small number of fatalities (20 and 60, respectively), but in London, high levels of smog were associated with 12,000 deaths in 1952 and 1,000 in 1956 (Hunt et al. 2003). Over 5 days in 1952, London's daily concentrations of total suspended particulate (TSP) peaked at about 7.0 $mg/m^3$ of air, with maximum concentrations of smoke at 4.46 $mg/m^3$ and sulfur dioxide at 1.34 ppm (Whittaker et al. 2004). Meanwhile, 98 % of the total particulate matter (PM) collected during a similar episode in London (1956) were respirable fine particles (<2.5 μm in diameter; $PM_{2.5}$), and

89 % were less than 1 μm (Whittaker et al. 2004). To put these levels in perspective, in 2005, the EPA recommended maximum exposure level for fine particles of 30–35 μg/m$^3$, 100-fold less than what was measured in London, and in 2006, 23 US cities had peak 24-h $PM_{2.5}$ levels in the range of 40 μg/m$^3$ (USEPA 2006).

The excess deaths in London occurred almost entirely from cardiopulmonary complications—especially among those with preexisting cardiopulmonary diseases (Whittaker et al. 2004). While some skeptics initially argued that increased deaths during high smog events resulted from displaced short-term deaths, several studies have since disproved these arguments (Biggeri et al. 2004; Zanobetti et al. 2003). Sulfur dioxide ($SO_2$) exposure was originally believed to be the cause of the adverse health responses seen in London, but more recent analyses have determined that PM was the dominant culprit (Schwartz 1996; Schwartz and Marcus 1990).

## Epidemiological Studies Linking PM with Cardiovascular Outcomes

Numerous epidemiological studies have associated ambient PM with increased mortality and morbidity (Biggeri et al. 2004; Zanobetti et al. 2002, 2003; Schwartz 1996; Schwartz and Marcus 1990; USEPA 2004), both in the long term (Dockery et al. 1993; Ostro et al. 2006; Pope et al. 2004a, b; Samet et al. 2000; Schwartz and Dockery. 1992) and short term (Ostro et al. 2006; Franklin et al. 2007, 2008; Franklin and Schwartz 2008; Zanobetti and Schwartz 2009). High levels of PM are associated with increased incidence of myocardial infarction (MI), heart failure, arrhythmia, and cardiac arrest (Ostro et al. 2006; Schwartz and Dockery 1992; Brook et al. 2004; Dockery et al. 2005; Le Tertre et al. 2002; Peters 2005; Peters et al. 2000, 2001a, b; Stenfors et al. 2004; Zanobetti and Schwartz 2005; Brook et al. 2010). In addition, PM exposure is associated with stroke and venous thrombosis (Baccarelli et al. 2008, 2009), and a prothrombotic status is presumed to contribute to cardiac and vascular effects (Kettunen et al. 2007; Villeneuve et al. 2006; Wallenborn et al. 2007b; Wellenius et al. 2005). EPA's *2004 Criteria Document for Particulate Matter* cites over 100 journal articles published between 1995 and 2004 that revealed positive associations between short-term PM exposure and cardiopulmonary and lung cancer mortality (USEPA 2004). Peters et al. (2001a, b) observed a 69 % increase in Boston-area heart attacks per 20 μg/m$^3$ increase in 24-h $PM_{2.5}$ on the preceding day.

In 2006, 23 US cities (accounting for 46 million people) had peak 24-h $PM_{2.5}$ levels of at least 40 μg/m$^3$ (USEPA 2006). Thus, acute fluctuations in fine particulate matter likely contribute to major surges in the national incidence of reported cardiovascular events. In addition to these acute short-term outcomes, others have observed stronger effects of PM on mortality and morbidity in humans with preexisting cardiovascular disease. Zanobetti and Schwartz recently (Zanobetti and Schwartz 2007) observed among heart attack survivors that a 10 μg/m$^3$ increase in annual $PM_{10}$ levels was linked with a 43 % increased occurrence of subsequent heart attacks and a 34 % increased mortality over 3 years. By comparing pollution records with data from implanted defibrillators, Dockery and colleagues (2005) found positive correlations between PM levels and potentially fatal ventricular tachyarrhythmias. Henneberger et al. (2005) revealed an association between elevated PM and impairments in ventricular repolarization by examining electrocardiograms (ECGs) of patients with coronary artery disease.

Diesel exhaust (DE) is a ubiquitous air pollutant that is strongly believed to contribute to adverse cardiovascular effects. Ischemic heart disease hospitalizations in eight European cities have been attributed to DE exposure (Le Tertre et al. 2002). In particular, Mills et al. (2007) found that DE exposure exacerbated exercise-induced electrocardiographic ST depression in human subjects with known coronary artery disease. Although many components of DE are suspected to play a role in DE-induced cardiovascular (CV) dysfunction, recent investigations using relatively healthy individuals have implicated particles as the predominant mediators (Lucking et al. 2011; Mills et al. 2011). Studies have demonstrated pathophysiologic effects on the CV system following acute exposure to either particle-containing whole diesel exhaust (wDE) (Mills et al. 2007; Anselme et al. 2007; Miller et al. 2009) or DE particles alone (Huang et al. 2010). Likewise, removal of particles by modern DE filters can prevent DE-induced thrombosis and vasoconstriction in healthy humans (Lucking et al. 2011; Mills et al. 2011).

## Potential Mechanisms Underlying PM Augmentation of Adverse Cardiovascular Responses

Observations of increased detrimental cardiovascular events such as cardiac arrhythmia, endothelial lipid peroxidation, ischemic myocardial lesions, MI, decompensation of heart failure, and changes in heart rate variability have guided many hypotheses about mechanistic pathways of air pollutant-induced cardiovascular insult, all of which concern neuroregulatory, vascular, cardiac, and/or pulmonary effects. Among the hypothesized mechanisms, the most substantiated include (1) dysfunction of the autonomic nervous system (ANS) resulting from chronic changes in responsiveness of lung irritant receptors, modifying lung receptor cardiopulmonary reflexes, and (2) inflammatory responses (systemic and pulmonary) that lead to vascular changes including procoagulant alterations of blood, endothelial malfunction, and structural deterioration of the endothelium (Schulz et al. 2005; Zareba et al. 2001). The assumption is that either of these can aggravate progression of underlying preexisting disease.

Autonomic control of heart function is frequently assessed by measuring heart rate variability (HRV)—the variation in time between successive heartbeats. Significant declines or increases in HRV parameters may indicate autonomic dysfunction. Decreased HRV has been associated with a risk of cardiovascular events such as myocardial infarct, cardiac arrhythmias, and sudden cardiac death as well as progression of heart failure and atherosclerosis (Ponikowski et al. 1996; Singh et al. 2003). PM exposure has been associated with significant decreases in HRV parameters among the elderly that intensify with preexisting arrhythmia, coronary heart disease, and hypertension (Devlin et al. 2003; Liao et al. 1999); however, air pollution's effects on autonomic function can vary with specific cardiopulmonary diseases. Wheeler et al. (2006) observed that increases in ambient $PM_{2.5}$ significantly increased HRV parameters in subjects with COPD but decreased HRV parameters in individuals with prior MI.

Currently, alterations in immune responsiveness are generating the greatest interest. The most consistent working premise is that PMs in the respiratory tree trigger an immune response of varying intensities. In cases of pulmonary diseases, the assumption is that the inflammatory trigger is contained within the lung but may, over time, alter the systemic sensitivity to subsequent challenges. Two competing arguments have been advanced in this regard. One suggests that exposure to PMs alters the phenotypic response of the immune system, decreasing its surveillance efficacy and increasing morbidity associated with exposure to opportunistic/infections or previously innocuous challenges. The other argument suggests that exposure to PMs generally, and perhaps nonspecifically, sensitizes the immune system. In that setting, any minor injuries that might otherwise have provoked a modest inflammatory response now generate exaggerated injury. In either case, it is known that a major component of an inflammatory response includes generation of free radicals and production of oxidative stress.

The role of metals in production of reactive oxygen and nitrogen intermediates is well known, and therefore, the involvement of metals is thought to be a key element of PM-mediated injury. Studies have associated the nickel and vanadium content of PM with adverse cardiovascular health effects (Lippmann et al. 2006; Lippmann 2007). Others have associated high levels of iron, copper, zinc, and lead content with increased pulmonary inflammation in human volunteers (Ghio and Devlin 2001), and the removal of the metals abolished inflammatory effects in a rodent model (Molinelli et al. 2002).

Nonmetal constituents of ambient PM also have been investigated for their potential role in cardiopulmonary toxicity (Li et al. 2008; Campen et al. 2010). Organic compounds associated with PM, such as polycyclic aromatic hydrocarbons (PAHs), can lead to the production of cytotoxic reactive oxygen species (ROS) (Nel et al. 2001). Fine and ultrafine PMs have been shown to contain the largest fraction of PAHs and therefore potentially can induce greater oxidant injury than coarse PM (Sioutas et al. 2005; Goulaouic et al. 2008). The role of oxidant burden cannot be ignored, but oxidant burden has been associated with many other disease processes, and in general, dietary antioxidant regimens have been ineffective in modulating outcome.

## Impact of Defined Particles on Cardiovascular Responses to Stress

Exposure of laboratory animals to ambient PM recapitulates many of the effects observed in humans during periods of high particulate pollution. For example, pulmonary exposure to ultrafine particles (<100 nm) isolated from ambient air doubles the size of a myocardial infarction induced by ischemia and reperfusion in mice, reduces endothelium-dependent relaxation of aortic smooth muscle, and alters hemostasis in ways that would enhance clot formation and reduce clot resolution (Cascio et al. 2007; Cozzi et al. 2006, 2007). This and other similar work has led to the exposure of laboratory animals to well-defined particles as a way of investigating the role of the physical and chemical characteristics of particles in biological responses.

Composition, size, and shape of particles contribute to the pathophysiology associated with respiratory exposures. The size effect is mediated, in part, by the depth to which the particles penetrate the respiratory tree, bypassing the normal biological air filtration systems of upper airways. Coarse particles greater than 10 μm in size are thought to be effectively cleared by impaction in the upper airways, while fine particles in the 10–2.5 μm size range deposit in the tracheal-bronchial trees and are capable of penetrating the alveolar regions (Kappos et al. 2004). Ultrafine airborne particles in the nanoscale range (<0.1 μm in size) can pass through the lung epithelial and pulmonary vascular endothelial barriers directly into the circulation (Nemmar et al. 2001; Ibald-Mulli et al. 2002; Kreyling et al. 2006).

Non-biological airborne particulates (particulate matter) most often are products of mechanical and combustion processes. Mechanical processes such as erosion and grinding lead to coarse particles that are high in minerals and metals. In contrast, combustion processes lead to fine and ultrafine particles high in organic and elemental carbon with traces of metals (Sioutas et al. 2005). Carbon black (CB) is a powdered form of elemental carbon resulting from controlled vapor-phase pyrolysis of gaseous or liquid hydrocarbons and represents the carbonaceous core of ambient PM. Inoue and co-workers have demonstrated that CB nanoparticles can induce modest lung inflammatory responses. When co-administered with a bacterial endotoxin it can act as an adjuvant and significantly aggravate the pulmonary inflammatory response to the infectious agent (Inoue et al. 2006). CB induces pulmonary inflammation, generates ROS (Dick et al. 2003a), and increases thrombogenic potential. CB exposure in humans has been associated with increased serum fibrinogen concentration (Zeka et al. 2006) and morbidity (Gardiner et al. 2001).

$TiO_2$ is a nonorganic nanomaterial that has been in commercial use for nearly 50 years in production of photocatalysts and surface coatings as well as cosmetics and sunscreens (Aitken et al. 2006). $TiO_2$ has been shown to alter blood vessel responsiveness and functional anatomy, ranging from impairments of vasodilatation to modification of the progression of atherosclerotic plaques (Mikkelsen et al. 2011; Nurkiewicz et al. 2009; Courtois et al. 2008). Cerium oxide ($CeO_2$) is another nonorganic nanomaterial used in a wide range of applications, such as solar cells, fuel cells, gas sensors, oxygen pumps, and fuel additives. It is currently listed as 1 of 5 nanomaterials under investigation by the US Environmental Protection Agency. $CeO_2$ is a metal oxide that possesses a cubic fluorite structure with oxygen vacancies which may potentially act as free radical scavengers (Schubert et al. 2006). Acute exposure of cells to $CeO_2$ in vitro has been shown to be relatively nontoxic (Schubert et al. 2006). However, $CeO_2$ persists in the lungs of humans up to 15 years after exposure (Pairon et al. 1995), and the long-term effects have not been defined. Recent work by our group, some of which is presented below, has demonstrated that $CeO_2$ nanoparticles activate mast cells, contributing to pulmonary inflammation,

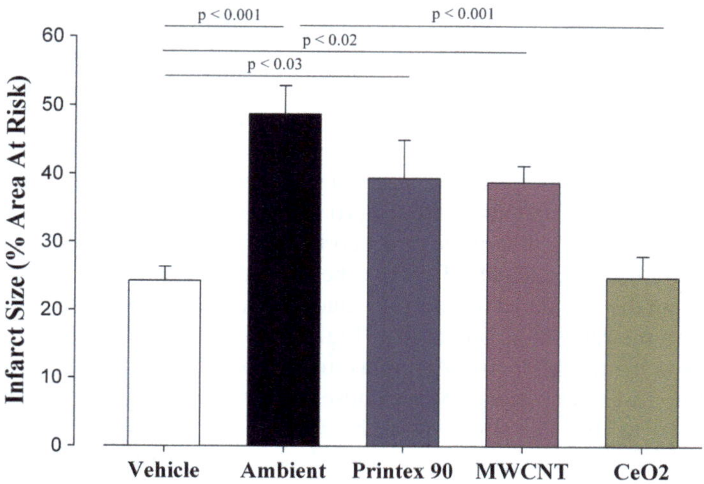


**Fig. 5.1** Comparison of the size of myocardial infarction in mice exposed to 100 μg of ambient or manufactured PM. 24 h after oropharyngeal aspiration of PM or vehicle, the LAD was ligated for 20 min and then reperfused for 2 h. The AAR was defined by religation of the LAD and retrograde perfusion of the myocardium with Evan's blue dye. The infarct was demarcated by incubating heart sections in 2,3,5-triphenyltetrazolium chloride (TTC). Areas were determined by morphometry in serial sections through the left ventricle. Values represent mean ± SE, $n = 21$ vehicle control-, 20 ambient-, 12 MWCNT-, 9 Printex 90-, and 8 $CeO_2$-exposed animals

impairment of vascular relaxation, and exacerbation of myocardial ischemia/reperfusion (I/R) injury (Wingard et al. 2011).

Carbon nanotubes (CNT) are graphite tubes created by adding energy (heat, light, or electricity) to a carbon source (Donaldson et al. 2006). Single-walled carbon nanotubes (SWCNT) are one graphite wall thick, while multi-walled carbon nanotubes (MWCNT) consist of multiple concentric carbon walls (Donaldson et al. 2006). CNT have high electrical conductivity as well as a large surface area that can be functionalized for attachment of diverse molecules. Recent studies have shown that intratracheal (i.t.) instillation of CNT can cause dose-dependent pulmonary epithelioid and collagen-rich granulomas (Lam et al. 2004; Muller et al. 2005; Huizar et al. 2011). In vitro studies have demonstrated that SWCNT stimulate TNF-β production in a murine macrophage cell line (Shvedova et al. 2005). Nemmar et al. have demonstrated that pulmonary instillation of CNT induces a mild lung inflammation and promotes platelet activation in the systemic circulation (Nemmar et al. 2007), while SWCNT promote atherosclerotic lesion progression and induce oxidative stress in the lung, heart, and aorta (Li et al. 2007).

We directly compared the effects of ambient PM, carbon black (Printex 90), $CeO_2$, and MWCNT on myocardial I/R injury in mice. As shown in Fig. 5.1, ambient PM increased I/R infarct size when compared to $CeO_2$ or vehicle control ($p < 0.001$) and to a greater extent than equivalent doses of Printex 90 and MWCNT ($p < 0.001$), for which infarct size was also significantly increased ($p < 0.03$). Infarct sizes in $CeO_2$- and vehicle-exposed mice were equivalent, indicating minimal effect of $CeO_2$ on ischemia-induced myocardial injury. Areas at risk (AAR) for ischemic injury were not different between the groups (data not shown). Thus, the specific particle properties define the extent of cardiovascular injury after ischemia.

Aortas were isolated from mice 24 h after exposure to the different particles to assess isometric force responses to applied constrictor and dilators. The ambient PM at the three concentrations examined (10, 30, and 100 μg) significantly impaired the ACh relaxation response of the intact aortas when compared to the vehicle control. There were no significant differences between the three doses in magnitude of relaxation, but the calculated mean $EC_{50}$ values revealed a progressive diminution in sensitivity to the relaxation agent ACh (Fig. 5.2a). Since we found no significant differences in the thoracic aorta Ach relaxation responses in animals instilled with the different doses of ambient PM we chose to examine the 100 μg dosage for all other particles to elucidate potential mechanisms of action.

Both ambient PM and $CeO_2$ reduced the relaxation response to ACh on the endothelial intact thoracic aortic rings. The response was associated with a statistically significant decrease in the magnitude of maximal relaxation in the ambient PM group and a decrease in the sensitivity to the ACh, as reflected by an increase in both the calculated $EC_{50}$ and Hill slope (Table 5.1, $p<0.05$). $CeO_2$ also appeared to inhibit the relaxation response to ACh as indicated by a rise in the calculated $EC_{50}$ value but did not affect the slope of the curve or the magnitude of maximal relaxation. The relaxation responses to ACh for vessels from animals exposed to MWCNT were statistically different from the vehicle control responses, while those for Printex 90 showed a trend toward significance (Fig. 5.2b), and both did appear to show a trend toward increased sensitivity to ACh by having lower calculated $EC_{50}$ values ($p=0.13$, Table 5.1).

Constrictor responses to the α-adrenergic agonist phenylephrine (PE), the β-adrenergic agonist norepinephrine (NE), and serotonin (5-HT) also were examined. There were no differences in the contractile response to PE or 5-HT in any of the tested particles (data not shown). Differences in contractile response to NE were seen only in denuded aorta rings of the MWCNT-exposed compared with the vehicle-exposed animals. The vehicle $EC_{50}$ was $0.06 \pm 0.03$ μM, and the MWCNT $EC_{50}$ was $0.12 \pm 0.09$ μM ($p<0.001$) (Fig. 5.1c). The modest differences in the maximal stress generation in response to 3 μM NE were $0.96 \pm 0.39$ and $0.76 \pm 0.16$ mN/mm$^2$ for vehicle and MWCNT group, respectively ($p=0.64$) (Fig. 5.2c), that are suggestive of sensitivity of mechanisms underlying control of vascular relaxation.

The impaired relaxation of aortic rings after ambient PM exposure shown here and previously by this group (Cozzi et al. 2006) is consistent with impaired dilation responses of rat arterioles following exposure to residual oil fly ash (ROFA) and titanium dioxide (Nurkiewicz et al. 2004). In addition, diesel exhaust, ambient PM, ROFA, and titanium dioxide have all been shown to alter vascular reactivity through impairment of endothelial function or free radical handling (Batalha et al. 2002; Hearse et al. 1985; O'Neill et al. 2005; Tzeng et al. 2003; Knuckles et al. 2008). It has also been postulated that particle-induced impairment of vascular relaxation is due to increases in endothelin (ET), ET-converting enzyme-1, prepro ET-1,

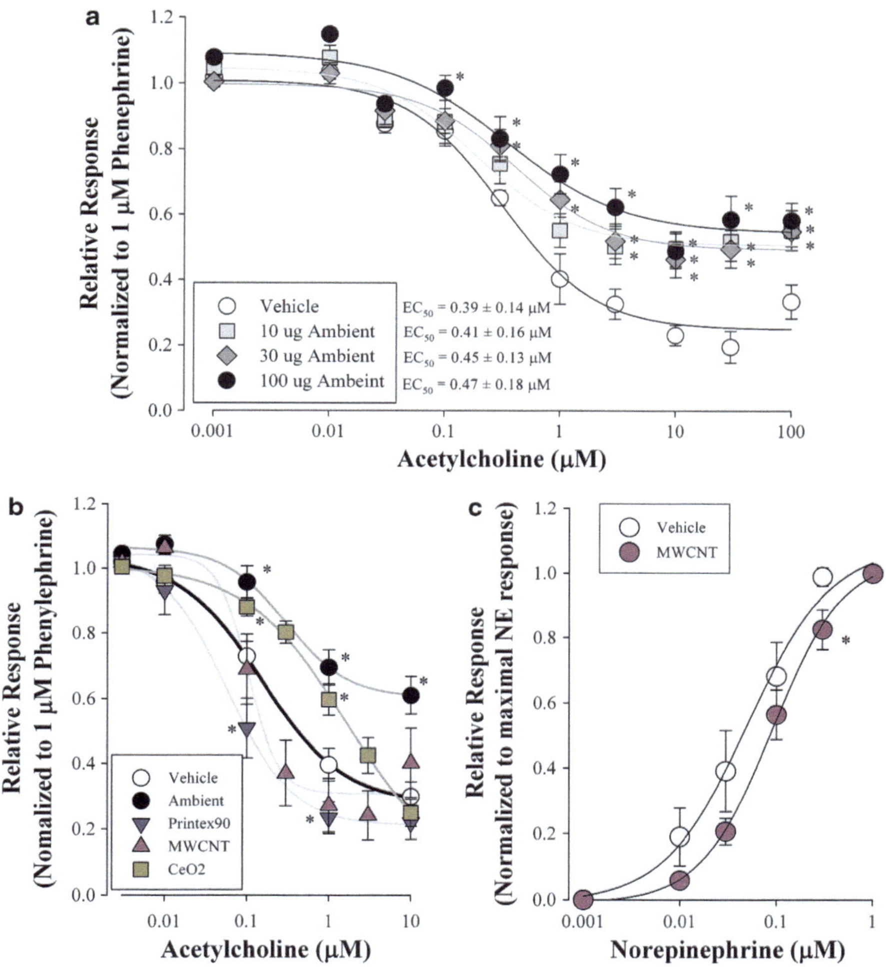


**Fig. 5.2** Thoracic aorta relaxation and constriction responses 24 h after particle instillation. All measurements were made in thoracic aortic rings obtained 24 h after oropharyngeal aspiration, and lines represent Hill fits to the mean data. *Asterisks* indicate statistical significance from vehicle values as determined by one-way ANOVA ($p<0.05$). *Panel A*: Effect of ambient particle dosing on acetylcholine-induced relaxation in rings with intact endothelium (values represent mean relative stress ± SE, $n=6$–16 animals). *Panel B*: Effect of ambient particle type at the same dose (100 μg) on acetylcholine-induced relaxation (values represent mean relative stress ± SE, $n\geq 7$ animals). *Panel C*: Constrictor response of denuded vessel to norepinephrine stimulation following MWCNT instillation (values represent mean relative stress ± SE, $n=6$–16 animals)

and depressed eNOS expression (Kang et al. 2002; Thomson et al. 2005). In contrast, Printex 90 and MWCNT exposure enhanced acetylcholine-induced aortic relaxation. Notably, none of the manufactured particles increased the ending active

**Table 5.1** Hill fit characteristics for acetylcholine relaxation of mouse thoracic aorta from vehicle- and nanoparticle-exposed mice

| Treatment | Ending active stress (mN/mm$^2$) | Calculated $EC_{50}$ (μM) | Hill slope | Count |
|---|---|---|---|---|
| Vehicle | 0.28±0.04 | 0.39±0.14 | 2.69±1.54 | 8 |
| Ambient PM | 0.62±0.06* | 0.47±0.18 | 6.71±3.92 | 16 |
| MWCNT | 0.31±0.09 | 0.12±0.03 | 3.49±0.57 | 8 |
| Printex 90 | 0.18±0.04 | 0.08±0.03 | 1.41±0.18 | 7 |
| $CeO_2$ | 0.28±0.16 | 1.23±0.38* | 1.04±0.23 | 7 |

*Indicates statistical significance from vehicle values as determined by one-way ANOVA ($p<0.05$). Data represented as means ± SE of the described characteristics for individual curve fits

stress relative to 10 μM acetylcholine relative to vehicle exposure (Table 5.1 and Fig. 5.2b).

The $EC_{50}$ value for response to acetylcholine was increased with $CeO_2$, but Printex 90 and MWCNT had increased sensitivity to acetylcholine when compared to vehicle control (Fig. 5.2). Bagate and colleagues have also demonstrated that particle exposure can enhance aortic relaxation to acetylcholine (Bagate et al. 2004). Thus, inhibition of cholinergic vascular smooth muscle relaxation and vessel dilation may be linked to the increased infarct size following ambient PM exposure relative to vehicle control and the manufactured particles.

## Particle Deposition and Lung Histology 24 h Post Instillation

Particle deposition in the lungs was assessed by histology 24 h post oropharyngeal instillation. Three to five serial sections were examined from each of the cephalic, middle, and caudal regions of the lung. Both Printex 90- and the MWCNT-exposed animals showed agglomerated particles in the lungs (Fig. 5.3, panels e–h arrows). Interestingly, some of the particles were closely associated with cells in the alveolar wall. Agglomerated particles were not observed in animals exposed to ambient PM and $CeO_2$. Twenty-four hours after exposure, lung sections from particle-exposed animals showed greater evidence of pulmonary inflammation compared with the vehicle-exposed animals (Fig. 5.3).

The increased inflammation identified in the representative micrograph specimens shown in Fig. 5.4 also was reflected in higher aggregate lung pathology scores. The degree of pneumonitis, edema, increased alveolar macrophages, subpleural lymphocyte aggregates, perivascular/peribronchial/peribronchiolar cuffing and pneumonia were assessed, and a semiquantitative scoring system was applied, where 0 = none, 1 = minimal, 2 = mild, 3 = moderate, and 4 = severe. The results are summarized in Fig. 5.4.

Pneumonitis scores were higher for all particle-exposed lungs, with more than 60 % of all the sections having scores of 1 or more, while only 37 % of vehicle-exposed lungs exhibited scores above 0. MWCNT exposure was associated with the

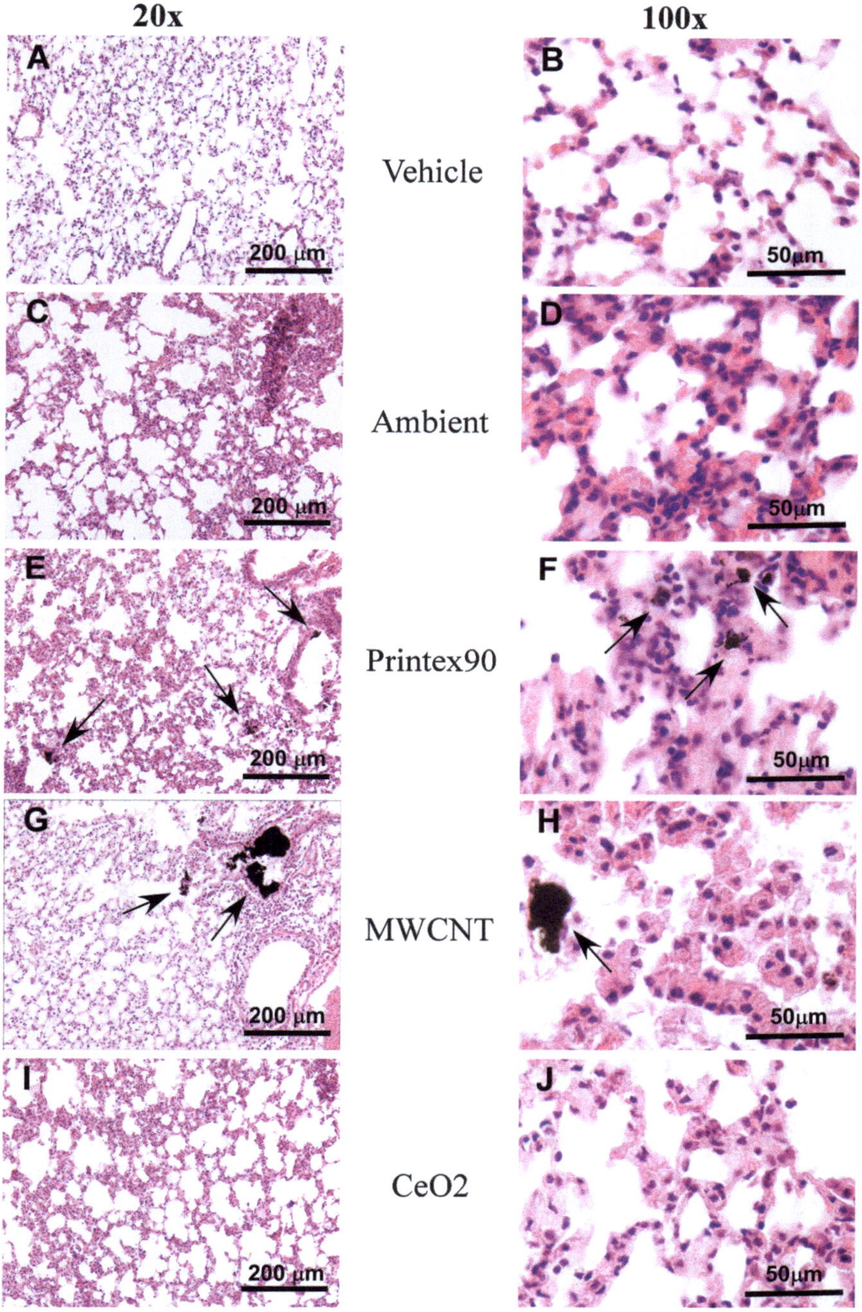


**Fig. 5.3** Lung histology 24 h after exposure to vehicle and particulate matter. Mice were exposed to vehicle (PBS) (**a**, **b**) or 100 μg of ambient PM (**c**, **d**), Printex 90 (**e**, **f**), MWCNT (**g**, **h**), or $CeO_2$ (**i**, **j**) by oropharyngeal aspiration. Lung sections were viewed by light microscopy (×20 or ×100 under oil) after staining with Harris' hematoxylin and eosin. Particle aggregation in the small airways and alveolar spaces were observed in Printex 90- and MWCNT-exposed lungs (*arrows*) but not in ambient PM- and $CeO_2$-exposed lungs. The micrographs are representative of each group ($n=4$ animals/group)

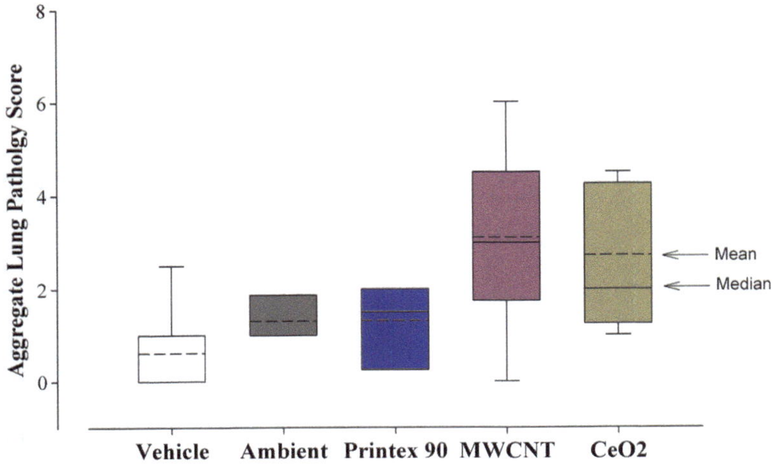


**Fig. 5.4** Aggregate incidence scores for all categories of lung pathology based on particle exposure. Multiple sections (6–12) from each of the three animals in each exposure group were analyzed. Cumulative score for each animals was complied and then plotted as box plot identifying mean (*dashed line*), median score (*solid line*), and then 90th percentiles with errors bars for each particle exposure

greatest inflammation, exhibiting scores of 1 or greater for all categories assessed. The particle with the next most frequently elevated scores was $CeO_2$, which had scores of 1 or greater in all categories except edema and subpleural lymphocyte aggregates, which were reported as 0. The histology of the ambient PM- and vehicle-exposed lungs was qualitatively similar to that previously reported by our group (Cozzi et al. 2006).

## Ambient and Manufactured PM Instillation Results in Unique Bronchial Alveolar Lavage Cell Profiles

To assess the potential in vivo toxicity of the different particles, we investigated pulmonary inflammation in bronchial alveolar lavage (BAL) obtained from ICR mice 24 h after equivalent mass instillations of the various particles. As shown in Fig. 5.5a, mice exposed to all particles displayed an increase in total inflammatory cell infiltrates within the lungs as compared to saline-instilled mice. The individual numbers of macrophages, neutrophils, and lymphocytes were increased. Mice instilled with ambient PM and MWCNT particles also exhibited elevations in the number of eosinophils. Yet, the relative proportion of the cell count was different among the various particle types. Printex 90 and MWCNT showed lower percentages of macrophages but increased neutrophils and eosinophils (Fig. 5.5b), and all particles resulted in a significantly lower percentage of epithelial cells than the vehicle control.

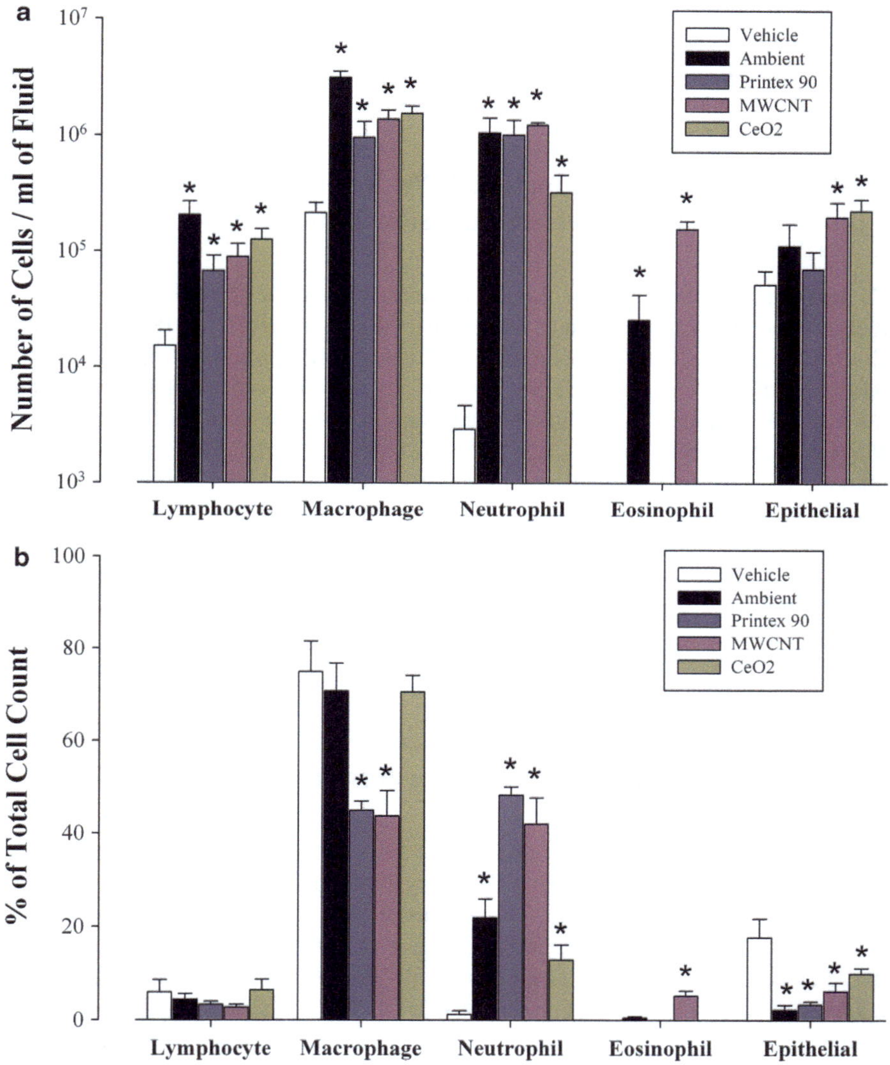


**Fig. 5.5** Bronchoalveolar lavage (BAL) cell counts 24 h after oropharyngeal aspiration of vehicle, ambient particulate matter, Printex 90, multiwall carbon nanotubes, or cerium oxide. The concentration of cells in the returned BAL fluid (**a**) and relative cell counts (**b**) are shown. Values represent mean ± SE, $n = 5–7$. *Asterisks* indicate statistical significance from vehicle values as determined by one-way ANOVA ($p < 0.05$)

Unrelated to the cardiovascular effects of nanoparticles, but interesting nonetheless, is the observation that ambient PM and MWCNT increased eosinophils in the BAL fluid (Fig. 5.5). Eosinophils are a prominent cell type in allergic asthma, and exacerbation of allergic asthma by ambient PM and CNT has been reported previously (Nygaard et al. 2009; Granum and Lovik 2002; Inoue et al. 2009). Our data demonstrate particle specificity of the effect. Furthermore, the results preclude the particles acting as an adjuvant since the effect was observed in the absence of overt allergen challenge and was not observed with Printex 90.

## Ambient PM and Manufactured PM Result in Nominal Changes in Serum Levels of Adhesion-Related Proteins

To further assess the ability of particles to induce systemic activation of the endothelium and thrombogenic state, we measured protein levels of tPAI-1, soluble E-selectin, soluble ICAM-1, soluble VCAM, and MMP-9 in serum from saline- and particle-instilled ICR mice. As shown in Fig. 5.6, protein levels of the thrombogenic marker tPAI-1 appeared slightly but not significantly elevated in the Printex90, MWCNT, and $CeO_2$ samples ($p = 0.153$ by ANOVA) (Fig. 5.6a). Likewise, for markers of activated endothelium, sE-selectin, and sICAM-1, only the MWCNT had slightly elevated levels compared to the other particles, but this also was not significant ($p = 0.15$ by ANOVA) (Fig. 5.6b, c). It is crucial to recognize that these results only represent a single snapshot of a continuum of a response profile and may not reflect peak or sustained levels of these molecules generated in response to the exposure.

## Ambient PM and Printex 90 Reduced Total Circulating Leukocytes Prior to Ischemia–Reperfusion Injury

Blood drawn from the tail vein 24 h after exposure to 100 μg of ambient PM but prior to the induction of myocardial I/R injury exhibited a reduction in total circulating leukocytes compared to the vehicle control (Fig. 5.7a, $p < 0.05$). These results are consistent with previous reports (Cozzi et al. 2006, 2007). For manufactured particles administered at the same dose, only Printex 90 reduced total leukocyte counts compared to vehicle (Fig. 5.6a, $p < 0.01$). This reduction may reflect leukocyte margination in the lungs as previously reported (Cozzi et al. 2006). It is useful to integrate the lung histology findings with the BAL findings and the circulating white cell counts. The histological evaluation of lung sections revealed particles and low-level inflammation in the distal airways and alveoli 24 h after the initial exposure, supporting the hypothesis that PM can contribute to inflammatory processes potentially impacting the cardiovascular system (Donaldson et al. 2005).

CBC results demonstrated that ambient PM and Printex 90 reduced total leukocyte counts 24 h after exposure as previously demonstrated (Fig. 5.7) (Cozzi et al. 2006, 2007). This reduction in circulating leukocytes was associated with increased pulmonary neutrophil infiltration, which also was observed for the other particles (Fig. 5.4b and Cozzi et al. 2006), indicating that, at this single time point, circulating and pulmonary neutrophils are regulated differently. Interestingly, Printex 90

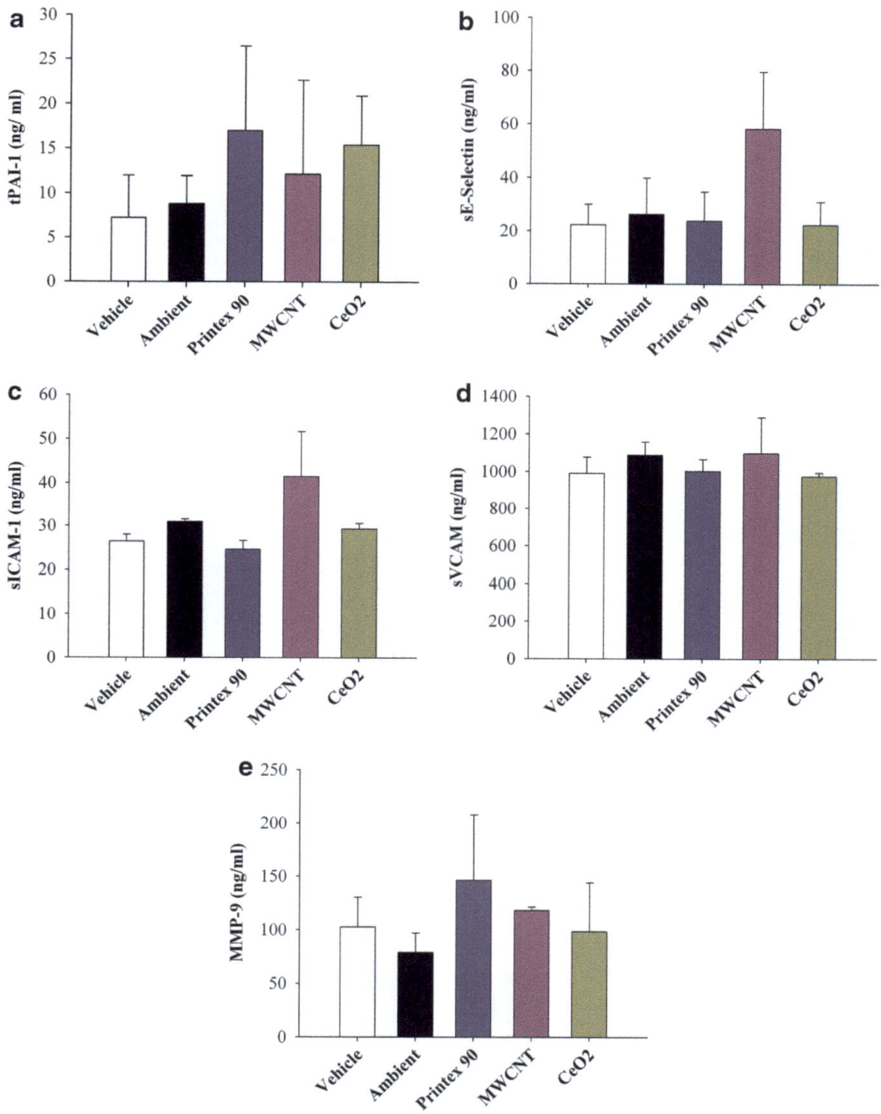


**Fig. 5.6** Concentration of soluble mediators in serum collected 24 h after particle administration. Animals received vehicle or were exposed to the same dose of (100 μg) ambient or manufactured PM by oropharyngeal aspiration. Serum was collected by cardiac puncture from animals that had not undergone myocardial ischemia and reperfusion. Values represent mean ± SEM, $n = 5$–7

reduced circulating leukocytes to a greater extent than ambient PM (Fig. 5.7a). Based on our current findings and previous studies, this reduction may reflect greater particle aggregation and subsequent lung retention of Printex 90 compared

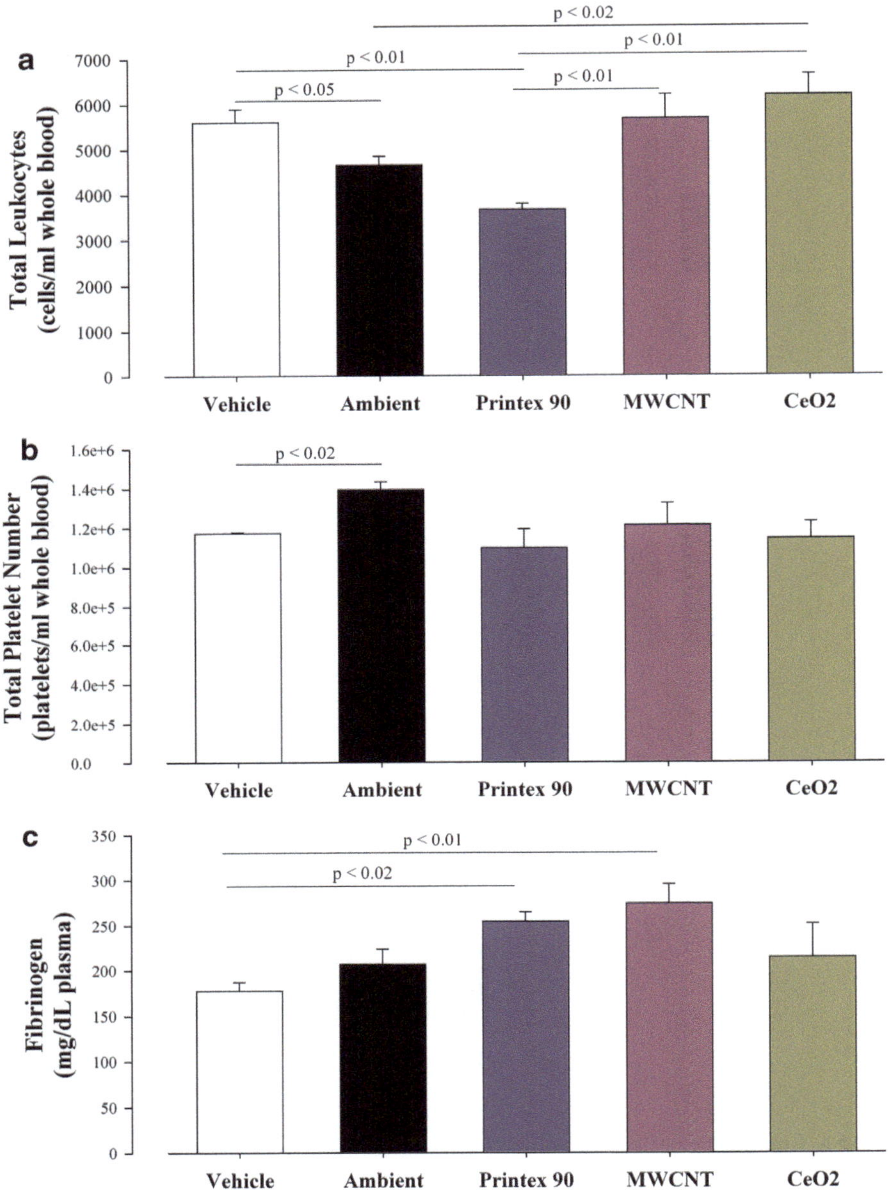


**Fig. 5.7** Total blood leukocyte counts, platelet number, and fibrinogen levels 24 h after ambient and manufactured PM administration. Blood leukocyte (*panel a*) and Platelet (*panel b*) values obtained from CBC analysis of a tail vein blood sample obtained 24 h after exposure to 100 μg of particle. Plasma fibrinogen levels (*panel c*) were determined by a modified thrombin time (Clauss 1957) on blood samples obtained by cardiac puncture 24 h post exposure. Values represent mean fibrinogen concentrations ± SE, $n = 24$–55 vehicle control-, 11–45 ambient-, 10–14 Printex 90-, 8–24 MWCNT-, and 6–18 $CeO_2$-exposed animals

to ambient PM. Therefore, Printex 90 may induce pulmonary inflammation for an extended period of time and thus promote greater pulmonary neutrophil infiltration and concomitant circulating leukocyte reduction compared to ambient PM. Interestingly, MWCNT also have been shown to aggregate extensively within the lungs in our studies as well as other animal studies (Donaldson et al. 2006; Lam et al. 2004). These nanoscale particles are predicted to have asbestos-like qualities and induce pulmonary epithelioid granulomas. In the present study we did not see a reduction in circulating leukocytes with MWCNT exposure (Fig. 5.6). This condition might be explained using a quantitative structure–activity relationship of these particles which could potentially demonstrate that there are less foci of inflammation within the lungs due to an increased propensity of MWCNT to aggregate higher in the airways as compared to Printex 90 and ambient PM (Duffin et al. 2007).

## Ambient and Manufactured PM Differentially Modulated Indices of Thrombogenic Potential

Blood was drawn from the tail vein of mice 24 h after PM exposure, and circulating platelet number was measured. Increased platelet number and plasma fibrinogen concentration are considered to be risk factors for cardiovascular events (Aukrust et al. 2001; Mueller et al. 2006). Only exposure to 100 μg ambient PM increased platelet number over vehicle control when compared to all other manufactured PM (Fig. 5.7b, $p<0.2$).

Thrombin acts on fibrinogen to form fibrin which polymerizes to form the fibrin clot (Toss et al. 1997). In these experiments plasma fibrinogen concentration was significantly elevated compared to control only after MWCNT and Printex 90 exposure (Fig. 5.7c, $p<0.02$). We have previously shown that ambient PM can alter factors involved in thrombus formation and resolution to promote a prothrombotic state (Cozzi et al. 2007). In the current study we extend these findings by demonstrating that ultrafine particles differentially affect hemostatic parameters. Only ambient PM was capable of significantly increasing circulating platelet numbers compared to vehicle control (Fig. 5.7). Alteration in platelet size, activity, and number have been shown to play an important role in acute coronary syndromes, such as myocardial infarction (Aukrust et al. 2001; Mueller et al. 2006; Weinberger et al. 1992; Kilicli-Camur et al. 2005; Yip et al. 2006; Reed et al. 2006). The results of this study are consistent with the increase in platelet number reported in rodents exposed to hardwood smoke by whole-body inhalation (Reed et al. 2006). However, other studies have failed to demonstrate an increase in circulating platelet number or activity with PM exposure (Pope et al. 2004a; Nemmar et al. 2004). This discrepancy could be due to differences in exposure methods, duration of administration, dose administered, or innate characteristics of PM utilized in those studies.

Alterations in plasma fibrinogen concentrations also appear to be particle dependent. We have shown previously that ambient PM exposure by intratracheal instillation increased plasma fibrinogen concentration 24 h after exposure

(Cozzi et al. 2007). In the present study, fibrinogen concentration increased at 24 h in response to ambient PM, did not reach statistical significance with instillation of Printex 90, and increased to the greatest extent with MWCNT when compared to vehicle control (Fig. 5.7). Increased plasma fibrinogen, an acute-phase reactant, has been associated with atherosclerotic lesion progression and future cardiovascular events (Toss et al. 1997). Increased fibrinogen concentration may be a consequence of particle aggregation. Printex 90 and MWCNT may aggregate within the lungs and cause pulmonary inflammation (Figs. 5.3 and 5.4), which is consistent with the reduction in circulating leukocytes we observed (Fig. 5.7). The increase in plasma fibrinogen may be secondary to particle-induced lung inflammation. As for $CeO_2$, an increased level of pulmonary inflammation, but not an increase in the extent of myocardial I/R injury or fibrinogen, may reflect the lack of a translocation of particle or soluble component to the myocardial tissue or the potential for free radical scavenging that can impact the systemic inflammatory state (Shvedova et al. 2005).

The ability of ambient PM, Printex 90, and MWCNT to increase infarct size after a myocardial I/R injury may be due to a common property: elemental carbon. $CeO_2$ contains no elemental carbon and did not increase the extent of myocardial injury over that of control animals. It appears that particle shape did not confer the cardiotoxicity of nanoscale particles. MWCNT and Printex 90 increased the induced infarct size to the same extent even though their shapes differed greatly. It is also possible that the common denominator for the effect of the different particles was their surface area rather than size or shape. Recent work by several investigators demonstrated changes in inflammatory and ROS signaling in in vitro models of nanoparticle exposure concluding that changes in nanomaterial primary size could result in significant inflammatory and oxidative stress responses (Stoeger et al. 2007; Hussain et al. 2009). Warheit and co-workers described results from pulmonary biohazard studies examining the impact of surface reactivity or surface coating effects and concluded that the differential toxicities are in large part based on surface reactivity characteristics rather than simply particle size or surface area (Warheit et al. 2009). Quantitative structural activity relationship (QSAR) as used in the pharmacology and toxicology fields could be used to categorize PM based on their physio-chemistry if they can be related to biological effects much like we illustrate here (Duffin et al. 2007).

Ambient PM increased the myocardial I/R injury to the largest extent when compared to the other particles, indicating that combustion by-products adsorbed the surface of the particles that might confer a greater cardiotoxicity. One possible explanation for this finding is that ambient particle constituents may indirectly or directly induce oxidative stress within the heart. Ambient PM is reported to induce pulmonary inflammation and subsequent oxidative stress within the lungs (Ghio and Devlin 2001; Cozzi et al. 2006; Dick et al. 2003a, b; Gurgueira et al. 2002). Likewise, metals from particles given by intratracheal instillation have been shown to exit the lung and enter the heart where they could potentially induce oxidative stress (Wallenborn et al. 2007a). While still subject to debate, particles in the size range studied here are reported to exit the lungs and enter the circulation where they could induce vascular oxidative stress (Nemmar et al. 2001, 2007). Overall, particles may lead to varying degrees of cardiopulmonary oxidative stress and a subsequent increased inflammatory state, thereby altering the substrate upon which an adverse cardiovascular event is superimposed. Any such increase in cardiopulmonary oxidative stress may be dependent on specific adsorbed particle constituents.

## Influence of Co-pollutants

PM levels frequently correspond with those of many co-pollutants, and it is often not possible for epidemiologists to assert a causal role for any single pollutant in an adverse health outcome. Common air pollutants of public health concern that are immediately derived from vehicular emissions include CO, $NO_2$, and $SO_2$. A recent study found the highest ambient concentrations of pollutants among 15 metropolitan areas reached an hourly upper quartile (75th percentile) of 0.65 ppm for CO, 32 ppb for $NO_2$, and 6 ppb for $SO_2$ (Bhaskaran et al. 2011). These values compared closely to those of ten Italian cities (Chiusolo et al. 2011) as well as Erfurt, Germany, the latter of which had comparable daily ambient concentrations and reported a peak CO level at 1.56 ppm (Berger et al. 2006). An additional study conducted over 126 US counties observed similar 24-h levels, with only a notable difference in CO concentrations (peak hourly observation = 9.7 ppm; peak daily = 2.5 ppm) (Bell et al. 2009). Yet, levels of these pollutants may reach much higher levels indoors, within traffic tunnels, or in occupational settings. For instance, while hourly $NO_2$ concentrations are unlikely to surpass 0.2 ppm outdoors, they can range from 0.4 to 1.5 ppm indoors during gas cooking (Hesterberg et al. 2009). In traffic tunnels, $NO_x$ levels (which are generally at higher levels than $NO_2$ in vehicular emissions) can reach 1.5–2.2 ppm, while CO has been shown to reach levels as high as 19–22 ppm (Gertler et al. 2002). Significant associations have been demonstrated between these pollutants and adverse health outcomes. Fluctuations in $NO_2$ and CO have both been shown to correspond with increased hospitalizations for cardiovascular disease across the USA (Bell et al. 2009; Mann et al. 2002), while cardiac mortality has been shown to increase with increasing $NO_2$ throughout Italy (Chiusolo et al. 2011). In a study spanning 15 cities within the United Kingdom, Bhaskaran et al. (2011) demonstrated an association between exposure to $NO_2$ and onset of myocardial infarction 1–6 h later. It is plausible that several of these pollutants exert toxicity in concert. Conversely, one pollutant may be the primary culprit, but it cannot be isolated from its co-pollutants in an epidemiologic setting. For example, Berger and colleagues (2006) found that three different size classes of PM (UFP, $PM_{2.5}$, and accumulation mode [1.0–0.1 μm]) as well as $NO_2$ concentrations correlated with episodes of ventricular tachycardia in men with coronary artery disease in Erfurt, Germany. Nonetheless, attention remains focused primarily on the PMs as the principal determinant in cardiopulmonary toxicity.

## PMs and Heart Failure

In Western countries, mortality from myocardial infarction has been decreasing for more than a decade, but the incidence of those living with chronic coronary artery disease and heart failure is increasing, and heart failure patients are particularly susceptible to the effects of PM. Elevated fine ambient PM levels have been associated more strongly with heart failure hospitalizations than hospitalizations for other cardiopulmonary diseases—including cerebrovascular disease, peripheral vascular disease, ischemic heart disease, COPD, heart rhythm problems, and respiratory tract infection (Dominici et al. 2006). Limited yet compelling evidence suggests that chronic particulate exposure promotes the development of heart failure. Among heart attack survivors, a 10 $\mu g/m^3$ increase in annual $PM_{10}$ levels corresponded with a 40 % increased incidence of development of heart failure over 3 years (Zanobetti and Schwartz 2007). Lastly, epidemiological studies have linked acute particulate exposure with acute exacerbation of heart failure. Schwartz and Morris (1995) observed that a 32 $\mu g/m^3$ increase in daily $PM_{10}$ was followed by a 3.2 % increase in daily heart failure hospital admissions among people over 64 years of age. There are striking commonalities in the blood profile of biomarkers following PM exposure and in patients with heart failure. Heart failure has been associated with elevations in circulating inflammatory markers (such as fibrinogen and C-reactive protein), endothelin 1 (ET-1), and the pro-inflammatory cytokines tumor necrosis factor alpha (TNF-α) and interleukin 6 (IL-6) (Seta et al. 1996). Similarly, short- and long-term air pollutant exposures have been shown to increase these markers (Brook et al. 2003; Calderon-Garciduenas et al. 2007; Peretz et al. 2008; Ruckerl et al. 2007; van Eeden et al. 2001). Researchers demonstrated a strong association between exposure to $PM_{2.5}$ and ET-1 as well as pulmonary arterial pressure, in children in Mexico City (Calderon-Garciduenas et al. 2007). Likewise, others detected an association between PM exposure and circulating IL-6 and fibrinogen in survivors of MI (Ruckerl et al. 2007). Heart failure and air pollutant exposure also both appear to increase natriuretic peptides, which are released upon myocardial stretch. Atrial and B-type natriuretic peptides (ANP and BNP) correlate closely with severity of cardiac dysfunction and heart failure (Clerico et al. 2006; de Denus et al. 2004) and have been demonstrated to increase upon short-term PM inhalation exposure (Tankersley et al. 2008).

TNF-α, a vasodepressor (decreases blood pressure) that promotes pulmonary edema and left ventricular dysfunction at high levels, is closely associated with myocyte hypertrophy and is believed to trigger cardiomyocyte apoptosis in conjunction with ANP (Francis 2001; Kang 2006). TNF-α may also induce IL-6, which is another vasodepressor that promotes myocardial dysfunction as well as myocyte atrophy (Seta et al. 1996). It must be noted that TNF-α and IL-6 both are products of immune system activity, again suggesting the potential for a linkage between immune-responsiveness, PM exposure, and progression of heart failure. As studies become more sophisticated, using both diesel particles and comparably sized manufactured nanoparticles, there is increasing attention of the immediate microenvironment of the particle that may help explain interactions with the immune system. For example, detailed high-resolution analysis indicates that physical and chemical characteristics of a particle cause a "corona" or an envelope to form, which has the potential to selectively sequester proteins and, presumably, convert a particle from a general irritant to something with possible antigenic characteristics, depending on the composition of the envelope (Mahmoudi et al. 2012; Arvizo et al. 2012; Walkey and Chan 2012). A great deal of work has yet to be done in this area, but it holds much promise.

## Conclusion

The cardiovascular complications following pulmonary exposure to a variety of unrelated forms of PM can manifest as adverse outcome events in both epidemiological and experimental settings. While the specific underlying mechanisms are yet to be fully elucidated it is apparent that the cardiovascular system response to the PM exposures is manifested as a more robust response to an imposed insult that is anticipated otherwise. The inherent complexity of ambient sources of PM and the growing diversity of specifically engineered PM that can be released into the environment reinforce the need to understand the impact of exposures to PMs on human health. Coupled with our increasing yet limited understanding of the integrative nature of the cardiovascular system with neural, humeral, and immune systems responses to PM only begins to hint at the importance of a hypersensitive state on human physiological and pathophysiological processes.

**Acknowledgments** The work supported in part by funding from NIH ES016246 and U19 ES019525 to CJW.

## References

Aitken RJ, Chaudhry MQ, Boxall AB, Hull M. Manufacture and use of nanomaterials: current status in the UK and global trends. Occup Med. 2006;56(5):300–6.

Anselme F, Loriot S, Henry JP, Dionnet F, Napoleoni JG, Thuillez C, et al. Inhalation of diluted diesel engine emission impacts heart rate variability and arrhythmia occurrence in a rat model of chronic ischemic heart failure. Arch Toxicol. 2007;81(4):299–307.

Arvizo RR, Giri K, Moyano D, Miranda OR, Madden B, McCormick DJ, et al. Identifying new therapeutic targets via modulation of protein corona formation by engineered nanoparticles. PLoS One. 2012;7(3):e33650.

Aukrust P, Waehre T, Damas JK, Gullestad L, Solum NO. Inflammatory role of platelets in acute coronary syndromes. Heart. 2001;86(6):605–6.

Baccarelli A, Martinelli I, Zanobetti A, Grillo P, Hou LF, Bertazzi PA, et al. Exposure to particulate air pollution and risk of deep vein thrombosis. Arch Intern Med. 2008;168(9):920–7.

Baccarelli A, Martinelli I, Pegoraro V, Melly S, Grillo P, Zanobetti A, et al. Living near major traffic roads and risk of deep vein thrombosis. Circulation. 2009;119(24):3118–24.

Bagate K, Meiring JJ, Gerlofs-Nijland ME, Vincent R, Cassee FR, Borm PJA. Vascular effects of ambient particulate matter instillation in spontaneous hypertensive rats. Toxicol Appl Pharmacol. 2004;197(1):29–39.

Batalha JR, Saldiva PH, Clarke RW, Coull BA, Stearns RC, Lawrence J, et al. Concentrated ambient air particles induce vasoconstriction of small pulmonary arteries in rats. Environ Health Perspect. 2002;110(12):1191–7.

Bell ML, Peng RD, Dominici F, Samet JM. Emergency hospital admissions for cardiovascular diseases and ambient levels of carbon monoxide: results for 126 United States urban counties, 1999–2005. Circulation. 2009;120(11):949–55.

Berger A, Zareba W, Schneider A, Ruckerl R, Ibald-Mulli A, Cyrys J, et al. Runs of ventricular and supraventricular tachycardia triggered by air pollution in patients with coronary heart disease. J Occup Environ Med. 2006;48(11):1149–58.

Bhaskaran K, Hajat S, Armstrong B, Haines A, Herrett E, Wilkinson P, et al. The effects of hourly differences in air pollution on the risk of myocardial infarction: case crossover analysis of the MINAP database. BMJ. 2011;343:d5531.

Biggeri A, Bellini P, Terracini B. Meta-analysis of the Italian studies on short-term effects of air pollution—MISA 1996–2002. Epidemiol Prev. 2004;28(4–5 Suppl):4–100.

Brook RD, Brook JR, Rajagopalan S. Air pollution: the "Heart" of the problem. Curr Hypertens Rep. 2003;5(1):32–9.

Brook RD, Franklin B, Cascio W, Hong Y, Howard G, Lipsett M, et al. Air pollution and cardiovascular disease: a statement for healthcare professionals from the Expert Panel on Population and Prevention Science of the American Heart Association. Circulation. 2004;109(21):2655–71.

Brook RD, Rajagopalan S, Pope 3rd CA, Brook JR, Bhatnagar A, Diez-Roux AV, et al. Particulate matter air pollution and cardiovascular disease: an update to the scientific statement from the American Heart Association. Circulation. 2010;121(21):2331–78.

Calderon-Garciduenas L, Vincent R, Mora-Tiscareno A, Franco-Lira M, Henriquez-Roldan C, Barragan-Mejia G, et al. Elevated plasma endothelin-1 and pulmonary arterial pressure in children exposed to air pollution. Environ Health Perspect. 2007;115(8):1248–53.

Campen MJ, Lund AK, Doyle-Eisele ML, McDonald JD, Knuckles TL, Rohr AC, et al. A comparison of vascular effects from complex and individual air pollutants indicates a role for monoxide gases and volatile hydrocarbons. Environ Health Perspect. 2010;118(7):921–7.

Cascio WE, Cozzi E, Hazarika S, Devlin RB, Henriksen RA, Lust RM, Van Scott MR, Wingard CJ. Cardiac and vascular changes in mice after exposure to ultrafine particulate matter. Inhal Toxicol. 2007;19 Suppl 1:67–73.

Chiusolo M, Cadum E, Stafoggia M, Galassi C, Berti G, Faustini A, Bisanti L, Vigotti MA, Dessi MP, Cernigliaro A, Mallone S, Pacelli B, Minerba S, Simonato L, Forastiere F. Short term effects of nitrogen dioxide on mortality and susceptibility factors in ten Italian cities: the EpiAir study. Environ Health Perspect. 2011.

Clauss A. Rapid physiological coagulation method in determination of fibrinogen. Acta Haemotol. 1957;17: 237–46.

Clerico A, Recchia FA, Passino C, Emdin M. Cardiac endocrine function is an essential component of the homeostatic regulation network: physiological and clinical implications. Am J Physiol Heart Circ Physiol. 2006;290(1):H17–29.

Courtois A, Andujar P, Ladeiro Y, Baudrimont I, Delannoy E, Leblais V, et al. Impairment of NO-dependent relaxation in intralobar pulmonary arteries: comparison of urban particulate matter and manufactured nanoparticles. Environ Health Perspect. 2008;116(10):1294–9.

Cozzi E, Hazarika S, Stallings 3rd HW, Cascio WE, Devlin RB, Lust RM, et al. Ultrafine particulate matter exposure augments ischemia-reperfusion injury in mice. Am J Physiol Heart Circ Physiol. 2006;291(2):H894–903.

Cozzi E, Wingard CJ, Cascio WE, Devlin RB, Miles JJ, Bofferding AR, et al. Effect of ambient particulate matter exposure on hemostasis. Transl Res. 2007;149(6):324–32.

de Denus S, Pharand C, Williamson DR. Brain natriuretic peptide in the management of heart failure: the versatile neurohormone. Chest. 2004;125(2):652–68.

Devlin RB, Ghio AJ, Kehrl H, Sanders G, Cascio W. Elderly humans exposed to concentrated air pollution particles have decreased heart rate variability. Eur Respir J Suppl. 2003;40:76s–80.

Dick CA, Brown DM, Donaldson K, Stone V. The role of free radicals in the toxic and inflammatory effects of four different ultrafine particle types. Inhal Toxicol. 2003a;15(1):39–52.

Dick CA, Singh P, Daniels M, Evansky P, Becker S, Gilmour MI. Murine pulmonary inflammatory responses following instillation of size-fractionated ambient particulate matter. J Toxicol Environ Health A. 2003b;66(23):2193–207.

Dockery DW, Pope 3rd CA, Xu X, Spengler JD, Ware JH, Fay ME, et al. An association between air pollution and mortality in six U.S. cities. N Engl J Med. 1993;329(24):1753–9.

Dockery DW, Luttmann-Gibson H, Rich DQ, Link MS, Mittleman MA, Gold DR, et al. Association of air pollution with increased incidence of ventricular tachyarrhythmias recorded by implanted cardioverter defibrillators. Environ Health Perspect. 2005;113(6):670–4.

Dominici F, Peng RD, Bell ML, Pham L, McDermott A, Zeger SL, et al. Fine particulate air pollution and hospital admission for cardiovascular and respiratory diseases. JAMA. 2006;295(10):1127–34.

Donaldson K, Mills N, MacNee W, Robinson S, Newby D. Role of inflammation in cardiopulmonary health effects of PM. Toxicol Appl Pharmacol. 2005;207(2 Suppl):483–8.

Donaldson K, Aitken R, Tran L, Stone V, Duffin R, Forrest G, et al. Carbon nanotubes: a review of their properties in relation to pulmonary toxicology and workplace safety. Toxicol Sci. 2006;92(1):5–22.

Duffin R, Mills NL, Donaldson K. Nanoparticles—a thoracic toxicology perspective. Yonsei Med J. 2007;48(4):561–72.

Francis GS. Pathophysiology of chronic heart failure. Am J Med. 2001;110 Suppl 7A:37S–46.

Franklin M, Schwartz J. The impact of secondary particles on the association between ambient ozone and mortality. Environ Health Perspect. 2008;116(4):453–8.

Franklin M, Zeka A, Schwartz J. Association between PM2.5 and all-cause and specific-cause mortality in 27 US communities. J Expo Sci Environ Epidemiol. 2007;17(3):279–87.

Franklin M, Koutrakis P, Schwartz P. The role of particle composition on the association between PM2.5 and mortality. Epidemiology. 2008;19(5):680–9.

Gardiner K, van Tongeren M, Harrington M. Respiratory health effects from exposure to carbon black: results of the phase 2 and 3 cross sectional studies in the European carbon black manufacturing industry. Occup Environ Med. 2001;58(8):496–503.

Gertler AW, Gillies JA, Pierson WR, Rogers CF, Sagebiel JC, Abu-Allaban M, Coulombe W, Tarnay L, Cahill TA. Real-world particulate matter and gaseous emissions from motor vehicles in a highway tunnel. Res Rep Health Eff Inst. 2002;107:5–56, discussion 79–92.

Ghio AJ, Devlin RB. Inflammatory lung injury after bronchial instillation of air pollution particles. Am J Respir Crit Care Med. 2001;164(4):704–8.

Goulaouic S, Foucaud L, Bennasroune A, Laval-Gilly P, Falla J. Effect of polycyclic aromatic hydrocarbons and carbon black particles on pro-inflammatory cytokine secretion: impact of PAH coating onto particles. J Immunotoxicol. 2008;5(3):337–45.

Granum B, Lovik M. The effect of particles on allergic immune responses. Toxicol Sci. 2002;65(1):7–17.

Gurgueira SA, Lawrence J, Coull B, Murthy GG, Gonzalez-Flecha B. Rapid increases in the steady-state concentration of reactive oxygen species in the lungs and heart after particulate air pollution inhalation. Environ Health Perspect. 2002;110(8):749–55.

Hazarika S, Van Scott MR, Lust RM. Myocardial ischemia-reperfusion injury is enhanced in a model of systemic allergy and asthma. Am J Physiol Heart Circ Physiol. 2004;286(5): H1720–5.

Hazarika S, Van Scott MR, Lust RM. Severity of myocardial injury following ischemia-reperfusion is increased in a mouse model of allergic asthma. Am J Physiol Heart Circ Physiol. 2007;292(1):H572–9.

Hazarika S, Van Scott MR, Lust RM, Wingard CJ. Pulmonary allergic reactions impair systemic vascular relaxation in ragweed sensitive mice. Vascul Pharmacol. 2010;53(5–6):258–63.

Hearse DJ, Erol C, Robinson LA, Maxwell MP, Braimbridge MV. Particle-induced coronary vasoconstriction during cardioplegic infusion. Characterization and possible mechanisms. J Thorac Cardiovasc Surg. 1985;89(3):428–38.

Henneberger A, Zareba W, Ibald-Mulli A, Ruckerl R, Cyrys J, Couderc JP, et al. Repolarization changes induced by air pollution in ischemic heart disease patients. Environ Health Perspect. 2005;113(4):440–6.

Hesterberg TW, Bunn WB, McClellan RO, Hamade AK, Long CM, Valberg PA. Critical review of the human data on short-term nitrogen dioxide (NO2) exposures: evidence for NO2 no-effect levels. Crit Rev Toxicol. 2009;39(9):743–81.

Huang CH, Lin LY, Tsai MS, Hsu CY, Chen HW, Wang TD, et al. Acute cardiac dysfunction after short-term diesel exhaust particles exposure. Toxicol Lett. 2010;192(3):349–55.

Huizar I, Malur A, Midgette YA, Kukoly C, Chen P, Ke PC, et al. Novel murine model of chronic granulomatous lung inflammation elicited by carbon nanotubes. Am J Respir Cell Mol Biol. 2011;45(4):858–66.

Hunt A, Abraham JL, Judson B, Berry CL. Toxicologic and epidemiologic clues from the characterization of the 1952 London smog fine particulate matter in archival autopsy lung tissues. Environ Health Perspect. 2003;111(9):1209–14.

Hussain S, Boland S, Baeza-Squiban A, Hamel R, Thomassen LC, Martens JA, et al. Oxidative stress and proinflammatory effects of carbon black and titanium dioxide nanoparticles: role of particle surface area and internalized amount. Toxicology. 2009;260(1–3):142–9.

Ibald-Mulli A, Wichmann HE, Kreyling W, Peters A. Epidemiological evidence on health effects of ultrafine particles. J Aerosol Med. 2002;15(2):189–201.

Inoue K, Takano H, Yanagisawa R, Hirano S, Sakurai M, Shimada A, et al. Effects of airway exposure to nanoparticles on lung inflammation induced by bacterial endotoxin in mice. Environ Health Perspect. 2006;114(9):1325–30.

Inoue K, Koike E, Yanagisawa R, Hirano S, Nishikawa M, Takano H. Effects of multi-walled carbon nanotubes on a murine allergic airway inflammation model. Toxicol Appl Pharmacol. 2009;237(3):306–16.

Kang YJ. Cardiac hypertrophy: a risk factor for QT-prolongation and cardiac sudden death. Toxicol Pathol. 2006;34(1):58–66.

Kang YJ, Li Y, Zhou Z, Roberts AM, Cai L, Myers SR, et al. Elevation of serum endothelins and cardiotoxicity induced by particulate matter (PM2.5) in rats with acute myocardial infarction. Cardiovasc Toxicol. 2002;2(4):253–61.

Kappos AD, Bruckmann P, Eikmann T, Englert N, Heinrich U, Hoppe P, et al. Health effects of particles in ambient air. Int J Hyg Environ Health. 2004;207(4):399–407.

Kettunen J, Lanki T, Tiittanen P, Aalto PP, Koskentalo T, Kulmala M, et al. Associations of fine and ultrafine particulate air pollution with stroke mortality in an area of low air pollution levels. Stroke. 2007;38(3):918–22.

Kilicli-Camur N, Demirtunc R, Konuralp C, Eskiser A, Basaran Y. Could mean platelet volume be a predictive marker for acute myocardial infarction? Med Sci Monit. 2005;11(8):CR387–92.

Knuckles TL, Lund AK, Lucas SN, Campen MJ. Diesel exhaust exposure enhances venoconstriction via uncoupling of eNOS. Toxicol Appl Pharmacol. 2008;230(3):346–51.

Kreyling WG, Semmler-Behnke M, Moller W. Ultrafine particle-lung interactions: does size matter? J Aerosol Med. 2006;19(1):74–83.

Lam CW, James JT, McCluskey R, Hunter RL. Pulmonary toxicity of single-wall carbon nanotubes in mice 7 and 90 days after intratracheal instillation. Toxicol Sci. 2004;77(1):126–34.

Le Tertre A, Medina S, Samoli E, Forsberg B, Michelozzi P, Boumghar A, et al. Short-term effects of particulate air pollution on cardiovascular diseases in eight European cities. J Epidemiol Community Health. 2002;56(10):773–9.

Li Z, Hulderman T, Salmen R, Chapman R, Leonard SS, Young SH, et al. Cardiovascular effects of pulmonary exposure to single-wall carbon nanotubes. Environ Health Perspect. 2007;115(3):377–82.

Li N, Xia T, Nel AE. The role of oxidative stress in ambient particulate matter-induced lung diseases and its implications in the toxicity of engineered nanoparticles. Free Radic Biol Med. 2008;44(9):1689–99.

Liao D, Creason J, Shy C, Williams R, Watts R, Zweidinger R. Daily variation of particulate air pollution and poor cardiac autonomic control in the elderly. Environ Health Perspect. 1999;107(7):521–5.

Lippmann M. Health effects of airborne particulate matter. N Engl J Med. 2007;357(23):2395–7.

Lippmann M, Ito K, Hwang JS, Maciejczyk P, Chen LC. Cardiovascular effects of nickel in ambient air. Environ Health Perspect. 2006;114(11):1662–9.

Lucking AJ, Lundback M, Barath SL, Mills NL, Sidhu MK, Langrish JP, et al. Particle traps prevent adverse vascular and prothrombotic effects of diesel engine exhaust inhalation in men. Circulation. 2011;123(16):1721–8.

Mahmoudi M, Saeedi-Eslami SN, Shokrgozar MA, Azadmanesh K, Hassanlou M, Kalhor HR, et al. Cell "vision": complementary factor of protein corona in nanotoxicology. Nanoscale. 2012;4(17):5461–8.

Mann JK, Tager IB, Lurmann F, Segal M, Quesenberry Jr CP, Lugg MM, et al. Air pollution and hospital admissions for ischemic heart disease in persons with congestive heart failure or arrhythmia. Environ Health Perspect. 2002;110(12):1247–52.

Mikkelsen L, Sheykhzade M, Jensen KA, Saber AT, Jacobsen NR, Vogel U, et al. Modest effect on plaque progression and vasodilatory function in atherosclerosis-prone mice exposed to nanosized TiO(2). Part Fibre Toxicol. 2011;8:32.

Miller MR, Borthwick SJ, Shaw CA, McLean SG, McClure D, Mills NL, et al. Direct impairment of vascular function by diesel exhaust particulate through reduced bioavailability of endothelium-derived nitric oxide induced by superoxide free radicals. Environ Health Perspect. 2009;117(4):611–6.

Mills NL, Tornqvist H, Gonzalez MC, Vink E, Robinson SD, Soderberg S, et al. Ischemic and thrombotic effects of dilute diesel-exhaust inhalation in men with coronary heart disease. N Engl J Med. 2007;357(11):1075–82.

Mills NL, Miller MR, Lucking AJ, Beveridge J, Flint L, Boere AJ, et al. Combustion-derived nanoparticulate induces the adverse vascular effects of diesel exhaust inhalation. Eur Heart J. 2011;32(21):2660–71.

Molinelli AR, Madden MC, McGee JK, Stonehuerner JG, Ghio AJ. Effect of metal removal on the toxicity of airborne particulate matter from the Utah Valley. Inhal Toxicol. 2002;14(10):1069–86.

Mueller C, Neumann FJ, Hochholzer W, Trenk D, Zeller T, Perruchoud AP, et al. The impact of platelet count on mortality in unstable angina/non-ST-segment elevation myocardial infarction. Am Heart J. 2006;151(6):1214–7.

Muller J, Huaux F, Moreau N, Misson P, Heilier JF, Delos M, et al. Respiratory toxicity of multiwall carbon nanotubes. Toxicol Appl Pharmacol. 2005;207(3):221–31.

Nel AE, Diaz-Sanchez D, Li N. The role of particulate pollutants in pulmonary inflammation and asthma: evidence for the involvement of organic chemicals and oxidative stress. Curr Opin Pulm Med. 2001;7(1):20–6.

Nemmar A, Vanbilloen H, Hoylaerts MF, Hoet PH, Verbruggen A, Nemery B. Passage of intratracheally instilled ultrafine particles from the lung into the systemic circulation in hamster. Am J Respir Crit Care Med. 2001;164(9):1665–8.

Nemmar A, Hoylaerts MF, Hoet PH, Nemery B. Possible mechanisms of the cardiovascular effects of inhaled particles: systemic translocation and prothrombotic effects. Toxicol Lett. 2004;149(1–3):243–53.

Nemmar A, Hoet PH, Vandervoort P, Dinsdale D, Nemery B, Hoylaerts MF. Enhanced peripheral thrombogenicity after lung inflammation is mediated by platelet-leukocyte activation: role of P-selectin. J Thromb Haemost. 2007;5(6):1217–26.

Nurkiewicz TR, Porter DW, Barger M, Castranova V, Boegehold MA. Particulate matter exposure impairs systemic microvascular endothelium-dependent dilation. Environ Health Perspect. 2004;112(13):1299–306.

Nurkiewicz TR, Porter DW, Hubbs AF, Stone S, Chen BT, Frazer DG, et al. Pulmonary nanoparticle exposure disrupts systemic microvascular nitric oxide signaling. Toxicol Sci. 2009;110(1):191–203.

Nygaard UC, Hansen JS, Samuelsen M, Alberg T, Marioara CD, Lovik M. Single-walled and multi-walled carbon nanotubes promote allergic immune responses in mice. Toxicol Sci. 2009;109(1):113–23.

O'Neill MS, Veves A, Zanobetti A, Sarnat JA, Gold DR, Economides PA, et al. Diabetes enhances vulnerability to particulate air pollution-associated impairment in vascular reactivity and endothelial function. Circulation. 2005;111(22):2913–20.

Ostro B, Broadwin R, Green S, Feng WY, Lipsett M. Fine particulate air pollution and mortality in nine California counties: results from CALFINE. Environ Health Perspect. 2006;114(1):29–33.

Pairon JC, Roos F, Sebastien P, Chamak B, Abd-Alsamad I, Bernaudin JF, et al. Biopersistence of cerium in the human respiratory tract and ultrastructural findings. Am J Ind Med. 1995;27(3):349–58.

Peretz A, Kaufman JD, Trenga CA, Allen J, Carlsten C, Aulet MR, et al. Effects of diesel exhaust inhalation on heart rate variability in human volunteers. Environ Res. 2008;107(2):178–84.

Peters A. Particles in the outside air increase the risk of cardiovascular diseases. Gesundheitswesen. 2005;67 Suppl 1:S79–85.

Peters A, Liu E, Verrier RL, Schwartz J, Gold DR, Mittleman M, et al. Air pollution and incidence of cardiac arrhythmia. Epidemiology. 2000;11(1):11–7.

Peters A, Frohlich M, Doring A, Immervoll T, Wichmann HE, Hutchinson WL, et al. Particulate air pollution is associated with an acute phase response in men. Results from the MONICA-Augsburg study. Eur Heart J. 2001a;22(14):1198–204.

Peters A, Dockery DW, Muller JE, Mittleman MA. Increased particulate air pollution and the triggering of myocardial infarction. Circulation. 2001b;103(23):2810–5.

Ponikowski P, Anker SD, Amadi A, Chua TP, Cerquetani E, Ondusova D, et al. Heart rhythms, ventricular arrhythmias, and death in chronic heart failure. J Card Fail. 1996;2(3):177–83.

Pope 3rd CA, Hansen ML, Long RW, Nielsen KR, Eatough NL, Wilson WE, et al. Ambient particulate air pollution, heart rate variability, and blood markers of inflammation in a panel of elderly subjects. Environ Health Perspect. 2004a;112(3):339–45.

Pope 3rd CA, Burnett RT, Thurston GD, Thun MJ, Calle EE, Krewski D, et al. Cardiovascular mortality and long-term exposure to particulate air pollution: epidemiological evidence of general pathophysiological pathways of disease. Circulation. 2004b;109(1):71–7.

Reed MD, Campen MJ, Gigliotti AP, Harrod KS, McDonald JD, Seagrave JC, et al. Health effects of subchronic exposure to environmental levels of hardwood smoke. Inhal Toxicol. 2006;18(8):523–39.

Ruckerl R, Greven S, Ljungman P, Aalto P, Antoniades C, Bellander T, et al. Air pollution and inflammation (interleukin-6, C-reactive protein, fibrinogen) in myocardial infarction survivors. Environ Health Perspect. 2007;115(7):1072–80.

Samet JM, Dominici F, Curriero FC, Coursac I, Zeger SL. Fine particulate air pollution and mortality in 20 U.S. cities 1987-1994. N Engl J Med. 2000;343(24):1742–9.

Schubert D, Dargusch R, Raitano J, Chan SW. Cerium and yttrium oxide nanoparticles are neuroprotective. Biochem Biophys Res Commun. 2006;342(1):86–91.

Schulz H, Harder V, Ibald-Mulli A, Khandoga A, Koenig W, Krombach F, et al. Cardiovascular effects of fine and ultrafine particles. J Aerosol Med. 2005;18(1):1–22.

Schwartz J. Air pollution and hospital admissions for respiratory disease. Epidemiology. 1996;7(1):20–8.

Schwartz J, Dockery DW. Increased mortality in Philadelphia associated with daily air pollution concentrations. Am Rev Respir Dis. 1992;145(3):600–4.

Schwartz J, Marcus A. Mortality and air pollution in London: a time series analysis. Am J Epidemiol. 1990;131(1):185–94.

Schwartz J, Morris R. Air pollution and hospital admissions for cardiovascular disease in Detroit, Michigan. Am J Epidemiol. 1995;142(1):23–35.

Seta Y, Shan K, Bozkurt B, Oral H, Mann DL. Basic mechanisms in heart failure: the cytokine hypothesis. J Card Fail. 1996;2(3):243–9.

Shvedova AA, Kisin ER, Mercer R, Murray AR, Johnson VJ, Potapovich AI, et al. Unusual inflammatory and fibrogenic pulmonary responses to single-walled carbon nanotubes in mice. Am J Physiol Lung Cell Mol Physiol. 2005;289(5):L698–708.

Singh RB, Cornelissen G, Weydahl A, Schwartzkopff O, Katinas G, Otsuka K, et al. Circadian heart rate and blood pressure variability considered for research and patient care. Int J Cardiol. 2003;87(1):9–28. discussion 29–30.

Sioutas C, Delfino RJ, Singh M. Exposure assessment for atmospheric ultrafine particles (UFPs) and implications in epidemiologic research. Environ Health Perspect. 2005;113(8):947–55.

Stenfors N, Nordenhall C, Salvi SS, Mudway I, Soderberg M, Blomberg A, et al. Different airway inflammatory responses in asthmatic and healthy humans exposed to diesel. Eur Respir J. 2004;23(1):82–6.
Stoeger T, Schmid O, Takenaka S, Schulz H. Inflammatory response to TiO2 and carbonaceous particles scales best with BET surface area. Environ Health Perspect. 2007;115(6):A290–1.
Tankersley CG, Champion HC, Takimoto E, Gabrielson K, Bedja D, Misra V, et al. Exposure to inhaled particulate matter impairs cardiac function in senescent mice. Am J Physiol Regul Integr Comp Physiol. 2008;295(1):R252–63.
Thomson E, Kumarathasan P, Goegan P, Aubin RA, Vincent R. Differential regulation of the lung endothelin system by urban particulate matter and ozone. Toxicol Sci. 2005;88(1):103–13.
Toss H, Lindahl B, Siegbahn A, Wallentin L. Prognostic influence of increased fibrinogen and C-reactive protein levels in unstable coronary artery disease. FRISC Study Group. Fragmin during instability in coronary artery disease. Circulation. 1997;96(12):4204–10.
Tzeng HP, Yang RS, Ueng TH, Lin-Shiau SY, Liu SH. Motorcycle exhaust particulates enhance vasoconstriction in organ culture of rat aortas and involve reactive oxygen species. Toxicol Sci. 2003;75(1):66–73.
USEPA. Air quality criteria for particulate matter, vol II. 2004.
USEPA. Air quality statistics by city, 2006 MSA factbook. 2006.
van Eeden SF, Tan WC, Suwa T, Mukae H, Terashima T, Fujii T, et al. Cytokines involved in the systemic inflammatory response induced by exposure to particulate matter air pollutants (PM(10)). Am J Respir Crit Care Med. 2001;164(5):826–30.
Villeneuve PJ, Chen L, Stieb D, Rowe BH. Associations between outdoor air pollution and emergency department visits for stroke in Edmonton, Canada. Eur J Epidemiol. 2006;21(9): 689–700.
Walkey CD, Chan WC. Understanding and controlling the interaction of nanomaterials with proteins in a physiological environment. Chem Soc Rev. 2012;41(7):2780–99.
Wallenborn JG, McGee JK, Schladweiler MC, Ledbetter AD, Kodavanti UP. Systemic translocation of particulate matter-associated metals following a single intratracheal instillation in rats. Toxicol Sci. 2007a;98(1):231–9.
Wallenborn JG, Schladweiler MC, Nyska A, Johnson JA, Thomas R, Jaskot RH, et al. Cardiopulmonary responses of Wistar Kyoto, spontaneously hypertensive, and stroke-prone spontaneously hypertensive rats to particulate matter (PM) exposure. J Toxicol Environ Health A. 2007b;70(22):1912–22.
Warheit DB, Reed KL, Sayes CM. A role for nanoparticle surface reactivity in facilitating pulmonary toxicity and development of a base set of hazard assays as a component of nanoparticle risk management. Inhal Toxicol. 2009;21(S1):61–7.
Weinberger I, Fuchs J, Davidson E, Rotenberg Z. Circulating aggregated platelets, number of platelets per aggregate, and platelet size during acute myocardial infarction. Am J Cardiol. 1992;70(11):981–3.
Wellenius GA, Schwartz J, Mittleman MA. Air pollution and hospital admissions for ischemic and hemorrhagic stroke among medicare beneficiaries. Stroke. 2005;36(12):2549–53.
Wheeler A, Zanobetti A, Gold DR, Schwartz J, Stone P, Suh HH. The relationship between ambient air pollution and heart rate variability differs for individuals with heart and pulmonary disease. Environ Health Perspect. 2006;114(4):560–6.
Whittaker A, BeruBe K, Jones T, Maynard R, Richards R. Killer smog of London, 50 years on: particle properties and oxidative capacity. Sci Total Environ. 2004;334–335:435–45.
Wingard CJ, Walters DM, Cathey BL, Hilderbrand SC, Katwa P, Lin S, et al. Mast cells contribute to altered vascular reactivity and ischemia-reperfusion injury following cerium oxide nanoparticle instillation. Nanotoxicology. 2011;5(4):531–45.
Yip HK, Chang LT, Sun CK, Chen MC, Yang CH, Hung WC, et al. Platelet activity is a biomarker of cardiac necrosis and predictive of untoward clinical outcomes in patients with acute myocardial infarction undergoing primary coronary stenting. Circ J. 2006;70(1):31–6.

Zanobetti A, Schwartz J. The effect of particulate air pollution on emergency admissions for myocardial infarction: a multicity case-crossover analysis. Environ Health Perspect. 2005;113(8):978–82.

Zanobetti A, Schwartz J. Particulate air pollution, progression, and survival after myocardial infarction. Environ Health Perspect. 2007;115(5):769–75.

Zanobetti A, Schwartz J. The effect of fine and coarse particulate air pollution on mortality: a national analysis. Environ Health Perspect. 2009;117(6):898–903.

Zanobetti A, Schwartz J, Samoli E, Gryparis A, Touloumi G, Atkinson R, et al. The temporal pattern of mortality responses to air pollution: a multicity assessment of mortality displacement. Epidemiology. 2002;13(1):87–93.

Zanobetti A, Schwartz J, Samoli E, Gryparis A, Touloumi G, Peacock J, et al. The temporal pattern of respiratory and heart disease mortality in response to air pollution. Environ Health Perspect. 2003;111(9):1188–93.

Zareba W, Nomura A, Couderc JP. Cardiovascular effects of air pollution: what to measure in ECG? Environ Health Perspect. 2001;109 Suppl 4:533–38.

Zeka A, Sullivan JR, Vokonas PS, Sparrow D, Schwartz J. Inflammatory markers and particulate air pollution: characterizing the pathway to disease. Int J Epidemiol. 2006;35(5):1347–54.

# Chapter 6
# Products of Tobacco Combustion

**Rebecca Bascom, Anne E.F. Dimmock, and Judie Ann Howrylak**

**Abstract** A growing body of research expands our knowledge of asthma and chronic rhinosinusitis (CRS) and how these common albeit heterogeneous conditions are impacted by active and passive tobacco smoke exposure. The syndromes of asthma and rhinitis have diverse endo-phenotypes, some including atopy. Chronic rhinosinusitis is defined through consensus endoscopic and CT criteria.

The risk of environmental tobacco smoke exposure parallels a country's active smoking rates, with wide variations in exposure risk related to socioeconomic status, education, region, and other demographic factors. Sites of exposure include home, work, travel, and private social gatherings.

This chapter reviews the impact of active and passive tobacco smoking on asthma incidence, prevalence, and severity as well as the response to asthma treatment. Also reviewed is the impact of active and passive smoking on allergic rhinitis, nonallergic rhinitis, and CRS.

While the integrated respiratory tract is an accepted concept for allergic respiratory tract disease, with a broad integrated body of animal and human data, there remain gaps in the information needed to determine whether active and/or passive smoking cause a common irritant respiratory tract disease. The diverse pathways

R. Bascom, M.D., M.P.H. • J.A. Howrylak, M.D.
Division of Pulmonary, Allergy and Critical Care Medicine,
Penn State College of Medicine, Milton S. Hershey Medical Center,
500 University Drive, MCH041, Hershey, PA 17033, USA

A.E.F. Dimmock, B.A. (✉)
Division of Pulmonary, Allergy and Critical Care Medicine,
Penn State College of Medicine, Milton S. Hershey Medical Center,
500 University Drive, MCH041, Hershey, PA 17033, USA

Penn State College of Medicine, MCH041, Room C6531A, 500 University Drive,
Hershey, PA 17033, USA
e-mail: adimmock@hmc.psu.edu

W.J. Meggs (ed.), *The Toxicant Induction of Irritant Asthma, Rhinitis, and Related Conditions*, DOI 10.1007/978-1-4614-9044-9_6,

that mediate these effects include effects on mucosal structure and function, allergy, epigenetic modulation, and bacterial pathogens.

**Keywords** Asthma • Rhinitis • Chronic rhinosinusitis • Tobacco smoke • Health effects • Inflammation • Inhalation toxicology

## Introduction

For a half-century the evidence has been sufficient to associate tobacco smoke with chronic bronchitis, emphysema, COPD, and cancers of the lung and oropharynx (US Department of Health, Education, and Welfare 1964). However, with regard to chronic rhinosinusitis (CRS) and asthma the available evidence was meager when the first 1964 Surgeon General's report was issued and was summed up in a brief statement that "cigarette smoking does not appear to cause asthma".

This initial conclusion has increasingly run counter to clinical experience. Pediatricians have long suspected parental smoking to be a risk factor for childhood asthma, and physicians commonly hear reports from nonsmoking asthmatic patients about symptoms being triggered by exposure to others' tobacco smoking. Patients with rhinosinusitis (and some otherwise healthy adults) frequently report exacerbations of nasal congestion and rhinorrhea from secondhand smoke (SHS).

The dearth of information relating to asthma, rhinitis, and tobacco has become increasingly problematic as asthma rates have increased, and scientists have sought to understand the roots of the asthma epidemic. While evidence has accrued that SHS is associated with increased asthma rates in children, as recently as 10 years ago there was a paucity of research data in key areas, particularly with respect to the relationship between secondhand tobacco smoke, rhinitis (Samet 2004), and asthma in adults.

Voluminous research has shifted the understanding of asthma, as evidenced by increasingly nuanced definitions (US Department of Health, Education and Welfare 1964; EPR 1991; EPR-2 1997; EPR-3 2007; Lotvall et al. 2011; Wenzel. 2006; Wenzel 2012a, b) (Table 6.1), the search for endo/phenotypes (Wenzel 2006; Wenzel 2012a, b), and the identification of multiple factors that could impact overall trends (Eder et al. 2006). Definitions of rhinitis and CRS have likewise evolved (International Rhinitis Management Working Group 1994; Lund and Kennedy 1995, 1997; Benninger et al. 2003) (Table 6.2), followed by the emerging hypothesis of an integrated pathogenesis for allergic asthma and rhinosinusitis (Togias 2003), resulting in the proposal that allergic rhinosinusitis and allergic asthma be considered to be one "common airway disease." Relationships among non-allergic rhinitis and asthma phenotypes continue to be investigated.

A further complication in the effort to understand associations between tobacco smoke, asthma, and rhinitis was the shifting profile of the cigarette (US Department of Health and Human Services 1981) and changing patterns of tobacco use.

**Table 6.1** History of definitions of asthma

| Year | 1964 | 1991 | 1997 | 2007 | 2013 |
|---|---|---|---|---|---|
| Asthma Document | American Thoracic Society definition, cited in Surgeon General's report | National Asthma Education Program(EPR) | National Asthma Education and Prevention Program<br>Expert Panel 2 | National Asthma Education and Prevention Program<br>Expert Panel 3 | Proposals for endotypes/phenotypes |
| Definition | Asthma is a disease characterized by an increased responsiveness of the trachea and bronchi to various stimuli and manifested by a widespread narrowing of the airways that changes in severity either spontaneously or as a result of therapy | Asthma is a lung disease with the following characteristics:<br>1. airway obstruction that is reversible (but not completely so in some patients) either spontaneously or with treatment;<br>2. airway inflammation; and<br>3. increased airway responsiveness to a variety of stimuli. | Asthma, whatever the severity, is a chronic inflammatory disorder of the airways.<br>The immunohistopathologic features of asthma include:<br>Denudation of airway epithelium<br>Collagen deposition beneath basement membrane<br>Edema<br>Mast cell activation<br>Inflammatory cell infiltration<br>Neutrophils (especially in sudden-onset, fatal asthma exacerbations)<br>Eosinophils<br>Lymphocytes (TH2-like cells)<br>Airway inflammation contributes to airway hyperresponsiveness, airflow limitation, respiratory symptoms, and disease chronicity.<br>Airway inflammation also contributes to several forms of airflow limitation, including acute bronchoconstriction, airway edema, mucus plug formation, and airway wall remodeling. These features lead to bronchial obstruction.<br>Atopy, the genetic predisposition for the development of an IgE-mediated response to common aeroallergens, is the strongest identifiable predisposing factor for developing asthma. | Asthma is a chronic inflammatory disorder of the airways.<br>The immunohistopathologic features of asthma include inflammatory cell infiltration:<br>Neutrophils (especially in sudden-onset, fatal asthma exacerbations; occupational asthma, and patients who smoke)<br>Eosinophils<br>Lymphocytes<br>Mast cell activation<br>Epithelial cell injury<br>Airway inflammation contributes to airway hyperresponsiveness, airflow limitation, respiratory symptoms, and disease chronicity<br>In some patients, persistent changes in airway structure occur, including sub-basement fibrosis, mucus hyper-secretion, injury to epithelial cells, smooth muscle hypertrophy, and angiogenesis<br>Gene-by-environment interactions are important to the expression of asthma<br>Atopy, the genetic predisposition for the development of an immunoglobulin E (IgE)-mediated response to common aeroallergens, is the strongest identifiable predisposing factor for developing asthma<br>Viral respiratory infections are one of the most important causes of asthma exacerbation and may also contribute to the development of asthma | "The common disease asthma is probably not a single disease, but rather a compels of multiple, separate syndromes that overlap."<br>Potential phenotypic categories (Wenzel 2006)<br>*Clinical or physiological phenotypes*<br>Severity-defined<br>Exacerbation-prone<br>Defined by chronic restriction<br>Treatment-resistant<br>Defined by age at onset<br>*Phenotypes related to the following triggers*<br>Aspirin or on-steroidal anti-inflammatory drugs<br>Environmental allergens<br>Occupational allergens or irritants<br>Menses<br>Exercise<br>*Inflammatory phenotypes*<br>Eosinophilic<br>Neutrophilic<br>Pauci-granulocytic<br>Lotvall et al. (2011)<br>Hereditary, early onset allergic asthma<br>Poorly reversible, very severe, neutrophilic asthma<br>Late onset eosinophilic asthma<br>Late onset, symptom dominant, obese minimal inflammation |

(continued)

**Table 6.1** (continued)

| Year | 1964 | 1991 | 1997 | 2007 | 2013 |
|---|---|---|---|---|---|
| Citations | US Department of Health (1964) | EPR | EPR-2 1997 | EPR-3 | Wenzel (2006), Lotvall (2011), Wenzel (2012) |

EPR-2 (1997). Expert panel report 2: guidelines for the diagnosis and management of asthma (EPR-2 1997). Bethesda, MD, US Department of Health and Human Services; National Institutes of Health; National Heart, Lung, and Blood Institute; National Asthma Education and Prevention Program

EPR-3 Expert Panel Report 3: Guidelines for the Diagnosis and Management of Asthma. Full Report 2007, US Department of Health and Human Services, National Institutes of Health, National Heart, Lung, and Blood Institute, National Asthma Education and Prevention Program

EPR Expert panel report: guidelines for the diagnosis and management of asthma (EPR 1991). Bethesda, MD, US Department of Health and Human Service; National Institutes of Health; National Heart, Lung, and Blood Institute; National Asthma Education and Prevention Program

Lotvall J, Akdis A. C., Bacharier LB, et al. (2011). Asthma endotypes: a new approach to classification of disease entities within the asthma syndrome. *J Allergy Clin Immunol* 127: 355–360

US Department of Health, Education, and Welfare, (1964). *Smoking and Health: Report of the Advisory Committee to the Surgeon General of the Public Health Service*. US Department of Health, Education, and Welfare, Public Health Service, Center for Disease Control. Washington

Wenzel, S. (2012). Severe asthma: from characteristics to phenotypes to endotypes. *Clinical & Experimental Allergy* 42(5): 650–658

Wenzel, S. E. (2006). Asthma: defining of the persistent adult phenotypes. *Lancet* 368(9537): 804–813

**Table 6.2** History of definitions of rhinitis, sinusitis and rhinosinusitis

| Year | 1993 | 1996–1997 | 2001 | 2003 |
|---|---|---|---|---|
| Document/ Organization | Allergic and Nonallergic Rhinitis Transatlantic Workshop | Multidisciplinary Rhinosinusitis Task Force | ARIA: Allergic Rhinitis and its Impact on Asthma | Task Force of the Sinus and Allergy Health Partnership; endorsed by the American Academy of Otolaryngology-Head and Neck Surgery, American Academy of Otolaryngic Allergy and the American Rhinologic Society |
| Definition | "It is very seldom that diseases are found pure and unmixed, as they are commonly described by authors; and there is almost an endless variety of constitutions"<br>The term rhinitis implies an inflammatory disease of the nasal mucous membrane. Demonstration of local inflammation is, however, not practical. Clinical diagnoses are based on the presence of symptoms…{which} may occur without inflammation…rhinopathy is strictly speaking, a more correct term—but it is rarely used.<br>There is no universally accepted system for the definition, classification or the terminology of rhinitis<br>"*Simple Classification*"<br>1. Infectious (purulent) rhinitis<br>2. Seasonal allergic rhinitis = hay fever = pollinosis<br>3. Perennial allergic rhinitis<br>4. Perennial non-allergic rhinitis (eosinophilic or non-eosinophilic) | *Major Factors:*<br>Facial pain/pressure<br>Nasal obstruction/blockage<br>Nasal discharge/purulence/ discolored postnasal drainage<br>Hyposmia/anosmia<br>Purulence in nasal cavity on examination<br>Fever(acute rhinosinusitis)<br>*Minor Factors*:<br>Headache<br>Fever (all nonacute)<br>Halitosis<br>Fatigue<br>Dental pain<br>Cough<br>Ear pain/pressure/fullness<br>*Distinct Clinical Categories of Rhinosinusitis*:<br>Acute: < 4 weeks<br>Subacute > 4- < 12 weeks<br>Chronic >12 weeks<br>Recurrent, Acute, >4/year<br>Acute exacerbations of chronic | Proposed to replace seasonal and perennial rhinitis with intermittent and persistent rhinitis | "*Rhinosinusitis* is replacing the term *sinusitis* because sinusitis is often preceded by rhinitis and rarely occurs without concurrent nasal airway inflammation" *Rhinosinusitis* is a group of disorders characterized by inflammation of the mucosa of the nose and paranasal sinuses. *Chronic rhinosinusitis* is rhinosinusitis of at least 12 weeks duration.<br>Chronic rhinosinusitis is a syndrome or symptom complex without regard to pathogenesis. Signs of inflammation must be present and identified in association with symptoms:<br>1. Discolored drainage, polyps or polypoid swelling<br>2. Edema or erythema of the middle meatus or ethmoid bulla by anterior rhinoscopy; generalized or localized erythema, edema or granulation tissue<br>3. CT scan showing isolated or diffuse mucosal thickening, bone changes, air fluid-level<br>Associated factors include<br>1. Systemic host factors (allergic, immunodeficiency, genetic/ congenital, mucociliary dysfunction, endocrine, neuromechanism)<br>2. Local host factors (anatomic, neoplastic, acquired mucociliary dysfunction)<br>3. Environmental factors (microorganisms, noxious chemicals, pollutants, smoke, medications, trauma and surgery)<br>Two leading scenarios of disease<br>1. Concurrent chronic rhinosinusitis and asthma: one airway disease<br>2. Unilateral or bilateral isolated chronic rhinosinusitis with no other evident respiratory tract involvement |

(continued)

**Table 6.2** (continued)

| Year | 1993 | 1996–1997 | 2001 | 2003 |
|---|---|---|---|---|
| Citation | Mygind and Naclerio (1993) | Lund, Kennedy et al. (1995), (1997); Lanza and Kennedy (1997) | Bousquet (2001) | Benninger et al. (2003) |

(1997). Report of the Rhinosinusitis Task Force Committee Meeting. Alexandria, Virginia, August 17, 1996. *Otolaryngology-Head and Neck Surgery* 117((3 Pt 2)): S1-68

Benninger, M. S., B. J. Ferguson, J. A. Hadley, D. L. Hamilos, M. Jacobs, D. W. Kennedy, D. C. Lanza, B. F. Marple, J. D. Osguthorpe, J. A. Stankiewicz, J. Anon, J. Denneny, I. Emanuel, and H. Levine (2003). Adult chronic rhinosinusitis: Definitions, diagnosis, epidemiology, and pathophysiology. *Otolaryngology-Head and Neck Surgery* 129(3): S1—32

Bousquet, J., Van Cauwenberge, P, Khaltaev, N (2001). Allergic rhinitis and its impact on asthma. *J Allergy Clin Immunol* 2001(108(5 suppl)): S147–S334

International Rhinitis Management Working Group (1994). International Consensus Report on Diagnosis and Management of Rhinitis. *Allergy* 49(19 suppl): 1–34

Lanza, D. C. and D. W. Kennedy (1997). Adult rhinosinusitis defined. *Otolaryngology-Head and Neck Surgery* 117(3 Pt 2): S1–7

Lund, V. J., D. Kennedy and a. t. S. a. T. Group (1995). Quantification for staging sinusitis. *Ann Otol Rhinol Laryngol* 167(Suppl): 17–21

Mygind N, Naclerio RM editors. Allergic and non-allergic rhinitis. 1993, Munksgaard, Copenhagen ISBN 87-16-10911-2 1996. pages

Despite these difficulties, there has been slow progress as evidenced by tables later in this chapter showing the gradually shifting history of conclusions regarding the relationship between tobacco combustion products and asthma (US Department of Health and Human Services 1964, 1986, 1990, 2004, 2006) (Table 6.3) and upper respiratory syndromes including rhinitis and CRS (US Department of Health and Human Services 1964, 1986, 1990, 2004, 2006) (Table 6.9). This chapter highlights key studies underlying our evolving understanding of tobacco smoke effects and also presents studies since the 2004 update on active smoking health effects (US Department of Health and Human Services 2004) and the 2006 update on passive smoking health effects (US Department of Health and Human Services 2006).

## Scope of the Chapter

This chapter aims to address tobacco smoke (both active and passive smoking) and its impact on asthma and rhinitis (including CRS). Included is data on international variation and trends in both active smoking rates and in environmental tobacco smoke exposure, demonstrating the wide range in exposure frequency among selected demographic groups and the importance of recognizing the diverse scenarios in which SHS occurs.

The impact of tobacco smoke on asthma and rhinitis/CRS is discussed in separate sections. Separate discussions address active smoking and passive smoking; associations with incident disease are distinguished from the impact on prevalent disease and the impact of smoking on current disease biomarkers.

Excluded from detailed presentation is the impact of environmental tobacco smoke on allergic sensitization and asthma in infants and children, with some review articles cited for general orientation. Excluded also is presentation of the data on middle ear disease and SHS exposure, although the mechanisms of SHS rhinitis may well contribute to mucosal abnormalities of the Eustachian tube and middle ear. A final exclusion is chronic bronchitis, fixed airflow obstruction, and COPD.

A review of recent literature shows new and important information on the interrelationships between active smoking, asthma, and rhinitis. This information is selectively discussed to point towards research needs, particularly as new mechanisms and biomarkers are defined.

A section highlights mechanistic studies supporting leading pathophysiologic hypotheses regarding the pathways of toxicity that lead from tobacco smoke exposure to asthma and rhinitis. Topics include immune dysregulation (immediate hypersensitivity, humoral and cellular immune pathways), epigenetic modification, altered mucosal histology (including muciliary structure and function), inflammation (including neurogenic inflammation), and direct effects on bacterial pathogens.

The final future directions will identify research needs.

**Table 6.3** History of conclusions regarding tobacco smoke, asthma, and asthma-like symptoms

| Year | 1964 | 1986 | 1990 | 2004 | 2006 |
|---|---|---|---|---|---|
| Organization | Smoking and Health: Report of the Advisory Committee to the Surgeon General of the Public Health Service | Office of the Surgeon General: Health Consequences of Involuntary Smoking | Office of the Surgeon General: The Health Benefits of Smoking Cessation | Office of the Surgeon General: The Health Consequences of Smoking | Office of the Surgeon General: The Health Consequence of Involuntary Exposure to Tobacco Smoke |
| No relationship specified | | SHS and asthma (adults or children) | | | |
| Evidence is insufficient | Cigarette smoking does not appear to cause asthma | | The importance of smoking-induced heightened airway reactivity in the pathogenesis of asthma is unknown | | Risk of Ig E-mediated allergy in children |
| Evidence is suggestive but not sufficient to infer a causal relationship between: | | | | | Acute respiratory symptoms among persons with asthma<br>Chronic respiratory symptoms<br>Acute decline in lung function in persons with asthma<br>Adult-onset asthma<br>A worsening of asthma control |
| Evidence is sufficient to infer a causal relationship between: | | | Smoking cessation and reduced rates of respiratory symptoms such as cough, sputum production, and wheezing | Active smoking and all major respiratory symptoms among adults, including coughing, phlegm, wheezing, and dyspnea<br>Active smoking and poor asthma control." | Onset of wheeze illness in early childhood<br>Onset of childhood asthma<br>Having asthma among children of school age<br>Cough, phlegm, wheeze and breathlessness among children of school age |

| Citation | US Department of Health (1964) | US Department of Health and Human Services (1986) | US Department of Health and Human Services (1990) | US Department of Health and Human Services (2004) | US Department of Health and Human Services (2006) |
|---|---|---|---|---|---|

US Department of Health, Education, and Welfare, (1964). *Smoking and Health: Report of the Advisory Committee to the Surgeon General of the Public Health Service*. U.S. Department of Health, Education, and Welfare, Public Health Service, Center for Disease Control. Washington
US Department of Health and Human Services (1986). *The Health Consequences of Involuntary Smoking. A Report of the Surgeon General*. US Department of Health and Human Services, Public Health Service, Centers for Disease Control, Center for Health Promotion and Education, Office on Smoking and Health. Rockville (MD), DHHS Publication No. (CDC) 87–8398
US Department of Health and Human Services (1990). *The Health Benefits of Smoking Cessation*, US Department of Health and Human Services. Public Health Service. Centers for Disease Control. Center for Chronic Disease Prevention and Health Promotion. Office on Smoking and Health
US Department of Health and Human Services (2004). *The Health Consequences of Smoking: A Report of the Surgeon General*. US Department of Health and Human Services, Centers for Disease Control and Prevention, National Center for Chronic Disease Prevention and Health Promotion, Office on Smoking and Health. Atlanta, GA
US Department of Health and Human Services (2006). The Health Consequences of Involuntary Exposure to Tobacco Smoke: A Report of the Surgeon General. US Department of Health and Human Services, Centers for Disease Control and Prevention, Coordinating Center for Health Promotion, National Center for Chronic Disease Prevention and Health Promotion, Office on Smoking and Health. Atlanta, GA

## Tobacco Smoke

Active smoking is the intentional inhaling of tobacco smoke, typically with a manufactured cigarette. In general, epidemiologic studies stratify by never, former, and current smoking, sometimes estimating pack-years. Most population-based studies do not seek to ascertain other sources of variation in active smoking such as cigarette brand or type (e.g., menthol vs. non-menthol (Muscat et al. 2002)), use of nicotine replacement products (Foulds et al. 1992), or smoking patterns, although these factors may be risk modifiers.

Several virtually interchangeable terms describe the inhalation of tobacco smoke by those who are in the vicinity of an active smoker: SHS, passive smoke or passive smoking (PS), involuntary tobacco smoke, or environmental tobacco smoke (ETS). Each of these terms has its proponents. In the tables, the chapter authors will use the term adopted by the primary researcher.

### *Prevalence and Usage Trends*

In the United States, more men (24 %) than women (18 %) currently smoke. Smoking rates vary with educational level, from around 6 % of adults with a graduate degree to nearly 50 % of the US adults who have a GED. The proportion of the US teenagers who smoke cigarettes decreased from 36 % in 1997 to 20 % in 2009; however, the rate of decline has slowed (Centers for Disease Control and Prevention 2010). Active smoking rates are higher among the US adults with mental illness (40 % men, 34 % women), including teenagers (42 %), leading to a recent focus by the CDC on smoking cessation in this group. Another subgroup recently highlighted was individuals with intellectual disability, many of whom had concomitant high body mass (Centers for Disease Control and Prevention 2013).

Overall, SHS exposure continues for an estimated 126 million Americans including 22 million children aged 3–11 years [19]. Broadly speaking, fewer people are smoking in the United States and there are more laws prohibiting smoking in public places, so fewer people are exposed to involuntary tobacco smoke. This can lead to a false perception that workplace ETS exposure is rare. Harris et al. (2011) looked at exposure to SHS in Missouri workers in 2007–2008. 11.5 % of respondents reported exposure to SHS at work within the past week. The highest exposure category in their results was young black men with earnings less than $15,000 annually, less than a high school education, and living in isolated areas; for this group the chance of being exposed to SHS in the workplace was 66 %.

Ecological analysis of multinational data by Janson et al. showed a significant correlation between the rates of active smoking in a community and the rates of passive smoking Janson et al. (2001) (Fig. 6.1). Internationally, there is wide variation in the rates of exposure to SHS across countries. The European Community Respiratory Health Survey, for example, reported workplace SHS exposure rates ranging from 2.5 % in Uppsala, Sweden, to 53.8 % in Gadalko, Spain (Janson et al. 2001). Similar data are beginning to be reported from South America (Gomez et al. 2009).

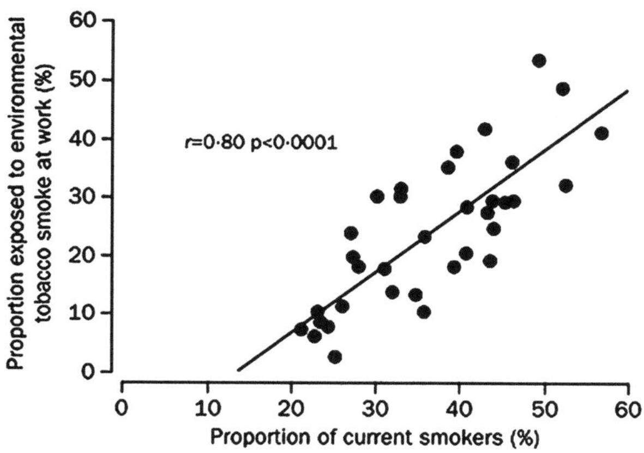


**Fig. 6.1** Ecological analysis of association between prevalence of smoking in all participants in a center and frequency of passive smoking in the workplace in occupationally active participants. Data are from Janson et al. 2001 "Effect of passive smoking on respiratory symptoms, bronchial responsiveness, lung function, and total serum IgE in the European Community Respiratory Health Survey: a cross-sectional study." The Lancet 358:2013–2109. (Used with permission of *Elsevier*)

Smoking patterns are shifting in Europe [27]; a more recent example is the longitudinal data from Sweden (Bjerg 2011).

Among patients with asthma, estimates of the rate of active smoking and passive smoking derive from cohort studies. Sippel et al. (1999) assessed patients with asthma (aged 15–55 years) by searching a US health maintenance organization database. Patients were included in the analysis if they had either been hospitalized or had two dispensings of asthma medications in the preceding year. Of the sample of 619 participants, 11 % self-identified as current smokers, 28 % as ex-smokers, and 61 % as lifetime nonsmokers. In the same cohort, 38 % reported regular exposure to other people's tobacco smoke either at home or at work. A study of asthmatics presenting to 64 US emergency rooms during a 2-week observation period indicated that 35 % were active smokers; ETS status was not mentioned (Silverman et al. 2003). Tables 6.4–6.7 reference other studies that provide exposure estimates in various cohorts.

## *Exposure Settings for Secondhand Smoke*

Researchers have defined five distinct settings in which SHS exposure occurs: home, work, public places, private social gatherings, and travel. Factors influencing tobacco smoke exposure in the home include the number of smokers in the home, intensity of the smoking habit, and size and ventilation system of the home. There is a developing literature on ETS in multiunit housing, particularly in public housing complexes in low-income urban areas (Levy et al. 2012; Wilson et al. 2010; Kraev et al. 2009).

Studies of workplace exposure stratify by hours of exposure, number of proximate smokers, and unique occupations such as waitresses and bartenders. Studies by

**Table 6.4** Summary of studies regarding active smoking and asthma or wheezing

| Authors | Population studied | Smoking status assessment | Outcome variable | Results | Observation | Reference |
|---|---|---|---|---|---|---|
| Higgins, 1977 | 4,699 adults Tecumseh, MI (USA) | Questionnaire | Chronic bronchitis, asthma, occupation, education, income | No significant associations between prevalence of asthma and smoking habits, occupation, education or income | Association noted with smoking and chronic bronchitis | Higgins et al. (1977) |
| Schenker et al., 1982 | 5,686 adult women | Questionnaire | Self-reported wheeze | Odds ratio for wheeze was 2.01 for >25 vs. 1–14 cigarettes per day. Tar content and smoke inhalation were not significant risk factors for wheeze (possibly more related to the vapor phase?) | | Schenker et al. (1982) |
| Vesterinen, 1988 | Finnish postal health surveys 1975 and 1981; *N*=10,416 | Questionnaire (nonsmoker <10 packs lifetime); Current smokers: 42.5 % of men and 22.4 % of women | Self-reporting of physician diagnosed asthma; record linkage to hospital records | Prevalence of diagnosed asthma in 1975 higher among male smokers vs. non-smokers (RR 1.73 95%CI 1.01–2.96); non-significant increase among female smokers vs. non-smokers (RR1.33 95%CI 0.78–2.26). Incidence of asthma among non-asthmatics (1981 vs. 1975) not related to current smoking: (Men 0.92 95%CI 0.44–1.93; Women 1.29 95%CI 0.69–2.40) | | Vesterinen et al. (1988) |
| McWhorter, 1989 | US population based survey or adults 25–74 years; (NHANES 1, *N*=14,404) | Questionnaire | Active doctor-diagnosed asthma (without COPD) | Asthma prevalence and incidence independent of age and smoking: (Ever Smoking and NHANESI Prevalent asthma OR 1.1 95%CI 0.9–1.4), Follow-up incidence hazard ratio (HR 1.1 95%CI 0.9–1.5) | Follow-up interview underestimated interim hospital diagnosis of asthma by 28 % | McWhorter et al. (1989) |

| | | | | | | |
|---|---|---|---|---|---|---|
| Flodin, 1995 | 79 adult onset asthma cases, 304 gender, age and community matched controls | Questionnaire | Cases identified from pharmacy beta agonist prescriptions; Physician confirmed | 3 years of smoking preceding the year of diagnosis increased risk of bronchial asthma (OR 1.9, 95 % CI 1.1–3.3); current smoking the year of diagnosis did not (OR 0.7, 95%CI 0.4–1.3), while being an ex-smoker did (OR 3.3, 95%CI 1.8–6.0) | Adjusted for age, gender, atopy (atopic dermatitis or hay fever in childhood) and air pollution at work | Flodin et al. (1995) |
| Troisi, 1995 | Nurses health study; 74,072 women; 671 incident asthma cases | Questionnaire | Physician diagnosed asthma; reported on questionnaire | Current smokers were at significantly lower risk for incident asthma (RR 0.57, 95 % CI 0.46–0.71) than women who never smoked. Risk increased in the first 2 years since quitting, then returned to baseline. | | |
| Sunyer, 1997 | Random sample, 16,884 adults from 5 areas of Spain | Face-to-face respiratory questionnaire | 35 % (1,169) underwent testing of methacholine bronchial responsiveness, total and specific IgE to mites, pets and moulds | Bronchial responsiveness greater in smokers than never smokers among non-atopic subjects only (Men aOR 3.52 95%CI 1.33–9.33; Women aOR 1.89 95%CI 1.06–3.29); Smoking did not increase responsiveness among atopics (Men 0.97 95%CI 0.4–2.39, Women 0.58 95%CI 0.2–1.9); Atopy had large effect on methacholine responsiveness at low levels. | Association between smoking and bronchial responsiveness varies with atopy | Sunyer (1997) |
| Siroux et al., 2000 | 200 adults asthmatics, 265 non-asthmatic controls, 586 relatives | Self-completed questionnaire | Physician diagnosed asthma, symptoms in last 12 months | Adult onset asthma and ever smoking: Males OR 1.21 (0.55–2.67); Females 1.19 (0.60–2.36) | | |

(continued)

**Table 6.4** (continued)

| Authors | Population studied | Smoking status assessment | Outcome variable | Results | Observation | Reference |
|---|---|---|---|---|---|---|
| Arif, 2003 | 18,825 US adults ≥20 years NHANES III (excluded 432 with physician diagnosed emphysema) | Self-report | Physician diagnosed asthma; wheezing | Using non-smokers as the reference group; Current smokers: asthma adjusted OR 1.27 (95 % CI 0.95–1.70); wheezing adjusted OR 3.62 (95 % CI 3.00–4.37)<br>Past smokers: asthma adjusted OR 1.19 (95 % CI 0.84–1.69), wheezing adjusted OR 1.39 (95 % CI 1.16–1.67) | | Arif et al. (2003) |
| Hersoug et al., 2010 | 3,471 adults (18–69 years); 773 current, 1,116 previous and 1,435 never smokers; excluded 113 occasional smokers | Self-administered questionnaire; smoking intensity categorized by grams tobacco per day | Wheeze, cough, spirometry | Prevalence of wheeze (vs. never smoking)<br>Adjusted odds ratio<br>Previous 1.37 (1.1–1.7)<br>Current<br>1–10 g 2.00 (1.31, 3.1)<br>10–15 g 2.1 (1.42, 3.23)<br>15–20 g 3.1 (2.1, 4.69)<br>>20 g 4.0 (2.85, 5.66) | Adjusted for gender, age, season, extensive environmental variables | Hersoug et al. (2010) |


Arif, A. A., G. L. Delclos, E. S. Lee, S. R. Tortolero and L. W. Whitehead (2003). Prevalence and risk factors of asthma and wheezing among US adults: an analysis of the NHANES III data. *Eur Respir J* 21(5): 827–833

Flodin, U., P. Jonsson, J. Ziegler and O. Axelson (1995). An epidemiologic study of bronchial asthma and smoking. *Epidemiology* 6(5): 503–505

Hersoug, L. G., L. L. Husemoen, T. Sigsgaard, F. Madsen and A. Linneberg (2010). Indoor exposure to environmental cigarette smoke, but not other inhaled particulates associates with respiratory symptoms and diminished lung function in adults. *Respirology* 15(6): 993–1000

Higgins, M. W., J. B. Keller and H. L. Metzner (1977). Smoking, socioeconomic status, and chronic respiratory disease. *Am Rev Respir Dis* 116(3): 403–410

McWhorter, W. P., M. A. Polis and R. A. Kaslow (1989). Occurrence, predictors, and consequences of adult asthma in NHANESI and follow-up survey. *Am Rev Respir Dis* 139(3): 721–724

Schenker, M. B., J. M. Samet and F. E. Speizer (1982). Effect of cigarette tar content and smoking habits on respiratory symptoms in women. *Am Rev Respir Dis* 125(6): 684–690

Sunyer, J. (1997). Smoking and bronchial responsiveness in nonatopic and atopic young adults. Spanish Group of the European Study of Asthma. *Thorax* 52(3): 235–238

Vesterinen, E., J. Kaprio and M. Koskenvuo (1988). Prospective study of asthma in relation to smoking habits among 14 729 adults. *Thorax* 43: 534–539

**Table 6.5** Summary of studies regarding active smoking and asthma severity/health burden/impact

| Authors | Population studied | Smoking status assessment | Outcome variable | Results | Reference |
|---|---|---|---|---|---|
| Sippel et al., 1999 | 619 subjects with physician-diagnosed asthma in a health maintenance organization; | Trained interviewer administered; self-reported smoking status as current, ex- or never smoker | Hospital-Based Asthma Care over 27.2 months | Active smoking associated with increased hospital-based care (RR 1.4, 95 % CI 1.01–1.95) adjusted for age, gender, severity, self-reported COPD, non-asthma medication use and self-reported income | |
| Silverman et al., 2003 | 64 US Emergency Departments, 1847 patients age 18–54 presenting with acute asthma; centers provided 24 h coverage for 2 weeks; 74 % participation rate | Structured questionnaire | Smoking status, demographics, medication use | 35 % were current smokers (median 10 pack years IQR 4–20 years), 23 % former smokers; factors associated with current smoking were age 30–39 years, white race, non-high school graduate, low income, lack of private insurance, lack of primary care doctor, no recent inhaled steroid use or systemic steroid use; 50 % reported smoking worsens their asthma symptoms; 4 % attributed current exacerbation to smoking | |
| Osborne et al., 2007 | 554 HMO adult asthmatics | Questionnaire; "omnibus" measures of cigarette smoke exposure included current smoking or SHS exposure | Acute care episodes; spirometry, skin prick testing | Stepwise regression into risk groups; FEV1 most significant predictor of risk (RR4.33); current cigarette smoke exposure also a risk (RR 1.6, 95 % CI 1.2–2.2) | |

(continued)

**Table 6.5** (continued)

| Authors | Population studied | Smoking status assessment | Outcome variable | Results | Reference |
|---|---|---|---|---|---|
| Chaudhuri et al. | Cross-sectional study Current ($n=60$) vs. never smokers ($N=74$) | Self-report | Juniper Asthma Control Questionnaire, Spirometry | Smokers had higher total score (poorer control) and increases in all component symptoms including nighttime awakening, morning symptoms, dyspnea, wheeze, activity limitation and rescue inhaler use. There was no difference in FEV1. | |
| Polosa et al., 2011 | Longitudinal 10-year study of 371 allergic rhinitis subjects (not diagnosed with asthma at first assessment); 152 of whom developed asthma | Self-report | Spirometry, skin test; GINA 2002 asthma severity class and level of control | Asthma was more severe (GINA Step III and IV) for 26 and 25 % of non-smokers and light smokers (1–10 pack years), 47 % of asthmatics with 11–20 pack years and 62.5 % of asthmatics with >20 pack-year smoking history. Current smoking >20 pack years a strong risk factor for uncontrolled asthma (multivariate odds ratio 5.59 95%CI 1.44–21.67) | |

**Table 6.6** Summary of studies regarding asthma biomarkers and tobacco smoke effects

| Sample | Biomarker | Asthma, Non-Smoker SN/ST | Asthma, Ex-smoker SN/ST | Asthma, Active Smoker SN/ST | Healthy, Non-smoker | Healthy, Ex-smoker | Healthy, Active Smoker | Citation |
|---|---|---|---|---|---|---|---|---|
| Exhaled Air | FeNO ppb (*N*) | 21.8/12.8 (29/19) | | 12.7/– (13/–) | 10.6 (18) | | 7.4 (16) | Verleden et al. (1999) |
| | FeNO ppb (*N*) | 25/7.1 (30/16) | | 7.7/5.4 (22/10) | 6.6 (22) | | 3.2 (20) | Horvath et al. (2004) |
| | FeNO ppb (*N*) | 14.3 (23) | 10.4 (13) | 4.3 (17) | 7.18 (20) | 6.08 (11) | 4.71 (20) | McSharry et al. (2005) |
| | FeNO ppb (*N*) | 33.7 (411) | | 18.1 (59) | | | | Michils et al. (2009) |
| | FeNO ppb<br>bronchial nl/s<br>Alveolar ppb | –/1<br>–/6.3<br>(–/66) | –/0.9<br>–/5.4<br>(–/46) | –/0.4<br>–/4.3<br>(–/35) | | | | Broekema et al. (2009) |
| Breath Condensate | Hydrogen peroxide | | | | | | Detected in only 47 % of all EBC samples | Van Hoydonck et al. (2004) |
| | 8-isoprostane | | | | | | Detected in only 36 % of samples | Van Hoydonck et al. (2004) |
| | pH | 7.31/7.56 (20/20) | | | | | | Kotsikos (2002) |
| | pH | | | | 7.6±0.2 | | 7.3±0.9 | Do et al. (2008) |
| | NH4+ | | | | 526±357 | | 456±355 | Do et al. (2008) |
| Expectorated Sputum | Eosinophils (%) Median (range) | 0.8 (0–67) | 0.5(0–38) | 1.4 (0.2– 6) | | | | Broekema et al. (2009) |

(continued)

**Table 6.6** (continued)

| Sample | Biomarker | | | | Citation |
|---|---|---|---|---|---|
| | Neutrophils% Median (range) | 47 (16–94) | 68 (22–94) | 56 (22–93) | Broekema et al. (2009) |
| | Lymphocytes(%) Median (range) | 0.9 (0–7) | 0.3 (0–3.3) | 0.2 (0–1.1) | Broekema et al. (2009) |
| | Macrophages (%) Median (range) | 42 (5–83) | 27 (5–75) | 38 (7–76) | Broekema et al. (2009) |
| | Neutrophil elastase | 1.4 (0.2–5) | 2.4 (0.3–5) | 0.8 (0.2–3) | Broekema et al. (2009) |
| | Eosinophil Cationic Protein | 35 (4–2,467) | 43 (4–1,363) | 17.4 (6–88) | Broekema et al. (2009) |
| | Histamine | 28 (0.2–130) | 29 (6–134) | 26 (0–215) | Broekema et al. (2009) |

*SN* Steroid Naïve, *ST* Steroid Treated

Broekema, M., N. H. T. ten Hacken, F. Volbeda, M. E. Lodewijk, M. N. Hylkema, D. S. Postma and W. Timens (2009). Airway Epithelial Changes in Smokers but Not in Ex-Smokers with Asthma. *American Journal of Respiratory and Critical Care Medicine* 180(12): 1170–1178

Do, R., K. H. Bartlett, W. Chu, H. Dimich-Ward and S. M. Kennedy (2008). Within- and between-person variability of exhaled breath condensate pH and NH4+ in never and current smokers. *Respir Med* 102(3): 457–463

Horvath I, D. L., Kiss A, Balint B, Kharitonov SA, Barnes PJ. (2004). Exhaled nitric oxide and hydrogen peroxide concentration in asthmatic smokers. *Respiration* 71: 463–468

McSharry, C. P., I. C. McKay, R. Chaudhuri, E. Livingston, I. Fraser and N. C. Thomson (2005). Short and long-term effects of cigarette smoking independently influence exhaled nitric oxide concentration in asthma. *Journal of Allergy and Clinical Immunology* 116(1): 88–93

Michils, A., R. Louis, R. Peché, S. Baldassarre and A. Van Muylem (2009). Exhaled nitric oxide as a marker of asthma control in smoking patients. *European Respiratory Journal* 33(6): 1295–1301

Van Hoydonck, P. G. A., W. A. Wuyts, B. M. Vanaudenaerde, E. G. Schouten, L. J. Dupont and E. H. M. Temme (2004). Quantitative analysis of 8-isoprostane and hydrogen peroxide in exhaled breath condensate. *European Respiratory Journal* 23(2): 189–192

Verleden GM, D. L., Verpeut AC, Demedts MG. (1999). he effect of cigarette smoking on exhaled nitric oxide in mild steroid–naive asthmatics. *Chest* 116: 59–64

**Table 6.7** Summary of studies regarding secondhand smoke and adult asthma

| Authors | Population studied | ETS exposure assessment | Outcome variable | Results | Observation | Reference |
|---|---|---|---|---|---|---|
| Greer et al., 1993 | 3,914 non-smoking adults completing standardized questionnaire in 1977 and 1987 | Self-administered questionnaire; home vs. work; years ever worked with smoker through 1987 | Incident asthma between 1977–1987 (definite asthma by reported symptoms or reported physician diagnosis) | Second-hand smoke exposure associated with development of asthma (RR 1.45, CI 1.21–1.75) (computed in increments of 10 years) | 20 % ex-smokers, passive smoking in workplace, past or present in 42 %; in home, 31 %; men only 1.5(1.12–2.01), women only 1.5 (1.17–1.92) | Greer et al. (1993) |
| Leuenberger et al., 1994 | 4,197 never-smoking adults, subsample of random sample from 8 areas of Switzerland | Questionnaire by trained examiners; passive smoker defined as work or home passive SHS exposure within the past 12 months; questions estimated duration in years and hours per day | Physician-diagnosed asthma; Wheezing apart from colds; specific IgE against pollen, dust mites, mold, animal epithelia | Passive smoking associated with elevated risk of physician-diagnosed asthma (OR 1.39, 95 % CI 1.04–1.89); elevated risk of wheezing apart from colds (OR 1.94, 95 % CI 1.39–2.70); evidence of dose response for both asthma and wheeze | Adjusted for age, sex, BMI, study area, atopy and parental and sibling history; unaffected by variables for low educational level, maternal smoking, paternal smoking or occupational exposure. | Leuenberger et al. (1994) |
| Dayal, 1994 | | | | | | |
| Flodin, 1995 | 79 adult onset asthma cases, 304 gender, age and community matched controls | Questionnaire | Cases identified from pharmacy beta agonist prescriptions; Physician confirmed | Three years or more of ETS exposure at work: OR 1.5, 95%CI 0.8–2.6; Three or more years of ETS exposure at home: OR 0.9, 95 % CI 0.5–1.9 | Adjusted for age, gender, atopy (atopic dermatitis or hay fever in childhood) and air pollution at work | Flodin et al. (1995) |

(continued)

**Table 6.7** (continued)

| Authors | Population studied | ETS exposure assessment | Outcome variable | Results | Observation | Reference |
|---|---|---|---|---|---|---|
| Hu, 1997 | 2,041 young adults; parental smoking assessed in 1986 and young adult asthma status in 1993 | Questionnaire; Mailed questionnaires | Physician reported asthma | Mother smoking (no or < vs. > ½ ppd), OR 1.8, 95%CI 1.1–3.0; Father smoking (no or <1/2 ppd vs. >1/2 ppd), OR 1.6, 95 % CI 1.1–2.4. Adjust OR for 2 vs. 0 smoking parents: 2.9 (1.6–5.6) | Adjusted for sex, race and education level; not adjusted for family history of asthma or visible mold (factors also significant) | Hu et al. (1997) |
| Janson et al., 2001 | 7,882 never smoking adults from 36 centers in 16 countries | Structured interview (workplace vs. home); validated at one center with cotinine | Asthma, symptoms, methacholine reactivity, spirometry | Passive smoking associated with nocturnal chest tightness, nocturnal breathlessness, breathlessness after activity and increased bronchial responsiveness | Passive smoking in the workplace associated with all types of respiratory symptoms and current asthma | Janson et al. (2001) |
| Larsson et al., 2001 | 8,008 randomly selected Swedish city residents, (15–69 years) | Questionnaire | ETS exposure, airway symptoms, respiratory history | Among never-smokers without a family history of asthma, physician-diagnosed asthma 6.8 % if childhood ETS exposure vs. 3.8 % if no childhood ETS exposure, $p<0.001$; relationship not present if family history of asthma | Does not distinguish age of asthma diagnosis; points to importance of family asthma history | Larsson et al. (2001) |

| | | | | | | |
|---|---|---|---|---|---|---|
| Thorn et al., 2001 | Nested case-referent study from random population sample ($n = 15,813$) 174 adult onset asthma cases/870 controls age 20–25 | Comprehensive mailed questionnaire about exposures in the home environment; considered only exposure before disease onset | Physician-diagnosed asthma, reported twice, beginning at age 16 or later; also analyzed asthma-like symptoms | Physician-diagnosed asthma associated with ETS in never smokers, OR 2.4, (95 % CI 1.4–4.0); Asthma-like symptoms also associated: OR 1.7, 95%CI 1.0–2.8 | Controlled for age, sex, smoking and atopy; ETS in 48 % of cases and 28 % of referents | Thorn et al. (2001) |
| Radon et al. 2002 | 1,890 adults, population based sample | Questionnaire, self-reported ETS exposure in home or workplace | Current asthma (defined as attack or nocturnal awakening in past year or use of asthma medication), wheezing, | Adjusted OR for asthma 1.51 (95%CI 0.99–2.32); for daily exposure >8 h, adjusted OR for asthma 2.06 (95%CI 1.07–3.97), and wheezing (OR2.12, 95%CI 1.25–3.58) | Adjusted for city, age, gender, active smoking, socioeconomic status, occupational exposure to dust or gases | Radon et al. (2002) |
| Larsson et al., 2003 | 4,995 females, 1,822 males, population based sample, never smokers | Postal questionnaire, ETS exposure inside and outside the home | Current symptom of wheeze, physician-diagnosed asthma | ETS exposure outside the home > 5 h daily, risk for wheeze OR 2.67 (95 % CI 1.98–3.61); Physician diagnosed asthma OR 1.79 (95%CI 1.02–3.16) | ETS at home did not show elevated OR | Larsson (2003) |
| Janson et al., 2004 IntJ Tub | | | | | | |

(continued)

**Table 6.7** (continued)

| Authors | Population studied | ETS exposure assessment | Outcome variable | Results | Observation | Reference |
|---|---|---|---|---|---|---|
| Gupta et al., 2006 | 62,109 non-smoking respondents, (<400 lifetime cigarettes); 52 % women, 4 sites; | IUATLD questionnaire translated into Hindi and Kannada; detailed section on tobacco exposure; 45 % with home ETS exposure | | Asthma prevalence higher in ETS exposed (2.2 %) vs. non-exposed (1.9 %), $p<0.05$; OR 1.22 (95 % CI 1.08–1.38); Exposure during childhood alone, or childhood and adulthood increased risk; | Adjusted for age, gender, usual residence, biomass fuel exposure and atopy | Gupta et al. (2006) |
| Simoni et al., 2007 | 2,195 non-smoking married or employed Italian women | Self-administered questionnaire, exposure validated with salivary cotinine | Respiratory symptoms, diagnosed asthma | Asthma diagnosis/ symptoms and exposure at work and to husband adjusted OR 1.5 (95%CI 1.09–2.08), PAR 10.3 | Similar results for recent wheeze | Simoni et al. (2007) |
| Hersoug et al., 2010 | 3,471 adults (18–69 years); 773 current, 1,116 previous and 1,435 never smokers; excluded 113 occasional smokers | Self-administered questionnaire; how many hours per day do you usually stay in rooms exposed to tobacco smoke (graded as 0, 0–1, 1–5,and >5 h/day) | Wheeze, cough, | Persons exposed to ETS for >5 h per day had significantly increased risk of wheeze and chronic cough as compared with those never exposed to ETS; results for physician-diagnosed asthma not significant | Effect of ETS appeared to be stronger in current smokers than never smokers | Hersoug et al. (2010) |

Flodin, U., P. Jonsson, J. Ziegler and O. Axelson (1995). An epidemiologic study of bronchial asthma and smoking. *Epidemiology* 6(5): 503–505

Greer, J. R., D. E. Abbey and R. J. Burchette (1993). Asthma related to occupational and ambient air pollutants in nonsmokers. *J Occup Med* 35(9): 909–915

Gupta, D., A. N. Aggarwal, K. Chaudhry, S. K. Chhabra, G. A. D'Souza, S. K. Jindal, S. K. Katiyar, R. Kumar, B. Shah and V. K. Vijayan (2006).Household environmental tobacco smoke exposure, respiratory symptoms and asthma in non-smoker adults: a multicentric population study from India. *Indian J Chest Dis Allied Sci* 48(1): 31–36

Hersoug, L. G., L. L. Husemoen, T. Sigsgaard, F. Madsen and A. Linneberg (2010). Indoor exposure to environmental cigarette smoke, but not other inhaled particulates associates with respiratory symptoms and diminished lung function in adults. *Respirology* 15(6): 993–1000

Hu, F. B., V. Persky, B. R. Flay and J. Richardson (1997). An epidemiological study of asthma prevalence and related factors among young adults. *J Asthma* 34(1): 67–76

Janson, C., S. Chinn, D. Jarvis, J.-P. Zock, K. Torén and P. Burney (2001). Effect of passive smoking on respiratory symptoms, bronchial responsiveness, lung function, and total serum IgE in the European Community Respiratory Health Survey: a cross-sectional study. *The Lancet* 358(9299): 2103–2109

Larsson, M. L., M. Frisk, J. Hallstrom, J. Kiviloog and B. Lundback (2001). Environmental tobacco smoke exposure during childhood is associated with increased prevalence of asthma in adults. *Chest* 120(3): 711–717

Leuenberger, P., J. Schwartz, U. Ackermann-Liebrich, K. Blaser, G. Bolognini, J. P. Bongard, O. Brandli, P. Braun, C. Bron, M. Brutsche and et al. (1994). Passive smoking exposure in adults and chronic respiratory symptoms (SAPALDIA Study). Swiss Study on Air Pollution and Lung Diseases in Adults, SAPALDIA Team. *Am J Respir Crit Care Med 150*(5 Pt 1): 1222–1228

Radon, K., K. Busching, J. Heinrich, H. E. Wichmann, R. A. Jorres, H. Magnussen and D. Nowak (2002). Passive smoking exposure: a risk factor for chronic bronchitis and asthma in adults? *Chest* 122(3): 1086–1090

Simoni, M., S. Baldacci, R. Puntoni, F. Pistelli, S. Farchi, E. Lo Presti, R. Pistelli, G. Corbo, N. Agabiti, S. Basso, G. Matteelli, F. Di Pede, L. Carrozzi, F. Forastiere and G. Viegi (2007). "Respiratory symptoms/diseases and environmental tobacco smoke (ETS) in never smoker Italian women." *Respir Med* 101(3): 531–538

Thorn, J., J. Brisman and K. Toren (2001). Adult-onset asthma is associated with self-reported mold or environmental tobacco smoke exposures in the home. *Allergy* 56(4): 287–292

Dimich-Ward correlated exposure history with biomarkers of exposure (hair nicotine and cotinine) showing the highest ETS exposure among employees of bars or private clubs (38 h/week ETS exposure) and moderate ETS exposure among housekeepers and office workers where smoking was permitted (21 h/week) (Dimich-Ward 1997).

Flight attendants are another unique group of workers in that they are in closed spaces, airline cabins, with airline passengers. For several decades flight attendants had regular occupational exposure to SHS. The ban on tobacco smoking on domestic airline flights occurred in 1988, followed by the smoking ban on international flights in 1995. This provided a natural comparison of the impact of smoking on the health status of this occupational group.

Tammemagi et al. (2010) developed a detailed SHS exposure questionnaire and used it to associate SHS exposure in the preceding 5 years with incident CRS. Their SHS exposure data demonstrated private social function SHS exposure as a risk factor for CRS (OR 2.6, 95 % CI 1.7–3.9); public SHS exposure was not a significant risk in this study.

Eisner and Blanc (2002) described travel-associated ETS; exposure in this setting within a 12-month period was reported by 30 % of a cohort of 374 non-smoking asthmatic adults, with over half reporting an asthma exacerbation and extra inhaled medication use as a result.

## Exposure Characterization

Exposure characterization begins with an understanding of the point source, its subsequent distribution in the environment, and then its update and deposition in the human target. ETS is generated by individual smokers and comprises exhaled mainstream smoke (the minor component) and sidestream smoke (the portion generated from the burning tip of the cigarette). In general, patients report more difficulty with a room of active smokers than a room of stale tobacco smoke—this may be a dose effect or may relate to the smaller particle size of fresh tobacco smoke. There is a wide particle size distribution of sidestream smoke measured minutes after smoke generation (US Department of Health and Human Services 1986, 2006). When the instrument used to measure particle size uses a light scattering technique (rather than a staged impactor method) the particle size can be overestimated at higher particle concentrations (Bascom et al. 1991).

ETS is a complex mixture that evolves as the smoke ages. Particles agglomerate and settle on surfaces. The volatile and semi-volatile species interact with the particles, and in enclosed spaces there is a back and forth of the ETS products and the indoor surfaces—a fact familiar to anyone who walks into a room and smells the smell of stale tobacco long after occupants have ceased to smoke.

Tobacco smoke contains endotoxin, the major glycolipid of the outer membrane of gram-negative bacteria and a potent initiator of airway inflammation. First demonstrated by Hasday et al. using the *Limulus* amebocyte lysate assay ("bioactive LPS") (Hasday et al. 1996), endotoxin was measured in smoke generated from a smoking machine using 1R4F experimental reference cigarettes and commercially

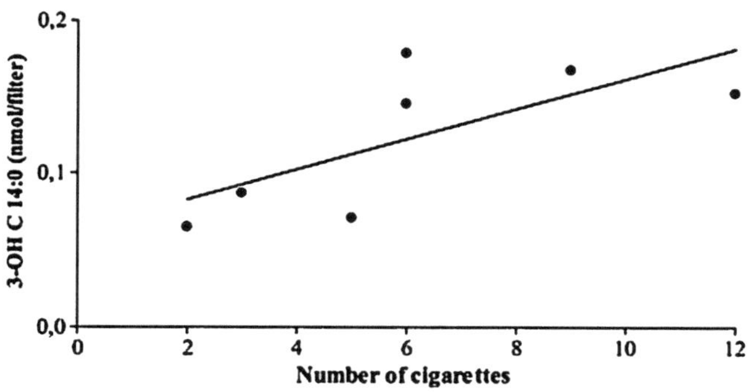


**Fig. 6.2** Amounts of 3-OH $C_{14:0}$ in airborne dust samples from student's rooms vs. the number of cigarettes smoked. Data are from Sebastien et al. 2006 "Elevated concentrations of endotoxin in inddor air due to cigarette smoking." J Environ Monitoring 8:519–522. (Used with permission of *Royal Society of Chemistry*)

available "lite" cigarettes; it was present in the tobacco portion of cigarettes and in the cigarette filter tip; bioactive LPS was found both in mainstream and sidestream smoke. Hasday et al. estimated that smoking one pack of cigarettes would provide an LPS dose equivalent to 13-day exposure at the workplace permissible exposure limit of 20 ng/m$^3$. Sebastian et al. performed active sampling of filtered dust drawn from the breathing zone of college dorm rooms occupied by nonsmokers and smokers and demonstrated a linear relationship between the number of cigarettes smoked and airborne levels of an LPS indicator (3-hydroxytetraenoic acid), assayed by gas chromatography/mass spectroscopy (Sebastian et al. 2006) (Fig. 6.2). Blanc et al. (2005) measured both indoor air endotoxin in vacuumed dust samples and serum cotinine in a panel of 226 asthmatics but did not correlate these measures. They did associate dust endotoxin levels with dog ownership (Blanc et al. 2005). Studies evaluating the effect of endotoxin (and susceptibility to endotoxin-induced inflammation) in asthma will need to be aware of both of these exposure pathways.

Tobacco smoke also contains nitric oxide (NO), a potential confounder when using exhaled NO as an asthma biomarker McSharry (2005). While tobacco smoke is a complex mixture, studies comparing the effects of exposure to different types of cigarettes or to the volatile fraction compared with unfiltered smoke can explore mechanisms of toxicants and strategies to produce modified risk tobacco products (Schenker et al. 1982; Bascom et al. 1996a, b; Rennard et al. 2002; CSSSMRF 2012).

## *Distribution, Uptake, and Deposition*

When a patient is adjacent to a smoker, the primary factors determining dose are the direction of the plume. As the distance from the point source increases, other factors such as the room size and ventilation become more important. Most humans at rest are nasal breathers. Exceptions include individuals with nasal congestion and people who are talking, laughing, and eating. The rate and depth of breaths alter the deposition pattern (Kesavanathan et al. 1998). Nostril shape is another determinant of particle uptake, with rounded nostrils delivering a higher fractional dose of particles to the nasopharynx when compared with more elliptical nostrils (Kesavan et al. 2000).

ETS components may remain in the airway or may be taken up and distributed by the circulation to distal targets. Brain scans demonstrate the uptake of nicotine from ETS in the brains of nonsmokers (Brody et al. 2011).

Vapor-phase deposition has been modeled in the upper and lower respiratory tracts, with some key insights: in the upper respiratory tract, the narrow nasal valve and extensive turbinates create turbulent flow and highly variable uptake. In the lower respiratory tract, the branching structure of the airways leads to rapid increases in cross-sectional area with a shift in deposition from impaction to diffusion.

The characteristics of the vapors themselves affect the uptake at the air–liquid interface (ALI). Vapors can be broadly divided into reactive and nonreactive materials and soluble and insoluble materials, with large differences in regional uptake based on these groups. For example, sulfur dioxide, a reactive, soluble gas, is 99 % taken up by the upper respiratory tract and does not reach the lower airway under conditions of quiet breathing. In contrast, ozone, a reactive but poorly soluble gas, is taken up only 40 % by the upper respiratory tract, with the remainder distributed along the lower airway (Bates et al. 2009).

The implication of the above information is that the individual components of tobacco smoke will be deposited nonuniformly throughout the respiratory tract. Larger particles and more reactive, soluble materials will be deposited more proximally, while the less reactive and less soluble materials will be deposited more distally.

## *Biomarkers of Exposure*

Self-reported tobacco exposures are strongly correlated with structured questionnaires (Carlsten et al. 2012; Biagini Mayers et al. 2012; Kvalvik et al. 2012; Wright et al. 2012). However, there is also evidence that in some situations, self-reported history might not be reliable (Lewis et al. 2003; Apseloff et al. 1994). In such cases it would be useful to have an available marker to ascertain the presence and degree of tobacco exposure.

To address issues associated with the reliability of self-reported smoking history, there has been a great deal of interest in identifying biomarkers of tobacco exposure. Cotinine, a metabolic by-product of nicotine, is an attractive option, especially in situations where there is a social stigma associated with cigarette smoking, such as during pregnancy, where discrepancies have been observed between reported cigarette smoking and measurements of cotinine in maternal blood (Dietz et al. 2010; Spencer and Cowans 2013; Shipton et al. 2009), saliva and urine (Aurrekoetxea et al. 2013), and fetal meconium (Himes et al. 2013; Spanier et al. 2011) or umbilical cord blood (Wright et al. 2011). However, one difficulty with using cotinine as a biomarker is that the rate of metabolism varies according to a variety of heredity factors, including race, which might incorrectly lead to assumptions of increased exposure among different demographic subgroups (Smith et al. 2013; Zhu et al. 2013).

## Impact of Tobacco Smoke on Asthma

Table 6.3 shows the evolution of the consensus view of the impact of tobacco smoke on asthma, beginning with the 1964 opinion that "cigarette smoking does not appear to cause asthma." In 1990, the early evidence linking tobacco to asthma was the reduced rate of wheezing following smoking cessation (USDHHD 1990). In 2004, the Surgeon General reported linked active smoking with wheezing and also with poor asthma control (of prevalent cases).

In 2006, the Surgeon General's report stated that evidence was sufficient for a causal link between passive smoking and onset of wheeze illness in early childhood and onset of childhood asthma as well as prevalent asthma, wheeze and breathlessness among children of school age. In contrast, evidence was insufficient to associate the risk of IgE allergy in children with passive smoking. The 2006 Surgeon General's report stated that evidence was suggestive but not sufficient to infer a causal relationship between passive smoking and acute respiratory symptoms among adults with asthma, chronic respiratory symptoms, acute decline in lung function in persons with asthma, adult-onset asthma, and a worsening of asthma control (Table 6.3).

### *Association of Active Smoking and Asthma*

Table 6.4 summarizes selected studies evaluating the association of active smoking and indicators of asthma including symptoms (wheeze, cough), physician-diagnosed asthma, pharmacy records, and biomarkers including methacholine challenge (Schenker et al. 1982; Higgins et al. 1977; Vesterinen et al. 1988; McWhorter et al. 1989; Flodin et al. 1995; Troisi et al. 1995; Arif et al. 2003; Hersoug et al. 2010; Siroux et al. 2000; Sunyer 1997). A comparison of two multi-country studies (ISAAC and ECHRS) indicates good overall agreement for using self-reported asthma and wheeze in the last 12 months as indicators for asthma (Pearce et al. 2000). An early community-based study was influential in steering interest away from smoking and asthma, as it associated active smoking with chronic bronchitis, but not asthma (Higgins et al. 1977). An interesting observation from another early study was the suggestion that the risk of wheeze (OR 2.01 for >25 vs. 1–14 cigarettes per day) was associated with the vapor of tobacco smoke (not the tar content) (Schenker et al. 1982). A Finnish postal survey noted a higher prevalence of physician-diagnosed asthma among male smokers (RR 1.73) but not female smokers (Vesterinen et al. 1988). McWhorter's US population-based First National Health and Nutrition Examination Survey (NHANES). I study indicated that asthma prevalence was independent of age and smoking (McWhorter et al. 1989). Flodin et al. demonstrated that 3 years of smoking preceding the year of diagnosis doubled the risk of bronchial asthma (OR 1.9, 95 % CI 1.1–3.3) (Flodin et al. 1995). Hersoug et al. demonstrated a dose–response relationship between the intensity of current smoking and prevalent wheeze, ranging from 2.0 for 1–10 g tobacco daily to 4.0 for >20 g daily (Hersoug et al. 2010). The study by Arif et al. of 18,825 US adults associated wheezing with current smoking (OR 3.62, 95 % CI 3–4.37); physician-diagnosed asthma was not associated (OR 1.27, 95 % CI 0.95-1.7) (Arif et al. 2003).

## Active Smoking and Asthma Severity/Impact/Health Burden

Table 6.5 summarizes studies examining the impact of active smoking on asthma severity, impact, and health burden (Sippel et al. 1999; Silverman et al. 2003; Osborne et al. 2007; Chaudhuri et al. 2008; Polosa et al. 2011). Sippel et al. (1999) examined the impact of active smoking on hospital-based asthma care over 27 months using health maintenance organization records and demonstrated increased hospital-based care (adjusted RR 1.4, 95 % CI 1.01–1.95). Chaudhuri et al. (2008) compared asthma control in a cross-sectional study of 60 current vs. 74 never smokers, using the validated Juniper asthma control questionnaire and spirometry. Smokers with asthma had a significantly higher total asthma control score (1.6, 95 % CI 1.1–2.3) vs. (2.8, 9.5 % CI 1.7–3.4), $P<0.0001$, indicating worse control. Polosa examined a group of well-characterized patients with allergic rhinitis who developed asthma during a 10-year longitudinal follow-up. In this group, asthma severity and lack of control were associated with current smoking (Polosa et al. 2011).

## Active Smoking and Asthma Biomarkers

Table 6.6 shows asthma biomarkers obtained through exhaled breath, exhaled breath condensates, and expectorated sputum (McSharry et al. 2005; Verleden et al. 1999; Horváth et al. 2004; Michils et al. 2009; Broekema et al. 2009; Van Hoydonck et al. 2004; Tanou et al. 2009; Do et al. 2008). Several biomarkers used to assess asthma severity and control are altered by tobacco exposure. For example, the fraction of nitric oxide in exhaled air ($FE_{NO}$) has long been explored as a potential biomarker for asthma diagnosis and management (Taylor et al. 2006), yet levels of $FE_{NO}$ are reduced in smokers relative to nonsmokers, making it difficult to generalize the results of $FE_{NO}$ testing to the clinical setting (Verleden et al. 1999; Horváth et al. 2004). An official ATS Clinical Practice Guideline: Interpretation of exhaled nitric oxide levels for clinical applications recently addressed the potential confounding by smoking and offered practical approaches to clinical interpretation (Dweik et al. 2011). Figure 6.3 shows data indicating a dose–response between cumulative tobacco dose and exhaled NO concentrations in patients with asthma (McSharry et al. 2005). Further refinement of the clinical interpretation algorithm will likely occur if this relationship is confirmed.

Another biomarker being investigated for its utility in asthma management is an induced sputum eosinophil count. Broekema et al. showed no effect of current or former smoking on sputum eosinophilia in a group of asthmatics (Broekema et al. 2009). Interestingly, median numbers of macrophages, neutrophils, and lymphocytes were decreased in asthmatics who were current smokers compared to nonsmokers; and levels of neutrophil elastase and eosinophil cationic protein were reduced as well. This is interesting because of the recognized association of active smoking with leukocytosis (van Eeden and Hogg 2000) and elevated macrophage and neutrophil counts on bronchoalveolar lavage samples of smokers compared with nonsmokers Costabel (1992). Many studies of asthma biomarkers (including

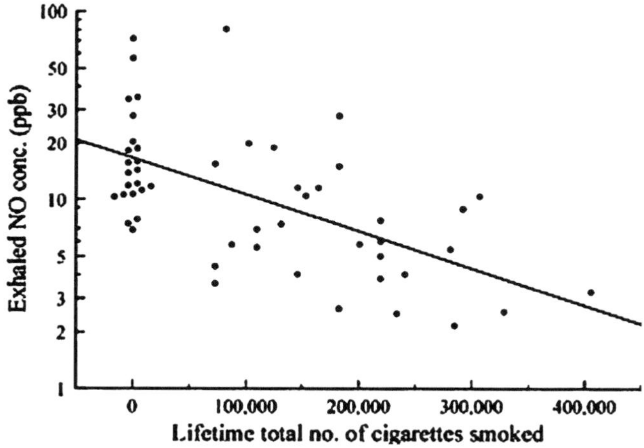


**Fig. 6.3** The long-term effect of smoking on exhaled NO concentration in patients with asthma. Reprinted from McSharry et al. 2005 "Short and long-term effects of cigarette smoking independently influence exhaled nitric oxide concentration in asthma." J Allergy Clin Immunol 116:88–93. (Used with permission of *Elsevier*)

those evaluating asthma severity) Jatakanon (1999) or novel cytokine biomarkers ascertain tobacco exposure status by self-report without verification using biomarkers of exposure (see discussion above). Active smoking was also associated with decreased pH and decreased $NH_4^+$ (Do et al. 2008).

## *Secondhand Smoke and Incident Asthma*

Extensive studies support a causal association between ETS exposure and childhood asthma as summarized in previous documents (Fig. 6.4) (CEPA 1997). This has been well documented and is not covered again here.

Table 6.7 presents studies examining the association of SHS exposure and adult asthma (Janson et al. 2006; Flodin et al. 1995; Hersoug et al. 2010; Greer et al. 1993; Leuenberger et al. 1994; Hu et al. 1997; Larsson et al. 2001; Thorn et al. 2001; Radon et al. 2002; Gupta et al. 2006; Simoni et al. 2007). Three large studies totaling over 8,000 adults and 2,000 young adults, published in the 1990s, demonstrated associations of SHS exposure with the risk of development of asthma. Greer et al. (1993) associated incident asthma and SHS exposure (both ascertained by self-administered questionnaire) and demonstrated a relative risk of 1.45 (CI 1.21–1.75), computed in increments of 10 years (CEPA 1997). Leuenberger et al. (1994) analyzed the SALPADIA data set, demonstrating an association of passive smoking with physician-diagnosed asthma (OR 1.39, 95 % CI 1.04–1.89) as well as wheezing apart from colds (OR 1.94, 95 % CI 1.39–2.70) with evidence of dose–response for both outcomes (Fig. 6.5) (Leuenberger et al. 1994). A smaller study using pharmacy records as the case source did not show an association (Flodin et al. 1995).

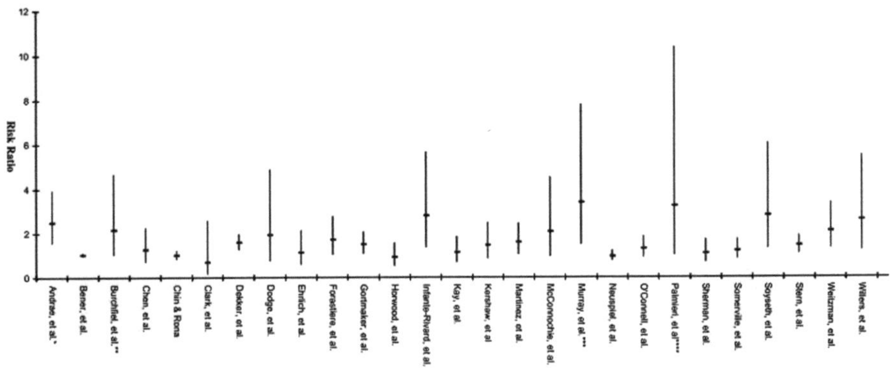


**Fig. 6.4** Reported risk ratios and 95% confidence intervals between ETS exposure and the occurrence of childhood asthma, for studies that used clinically recognized asthma as an outcome. Reprinted fig. 6.1 of California Environmental Protection Agency, Health Effects of Exposure to Environmental Tobacco Smoke http://www.calepa.ca.gov Office of Environmental Health Hazard Assessment 1997. (Public Domain)

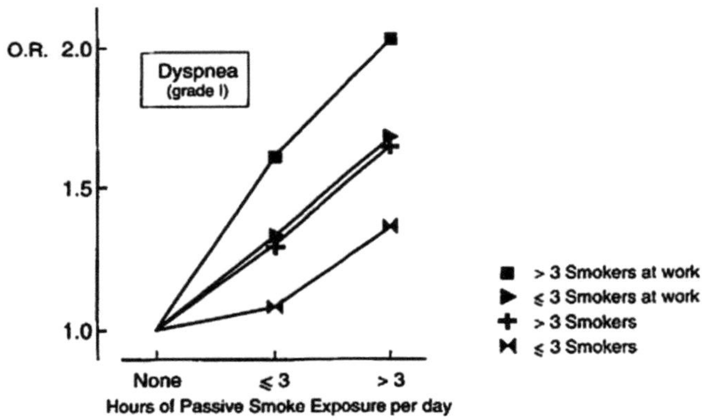


**Fig. 6.5** Relative odds of physician diagnosed asthma in passive smoking exposure. Reference category is 'no passive smoking exposure' (OR 1.0/None). Passive smoking exposure is at home and/or the workplace. Data are from Leuenberger et al. 1994 "Passive smoking exposure in adults and chronic respiratory symptoms (SAPALDIA Study). Swiss Study on Air Pollution and Lung Diseases in Adults, SAPALDIA Team." Am J Respir Crit Care Med 150:1222–1228. (Reprinted with permission of the American Thoracic Society. Copyright © 2013 American Thoracic Society)

Eight studies published between 2001 and 2010 drew their data from over 50,000 subjects and are also summarized in Table 6.7 (Janson et al. 2006; Flodin et al. 1995; Hersoug et al. 2010; Greer et al. 1993; Leuenberger et al. 1994; Hu et al. 1997; Larsson et al. 2001; Thorn et al. 2001; Radon et al. 2002; Gupta et al. 2006; Simoni et al. 2007). These studies, taken together, address the spectrum of ETS exposures from childhood to adulthood (at home and work). Janson et al. (2006) ascertained exposure through structured interviews, in a multicenter ($N=36$), multi-country

($N$=16) study with validation (at one site) of the exposure questionnaire (Janson et al. 2006). A further strength of the Janson study was performance both of spirometry and methacholine reactivity. The authors associated passive smoking in the workplace with all types of respiratory symptoms and with current asthma. A strength of Simoni et al.'s study of Italian women was the validation of exposure with salivary cotinine. This study associated asthma diagnosis and symptoms with exposure at work and a smoking husband (Simoni et al. 2007).

A large multinational European survey ($n$=7,882, ages 20–48, 36 centers in 16 countries) demonstrated that passive smoking in the workplace was significantly associated with current asthma (OR 1.9, 95 % CI 0.9–2.88) as well as asthma-like respiratory symptoms and bronchial hyperreactivity (Janson et al. 2006). Beatty et al. (2011) found similar rates of physician-diagnosed asthma in non-smoking flight attendants with occupational SHS exposure (pre-aircraft smoking ban) and an age-matched NHANES population control (16.3 and 15 %, $p$=NS). In the same population, physician-diagnosed chronic bronchitis was increased (11.7 vs. 7.2 %, $p<0.002$) as was emphysema/COPD (3.2 vs. 0.9 %, $p<0.03$).

Hersoug et al. (2010) demonstrated the novel concept that ETS exposure was harmful to active smokers. This had not been investigated heretofore, based on the notion (evidently erroneous) that the toxicity of active smoking would vastly outweigh any impact of ETS (Hersoug et al. 2010).

## *Secondhand Smoke and Prevalent Asthma*

As shown in Table 6.8, ETS exposure among adults with physician-diagnosed asthma, physician-treated asthma, and self-reported breathlessness, wheeze, or cough showed increased episodes of care and ETS-associated increased medication use and increased symptoms (Sippel et al. 1999; Eisner 2002a; Eisner and Blanc 2002; Larsson et al. 2001).

Passive smoking (at home and/or work) was significantly associated with nocturnal chest tightness (odds ratio 1.28, 95 % CI 1.02–1.60), nocturnal breathlessness (1.30, 95 % CI OR 1.01–1.67), breathlessness after activity (1.25 [1.07–1.47]), and increased bronchial responsiveness (effect –0.18, 95 % –0.30 to –0.05). Passive smoking at work only was significantly associated with nocturnal chest tightness: (OR 1.60, 95 % 1.14–2.25) nocturnal breathlessness (1.56, 95 % 1.12–2.18) as well as breathlessness after activity (OR 1.31, 95 % CI 1.06–1.62) (Janson et al. 2006).

## *Tobacco Exposure and Response to Asthma Therapy*

Additional studies have determined that tobacco exposure can affect subsequent response to medical therapy, particularly with corticosteroids. Cohen and colleagues observed that intrauterine exposure to tobacco was associated with decreased responsiveness to inhaled corticosteroids among children with asthma (Cohen et al. 2010). A similar observation was made among adults with asthma, with a diminished

**Table 6.8** Summary of studies regarding secondhand smoke and prevalent asthma

| Authors | Population studied | ETS Exposure Assessment | Outcome Variable | Results | Observation | Reference |
|---|---|---|---|---|---|---|
| Sippel et al., 1999 | 619 subjects with physician-diagnosed asthma in a health maintenance organization | Trained interviewer administered; self-reported regular exposure either at home or work | Hospital-Based Asthma Care over 27.2 months | Baseline ETS exposure associated with increased episodes of care (28 vs. 10 episodes per 100 person-years of observation; adjusted RR 2.34 (95%CI 1.80–3.05) | | Sippel et al. (1999) |
| Eisner et al., 2002 | 374 nonsmoking adults with physician-treated asthma | Structured interview | ETS exposure during travel; associated symptoms and medication use | 30 % self-reported ETS exposure during travel in last 12 months; ETS-related cough, wheezing or chest tightness (66 %), eye irritation (46 %) nose irritation (43 %); extra medication use (55 %) | | Eisner and Blanc (2002) |
| Larsson et al., 2001 | 8,008 randomly selected Swedish city residents, (15–69 years) | Questionnaire | Self-reported breathlessness, wheeze or cough with ETS exposure | 50 % of asthmatics reported ETS associated lower respiratory symptoms vs. 21 % of all subjects | | (Larsson, Frisk et al. 2001) |
| Eisner et al., 2002 | 349 adults with physician-treated asthma | Structured telephone interview | ETS exposure at baseline interview; longitudinal health status | Higher level ETS exposure ≥3 h/week associated with worse severity of asthma scores; greater risk of ER visits (OR3.4 95%CI 1.1–10.3) or hospital admission (OR 12.2, 95%CI 1.5–102) | Controlled for baseline asthma severity, age, sex, race, income, education | Eisner et al. (2002) |

Jindal, 1994
Jindal, 1997

Jindal SK, Gupta D, Singh AJ. Indices of morbidity and control of asthma in patients exposed to environmental tobacco smoke. Chest 1994; 106: 746–9

Jindal SK, Gupta D, Chattopadhaya S, Kumar L. Environmental tobacco smoke exposure precipitates acute exacerbation in nonsmoker asthmatics. Lung India 1997; 15: 168–72

Jindal SK, Gupta D, D' Souza GA, Kalra S. Bronchial responsiveness of non-smoking women exposed to environmental tobacco smoke or biomass fuel combustion. Indian J Med Res 1996; 104: 359–64

Jindal SK, Jha LK. Gupta D. Bronchial hyper-responsiveness of women with asthma exposed to environmental tobacco smoke. Indian J Chest Dis Allied Sci 1999; 41: 75–82

Aggarwal AN, Chaudhry K, Chhabra SK, D'Souza GA, Gupta D, Jindal SK, et al. Prevalence and risk factors for bronchial asthma in Indian adults: a multicentre study. Indian J Chest Dis Allied Sci 2006; 48: 13–22

Eisner, M. D. and P. D. Blanc (2002). "Environmental tobacco smoke exposure during travel among adults with asthma." Chest 122(3): 826–828

Eisner, M. D., E. H. Yelin, P. P. Katz, G. Earnest and P. D. Blanc (2002). "Exposure to indoor combustion and adult asthma outcomes: environmental tobacco smoke, gas stoves, and woodsmoke." *Thorax* 57(11): 973–978

Larsson, M. L., M. Frisk, J. Hallstrom, J. Kiviloog and B. Lundback (2001). "Environmental tobacco smoke exposure during childhood is associated with increased prevalence of asthma in adults." *Chest* 120(3): 711–717

Sippel, J. M., K. L. Pedula, W. M. Vollmer, A. S. Buist and M. L. Osborne (1999). "Associations of smoking with hospital-based care and quality of life in patients with obstructive airway disease." *Chest* 115(3): 691–696 therapeutic response to inhaled corticosteroids (Lazarus et al. 2007) and oral corticosteroids (Chaudhuri et al. 2003) among smokers. These observations correspond to those observed at the molecular level, where the effects of inhaled corticosteroids are associated with changes in the activity levels of neutrophils and eosinophils among nonsmokers, while the levels of activity in smokers are unaffected (Pedersen et al. 1996). The mechanism behind this altered response has been ascribed to a reduction in the histone deacetylase 2 (HDAC2) enzyme system (Ito et al. 2000; Barnes 2006). Another mechanism that has been put forward includes a tobacco-induced increase in pro-inflammatory cytokines, such as IL-2, 4, and 8 and TNF-α (Chalmers et al. 2002; Byron et al. 1994; Churg et al. 2002) which has been postulated to lead to the overexpression of glucocorticoid receptor beta (GR-β) (Strickland et al. 2001; Webster et al. 2001).

## Impact of Tobacco Smoke on the Upper Respiratory Tract

Table 6.9 shows the history of conclusions regarding tobacco smoke, upper respiratory symptoms, acute rhinitis, and CRS. Expert panels (USDHHD 1986, 2006; CEPA 1997) and review articles (Samet 2004) through 2005–2006 focused on SHS-associated acute upper respiratory symptoms and identified a need for epidemiologic studies focused on the association between tobacco smoke and chronic upper respiratory conditions including rhinitis, allergic rhinitis, and CRS. Tables 6.10 and 6.11 summarize recent studies that address this knowledge gap (Samet 2004; USDHHD 1986, 2006; Janson et al. 2006; Tammemagi et al. 2010; CEPA 1997; Leuenberger et al. 1994; Simoni et al. 2007; Beatty et al. 2011; Wieslander et al. 2000; Topp et al. 2005; Miyake et al. 2005; Ho et al. 2007; Lin et al. 2011; Montano-Velazquez et al. 2011; Ebbert et al. 2007; Reh et al. 2009).

### *Active Smoking and Chronic Rhinosinusitis*

Acute sinusitis is reported by 35 % of the US adult population in a 12-month period, and chronic sinusitis is reported by 14 % of the US adult population (Lieu and Feinstein 2000). Lieu and Feinstein associated direct use of tobacco with increased prevalence of any sinusitis in an analysis of data from the Third National Health and Nutrition Examination Survey (NHANES III); cigarette smoking increased the risk of any sinusitis (aRR 1.14, 95 % CI 1.06–1.22) as well as risks of acute sinusitis (RR 1.18, 95 % CI 1.05–1.30) and recurrent or chronic sinusitis (RR 1.22, 95 % CI 1.05–1.39). Other tobacco products (chewing tobacco, snuff, pipe, and cigar) taken as a group also increased sinusitis risk (RR 1.37, 95 % CI 1.21–1.54); sample numbers were too small to examine risks related to individual non-cigarette products.

Annesi-Maesano et al. (1997) prospectively studied a cohort of 191 men twice at an interval of 5 years to evaluate the role of tobacco smoking on upper airway disease and found an odds ratio of 5.4 and 4.9 for current smoking and chronic rhinitis, with a dose–response between the amount smoked and the likelihood of chronic rhinitis. A limitation of both studies is the reliance on disease self-report.

**Table 6.9** History of conclusions regarding tobacco smoke, upper respiratory symptoms, rhinitis, and chronic rhinosinusitis

| Year | 1964 | 1986 | 1990 | 2004 | 2006 |
|---|---|---|---|---|---|
| Organization | Smoking and Health: Report of the Advisory Committee to the Surgeon General of the Public Health Service | Office of the Surgeon General: Health Consequences of Involuntary Smoking | Office of the Surgeon General: The Health Benefits of Smoking Cessation | Office of the Surgeon General: The Health Consequences of Smoking | Office of the Surgeon General: The Health Consequence of Involuntary Exposure to Tobacco Smoke |
| No Relationship Specified | | SHS and rhinitis | | | |
| Evidence is insufficient | | | | | |
| Evidence is suggestive but not sufficient to infer a causal relationship between exposure and… | | | | | Persons with nasal allergies or a history of respiratory illnesses are more susceptible to developing nasal irritation |
| Evidence is sufficient to infer a causal relationship between exposure and… | | | | | Odor annoyance<br>Nasal irritation |
| Citation | US Department of Health (1964) | US Department of Health and Human Services (1986) | US Department of Health and Human Services (1990) | US Department of Health and Human Services (2004) | US Department of Health and Human Services (2006) |

US Department of Health, Education, and Welfare, (1964). *Smoking and Health: Report of the Advisory Committee to the Surgeon General of the Public Health Service*. U.S. Department of Health, Education, and Welfare, Public Health Service, Center for Disease Control. Washington

US Department of Health and Human Services (1986). *The Health Consequences of Involuntary Smoking. A Report of the Surgeon General*. US Department of Health and Human Services, Public Health Service, Centers for Disease Control, Center for Health Promotion and Education, Office on Smoking and Health. Rockville (MD), DHHS Publication No. (CDC) 87–8398

US Department of Health and Human Services (1990). *The Health Benefits of Smoking Cessation*, US Department of Health and Human Services. Public Health Service. Centers for Disease Control. Center for Chronic Disease Prevention and Health Promotion. Office on Smoking and Health

US Department of Health and Human Services (2004). *The Health Consequences of Smoking: A Report of the Surgeon General*. US Department of Health and Human Services, Centers for Disease Control and Prevention, National Center for Chronic Disease Prevention and Health Promotion, Office on Smoking and Health. Atlanta, GA

US Department of Health and Human Services (2006). The Health Consequences of Involuntary Exposure to Tobacco Smoke: A Report of the Surgeon General. US Department of Health and Human Services, Centers for Disease Control and Prevention, Coordinating Center for Health Promotion, National Center for Chronic Disease Prevention and Health Promotion, Office on Smoking and Health. Atlanta, GA

**Table 6.10** Summary of studies regarding environmental tobacco smoke and rhinitis

| Authors | SHS and rhinitis | | | | |
|---|---|---|---|---|---|
| | Population studied | ETS exposure assessment | Outcome variable | Results | Reference |
| Leuenberger et al., 1994 | 4,197 never-smoking adults, subsample of random sample from 8 areas of Switzerland | Questionnaire by trained examiners; passive smoker defined as work or home passive SHS exposure within the past 12 months; questions estimated duration in years and hours per day | Do you have any nasal allergies including hay fever | Passive smoking not a risk factor for allergic rhinitis. Prevalence of allergic rhinitis among "true never smokers" 21.1(SD 19.6–22.6); prevalence among passive never smokers 20.5 (SD 18.2–22.7) | Leuenberger et al. (1994) |
| Wieslander et al., 2000 | 51 air crew members traveling Stockholm to Tokyo: 27 pre and 24 post smoking ban | Particle concentrations were 66 ± 56 mcg/m3 in flight pre smoking ban and 3 ± 0.8 post smoking ban ($p < 0.001$) | Eye and nasal symptoms and signs (ocular tear film stability and acoustic rhinometry—nasal cavity dimensions) | In-flight runny nose decreased from 25 % to 11 %, "irritative cough" decreased from 15 % to 0 %. "Sensation of getting a cold" decreased from 20 % to 0 %. Post-flight anterior nasal volume was greater after the smoking ban (pre ban vol1 3.9 ± 0.5 cm3, post ban vol1 4.4 ± 0.8 cm3, $P = 0.03$) ; In-flight tear film stability also increased from a break-up time of 10–25 s, $p = 0.01$ | Wieslander et al. (2000) |
| Janson et al., 2001 | 7,882 never smoking adults(20–48) from 36 centers in 16 European countries | Interview-led questionnaire; passive smoking at work and home; quantified from 0 to >8 h daily | "Do you have hay-fever or any other kind of allergic rhinitis" | No association between passive smoking and current allergic rhinitis (OR 1.02, 95 % CI 0.81–1.20); Stratified by daily passive smoking exposure intensity: 1 to < 4 h OR 1.00 (0.84–1.18), 4 to < 8 h 0.99 (0.78–1.25); >8 h 0.93 (0.71–1.20). | Janson et al. (2001) |

| | | | | | |
|---|---|---|---|---|---|
| Topp et al., 2005 | 4,093 non-smoking German adults (17–79 years) | Self-administered questionnaire; ETS exposure at work (17 %), home (8 %), or both (5 %) | "have you ever had.. hay fever, allergic conjunctivitis" (yes = 17 %); specific IgE to mite, cat, dot, cladosporium and pollens (29 % positive) | Allergic sensitization and allergic rhinoconjunctivitis significantly associated with workplace but not home ETS for crude odds ratio, but not when adjusted for gender, age group social class and residential region: (AS OR 0.96; 95%CI 0.69–1.33), AR-C OR 0.89, 95%CI 0.59–1.35) | Topp et al. (2005) |
| Miyake et al., 2005 | 1,002 pregnant Japanese women | | Allergic rhinitis (medication use) | Prevalence of current allergic rhinitis significantly associated with current passive smoking exposure at home (adjusted OR, 1.89; 95 % CI, 1.10–3.30) and at work (adjusted OR, 2.50; 95 % CI, 1.29–4.76); Not associated with active smoking | Miyake et al. (2005) |
| Simoni et al., 2007 | 2,195 non-smoking married or employed Italian women | Self-administered questionnaire, exposure validated with salivary cotinine | Any rhinoconjunctivitis | Adjusted OR showed increased symptoms with ETS exposure only to husband(OR 1.3 95%CI 1.02–1.65), PAR 9.5 %; or both at work and to husband (OR 1.48, 95%CI 1.13–1.94); PAR 17 %; Adjusted for age, education, residence, age-residence interaction | Simoni et al. (2007) |

(continued)

**Table 6.10** (continued)

| Authors | SHS and rhinitis | | | | |
|---|---|---|---|---|---|
| | Population studied | ETS exposure assessment | Outcome variable | Results | Reference |
| Ho et al., 2007 | 7,336 never-smoking Hong Kong workers; 2 year follow-up for 2,213 workers with consistent SHS exposure | Telephone questionnaire | "Rhinitis"; 2 year follow-up analysis included only subjects with no baseline rhinitis | No association with rhinitis and workplace SHS (OR 0.87, 95%CI 0.71–1.05), adjusted for age, sex, educational attainment and occupational exposure to chemicals, chemical gases and dust; 2-year incident rhinitis also not significantly associated with workplace SHS exposure (OR 1.29, 95 % CI 0.93–1.8) | Ho et al. (2007) |
| Lin et al., 2011 | 83 subjects with AR (58 years old, 69 % female); 117 nonallergic subjects (age and gender-matched community controls) | Interview | 78 % of the AR subjects reported chronic rhinosinusitis vs. 30 % of the nonallergic participants | AR subjects had longer current SHS exposure (adjusted mean difference 1.6 h/week, $p=0.01$) and 20 years ago (2.9 h /week, $p=0.03$) | Lin et al. (2011) |
| Montano-Velazquez et al., 2011 | 50 youths (age 10–19) with perennial allergic rhinitis | Questionnaire verified by cotinine:creatinine ratio; 25 not exposed, 25 exposed (13 active and passive smoke, 12 passive smoke only) | Symptom questionnaire, nasal airway resistance (anterior rhinomanometry) | PAR patients with tobacco smoke exposure had higher total nasal airway resistance despite similar symptom scores | Montano-Velazquez et al. (2011) |

*AR* allergic rhinitis, *A-RC* allergic rhinoconjunctivitis, *AS* allergic sensitization

Ho, S. Y., T. H. Lam, S. F. Chung and T. P. Lam (2007). Cross-sectional and prospective associations between passive smoking and respiratory symptoms at the workplace. *Ann Epidemiol* 17(2): 126–131

Janson, C., S. Chinn, D. Jarvis, J.-P. Zock, K. Torén and P. Burney (2001). Effect of passive smoking on respiratory symptoms, bronchial responsiveness, lung function, and total serum IgE in the European Community Respiratory Health Survey: a cross-sectional study. *The Lancet* 358(9299): 2103–2109

Leuenberger, P., J. Schwartz, U. Ackermann-Liebrich, K. Blaser, G. Bolognini, J. P. Bongard, O. Brandli, P. Braun, C. Bron, M. Brutsche and et al. (1994). Passive smoking exposure in adults and chronic respiratory symptoms (SAPALDIA Study). Swiss Study on Air Pollution and Lung Diseases in Adults, SAPALDIA Team. *Am J Respir Crit Care Med* 150(5 Pt 1): 1222–1228

Lin, S. Y., D. D. Reh, S. Clipp, L. Irani and A. Navas-Acien (2011). Allergic rhinitis and secondhand tobacco smoke: a population-based study. *Am J Rhinol Allergy* 25(2): e66-71

Miyake, Y., S. Miyamoto, Y. Ohya, S. Sasaki, I. Matsunaga, T. Yoshida, Y. Hirota and H. Oda (2005). Association of active and passive smoking with allergic disorders in pregnant Japanese women: baseline data from the Osaka Maternal and Child Health Study. *Annals of Allergy, Asthma & Immunology* 94(6): 644–651

Montano-Velazquez, B. B., R. C. Navarrete, M. D. Mogica Martinez, M. Becerril-Angeles and K. Jauregui-Renaud (2011). Rhinomanometry in young patients with perennial allergic rhinitis with/without recent exposure to tobacco smoke. *Clin Otolaryngol* 36(4): 320–324

Simoni, M., S. Baldacci, R. Puntoni, F. Pistelli, S. Farchi, E. Lo Presti, R. Pistelli, G. Corbo, N. Agabiti, S. Basso, G. Matteelli, F. Di Pede, L. Carrozzi, F. Forastiere and G. Viegi (2007). Respiratory symptoms/diseases and environmental tobacco smoke (ETS) in never smoker Italian women. *Respir Med* 101(3): 531–538

Topp, R., W. Thefeld, H. E. Wichmann and J. Heinrich (2005). The effect of environmental tobacco smoke exposure on allergic sensitization and allergic rhinitis in adults. *Indoor Air* 15(4): 222–227

Wieslander, G., T. Lindgren, D. Norback and P. Venge (2000). Changes in the ocular and nasal signs and symptoms of aircrews in relation to the ban on smoking on intercontinental flights. *Scand J Work Environ Health* 26(6): 514–522

**Table 6.11** Summary of studies regarding environmental tobacco smoke and chronic rhinosinusitis

| Authors | Population studied | ETS exposure assessment | Outcome variable | Results | Citation |
|---|---|---|---|---|---|
| Ebbert et al., 2007 | 1,007 never smoking flight attendants | Self-administered, mailed survey; calculated hours spent in smoking cabin | "..ever taken medication for, had survey for, or been told by a doctor…"sinusitis, allergies | Overall frequency: Sinusitis: 43.4 %(40.9 % for lower quartile exposure, 47-5 % for third and fourth quartile exposures); allergies 40.3 %; hay fever 13.4 %; Adjusted odds ratio 1.21 for sinusitis by hours of smoky cabin exposure | Ebbert et al. (2007) |
| Reh et al., 2009 | Case Control Study; 100 CRS, 100 age, sex and smoking status matched | Validated SHS questionnaire (Non SHS vs. current or childhood SHS) | Disease specific quality of life measures | Significantly increased CRS risk for current or childhood SHS vs. never SHS (OR 2.33 95 % CI 1.02–5.34). CRS cases exposed to SHS had worse mean scores in nasal obstruction/blockage, nasal discharge, headaches and cough; also more likely to use nasal decongestants. | Reh et al. (2009) |
| Tammemagi et al., 2010 | 306 nonsmoking patients with incident CRS (Henry Ford Hospital Otolaryngology practice) and 306 age, sex and race/ethnicity matched non-smoking controls selected from the Henry Ford Hospital database | Structured telephone questionnaire | SHS exposure 5 years before diagnosis at home, work, public places and private social function | Odds ratio for CRS: 1.69 (95 % CI 0.92–3.1) for SHS exposure at home, 2.81 (1.42–5.57) for exposure at work, 1.48 (0.88–2.49) for exposure in public places, and 2.6 (1.74–3.89) for exposure at private functions | Tammemagi et al. (2010) |

| | | | | | |
|---|---|---|---|---|---|
| Beatty et al., 2011 | 362 flight attendants; age and smoking history-matched population sample from NHANES 2005–2006 | On-line questionnaire | Physician diagnosed sinus problems (also other medical illnesses) | Higher rate of sinus problems among flight attendants 31.5 % vs. 20.9 % NHANES, $p<0.002$; lower rates of high blood pressure, diabetes, high cholesterol, heart failure; Dose response for pre smoking ban flight time and symptoms for nasal congestion, throat or eye irritation (but not post smoking ban) | Beatty et al. (2011) |

## Active Smoking and Prevalent Allergic Rhinitis

Two studies, published as a single paper, examined the impact of active smoking on untreated allergic rhinitis and concluded that there was no impact on nasal symptoms or nasal-specific quality of life (Bousquet et al. 2009). These two French studies have complementary designs that increase the generalizability of the findings. One study recruited patients from primary care physicians ($N=472$); the other recruited from specialists including allergists, pulmonologists, and otorhinolaryngologists ($N=672$). Patients were well characterized with recent (within 5 years) skin prick tests (SPT) or allergen-specific IgE that correlated with symptoms and physician-diagnosed allergic rhinitis using 1994 consensus criteria (Table 6.2). Study endpoints were well standardized and included the Rhinoconjunctivitis Quality of Life Score (Juniper 1997) (a validated instrument) and stratification of rhinitis severity using the ARIA classification (Allergic Rhinitis and Its Impact on Asthma Initiative) (Bousquet et al. 2001) as well as individual symptoms. A limitation of the study was its lack of objective assessment of mucosal function.

In contrast, Tanou et al. (2000) demonstrated differences in inflammatory and oxidative stress biomarkers obtained from patients with allergic rhinitis, stratified by smoking status (Table 6.12) (Tanou et al. 2009). Smokers with allergic rhinitis presented with higher EBC $LTB_4$ levels (Fig. 6.6) and lower EBC pH levels (Fig. 6.7), suggesting evidence for an interaction between allergic upper airway disease and susceptibility to lower airway injury. Tanou's study points to the importance of developing biomarkers to use in understanding the interactions between tobacco smoke exposure and airway diseases.

## SHS and Risk of Allergic Rhinitis

Several population-based studies indicated that passive smoking was not a risk factor for allergic rhinitis. Leuenberger et al. (1994) showed a similar prevalence of allergic rhinitis among Swiss never smokers with (21 %) and without (20.5 %) a passive smoking history. Janson et al.'s multi-country European study (Janson et al. 2006) showed no association between passive smoking and current allergic rhinitis (including examination of three levels of exposure intensity).

Topp et al. (2005) assessed the association between exposure to ETS at home or at work and allergic sensitization in 4,093 German adults (aged 17–79 years) using logistic regression models and found a statistically nonsignificant tendency for workplace ETS to increase allergic sensitization (adjusted OR 1.17, 95 % CI 0.97–1.41) and allergic rhinitis (adjusted OR 1.20, 95 % CI 0.96–1.51); a similar tendency was *not* found with ETS exposure at home for either allergic sensitization (adjusted OR 0.99, 95 % CI 0.76–1.29) or allergic rhinoconjunctivitis (adjusted OR 1.05, 95 % CI 0.76–1.43).

**Table 6.12** Summary of studies regarding tobacco smoke, rhinitis, and biomarkers

| | Biomarker | Rhinitis, non-Smoker SN/ST | Rhinitis, ex-smoker SN/ST | Rhinitis, SHS SN/ST | Rhinitis, active smoker SN/ST | Healthy, non-smoker | Healthy, ex-smoker | Healthy, SHS | Healthy, active smoker | Citation |
|---|---|---|---|---|---|---|---|---|---|---|
| Exhaled air | FeNO ppb (*N*) | 29 (20) | | | 15 (20) | 9.5 (15) | | | 9(est) (15) | Tanou et al. (2009) |
| Exhaled Breath Condensate | LTB4, pg/ml | 61.9 | | | 202.4 | 55.2 | | | 50.3 | Tanou et al. (2009) |
| | pH | 7.47 | | | 7.67 | 7.67 | | | 7.67 | Tanou et al. (2009) |
| | Eosinophils | | | | | | | | | |
| | Neutrophils | | | | | | | | | |
| | TGF beta | | | | | | | | | |
| | IL-11 | | | | | | | | | |
| | TNF-alpha | | | | | | | | | |
| | IL-b | | | | | | | | | |
| | ADAM33 | | | | | | | | | |
| | IL-4 | | | | | | | | | |
| | IL-4R | | | | | | | | | |
| | IL-8 | | | | | | | | | |
| | Neutrophil elastase | | | | | | | | | |
| | HMW matrix metalloproteinase 9 showing reduced inhibitor by TIMP | | | | | | | | | |

*SN* Steroid Naïve, *ST* Steroid Treated

Tanou, K., A. Koutsokera, T. S. Kiropoulos, M. Maniati, A. I. Papaioannou, K. Georga, S. Zarogiannis, K. I. Gourgoulianis and K. Kostikas (2009). "Inflammatory and oxidative stress biomarkers in allergic rhinitis: the effect of smoking." *Clinical & Experimental Allergy* 39(3): 345–353

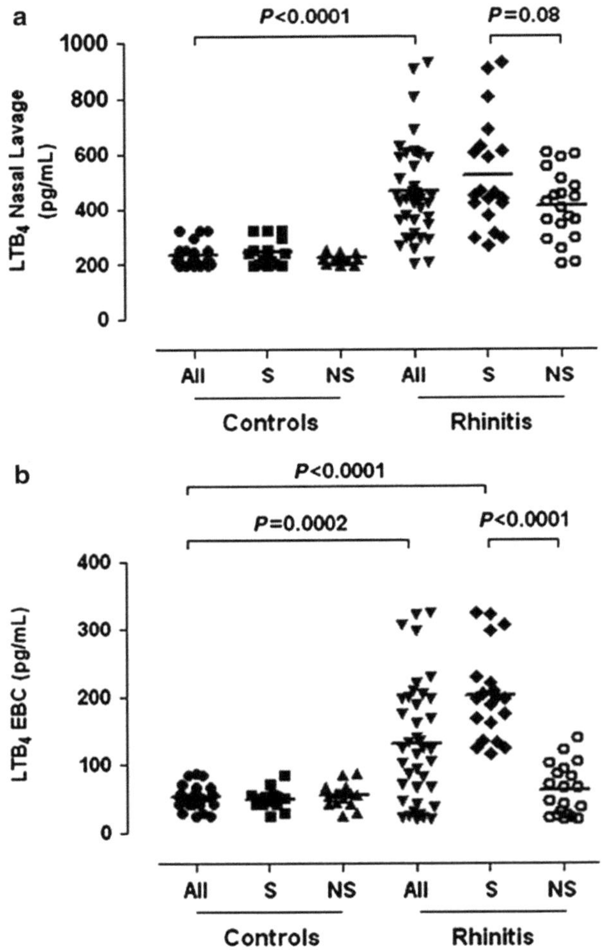


**Fig. 6.6** Comparison of leukotriene B4 ($LTB_4$) levels between healthy subjects (smokers and nonsmokers) and patients with allergic rhinitis (smokers and non-smokers) in nasal lavage (upper figure) and in exhaled breath condensate (lower figure). Horizontal bars represent mean values. Figure is from Tanou et al. 2009 "Inflammatory and oxidative stress biomarkers in allergic rhinitis: the effect of smoking." Clin Exp Allergy 39:345–353. (Used with permission of *John Wiley and Sons*)

## *SHS and Acute Rhinitis*

A questionnaire administered to 77 healthy non-smoking young adults showed that 34 % reported one or more rhinitis symptoms (congestion, rhinorrhea, or sneezing) following ETS exposure while 66 % reported no history of ETS rhinitis (Bascom et al. 1991). A series of controlled human exposure studies then characterized the subjective and objective upper respiratory response of healthy nonsmokers to sidestream tobacco smoke (STS), chosen as a reasonable surrogate for SHS. In an effort to understand the mechanisms of the response to ETS, subjects were stratified and compared based on their ETS symptom history. Exposure to 15 min of clean air followed by 15 min of STS (45 ppm CO, akin to levels in a smoky bar or tavern) caused eye, nose, and throat irritation. Subjects with a history of ETS rhinitis demonstrated increased nasal airway resistance, measured by posterior

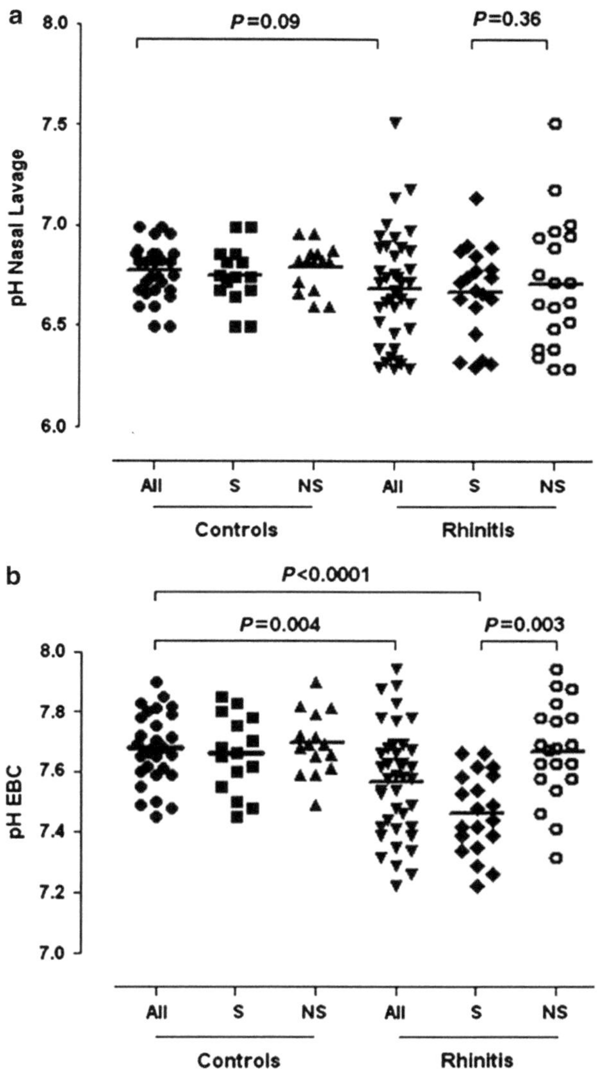


**Fig. 6.7** Comparison of pH between healthy subjects (smokers and non-smokers) and patients with allergic rhinitis (smokers and non-smokers) in nasal lavage and exhaled breath condensate. Horizontal bars represent mean values. Figure is from Tanou et al. 2009 "Inflammatory and oxidative stress biomarkers in allergic rhinitis: the effect of smoking." Clin Exp Allergy 39:345–353. (Used with permission of *John Wiley* and *Sons*)

rhinomanometry, while subjects without a history of ETS rhinitis did not show a change in nasal resistance (Bascom et al. 1991). Analysis of nasal lavage fluid showed no evidence of histamine, albumin, kinin, or TAME esterase, providing evidence against an allergic mechanism and against plasma transudation as the mechanism of the congestion. Subsequent studies showed an increased congestive response to intranasal capsaicin in the ETS-sensitive subjects, suggesting that c-fiber/chemosensitive neuronal mechanisms were involved in the differential response (Bascom et al. 1991).

Dose–response studies, conducted at 1, 5, and 15 ppm CO for 2 h, demonstrated increased nasal airway resistance by posterior rhinomanometry in both groups at the 15 ppm exposure level, with differential dose–response curves between the ETS-sensitive and ETS-nonsensitive groups (Bascom et al. 1996a, b).

In a separate study, the effect of acute STS exposure on nasal mucociliary clearance was measured in health young adults (Bascom et al. 1995). A 1-h challenge with clean air or STS (15 ppm CO) was followed by a 1-h hiatus, while the initial congestive response subsided. A radiolabelled tracer was then aerosolized and monitored for another hour. STS accelerated mucociliary clearance in 9 of the 12 subjects, as was expected. Three subjects, however, demonstrated a marked slowing of mucociliary clearance, with two subjects showing over 90 % of the tracer remaining. The importance of this finding is that it suggests a susceptibility of the mucosa to an injury response. Because impaired mucociliary clearance is a hallmark of CRS, understanding the basis for this differential response may provide insights into the pathogenesis of CRS.

## *Impact of SHS on Existing (Prevalent) Allergic Rhinitis*

Beatty et al. (2011) examined associations between flight attendant SHS exposure and upper respiratory symptoms using an online questionnaire for flight attendants ($N=362$, mean age 58.2 years; analysis was of 235 never smokers). Exposure burdens were estimated for decades of service before and after flight smoking bans (1,988 domestic, 1,995 international flights). Odds ratios for a composite upper respiratory variable ("nasal congestion, throat or eye irritation") showed a significantly higher risk of daily symptoms vs. no symptoms per decade of pre-ban service (OR 2.14, 95 % CI 1.41–3.24); the risk of daily symptoms did not change with increasing time of post-ban service.

Montano-Velazquez et al. demonstrated increased nasal resistance in young adults with perennial allergic rhinitis with exposure to SHS as compared to those without SHS exposure (Montano-Velazquez et al. 2011). Unilateral and total nasal resistance was measured with anterior rhinomanometry, and SHS exposure was ascertained by questionnaire and confirmed by cotinine/creatinine ratios. Rhinitis symptoms (sneezing, rhinorrhea, itching, and congestion) were reported by 65–85 % regardless of exposure, as would be expected based on their primary clinical diagnosis of perennial allergic rhinitis. In this group, the frequency of having perennial allergic rhinitis associated with other atopic disease was 92 % in the tobacco-exposed group but 64 % in the non-tobacco-exposed group ($p<0.05$).

In a community-based study, Lin et al. (2011) demonstrated that patients with physician-diagnosed allergic rhinitis who were exposed to SHS reported higher rates of nasal decongestant use compared to those who were not exposed to SHS (56 vs. 29 %, $p=0.012$). An extensive comparison of self-reported symptoms (rated on a six-point Likert scale) for time frames over the last 2 weeks and, separately, over the past 3 months showed similar intensity of upper respiratory symptoms in the two groups. A limitation of the study was the reliance on the physician diagnosis of allergy without independent verification. The study does provide a detailed description of the substantial burden of allergic rhinitis with respect to symptoms, medication use, and disease impact on the quality of sleep and daytime function.

## SHS and Chronic Rhinosinusitis

Tammemagi et al. (2010) demonstrated that SHS was independently associated with incident CRS in a study of patients seen by otolaryngologists at a single institution. A strength of the study was the use of a case definition using well-established clinical criteria, specifically by computerized tomography, or nasal endoscopy, criteria recommended by recent consensus documents (Benninger et al. 2003). The authors noted that private social functions were not previously recognized as an exposure venue and that epidemiologic studies of SHS typically focus on home or workplaces as exposure venues. The risk of CRS increased with increasing total SHS score in a model adjusted for socioeconomic status, exposure to air pollution, and worksite and hobby exposure to chemicals and respiratory irritants.

Beatty et al. (2011) associated flight attendant SHS exposure and the development of sinus disease using an online questionnaire. Rates of physician-diagnosed sinus disease were 31.5 % for the flight attendants and 20.9 % ($p<0.002$) for the age-matched comparator group, the National Health and Nutrition Examination Survey (NHANES 2007) 2005–2006. The rates of an array of cardiovascular conditions were lower, as might be predicted for a healthy worker effect. Evidence of a dose–response relationship was sought by calculating odds ratios of reported medication conditions for each decade (10-year increase) of pre-ban service. There was a nonsignificant association between years of service as a flight attendant with sinus problems (OR 1.27, 95 % CI 0.98–1.64) and ear infections (OR 1.20, 95 % CI 0.86–1.69). Adjustment for age, living with a smoker as an adult, and living with a smoker as a child did not attenuate this association.

## SHS and Laryngopharyngitis

The throat (laryngopharynx) is an essential structure that is infrequently assessed in studies of tobacco smoke health effects, despite its location between sinonasal structures and the lung. The narrow cross-sectional area of the larynx increases local airflow, resulting in impaction of inspired toxicant particles, and in active smokers, laryngeal cancers are a recognized health risk. Evaluated the effect of workplace SHS exposure on "frequent throat problem" in a random digit dialed survey of never-smoking Hong Kong workers (Ho et al. 2007). There was a significant association (OR 1.88, 95 % CI 1.63–2.15) when adjusted for age, sex, education attainment, and occupational exposures. A dose–response relationship was present comparing workers with ≤2 years' SHS exposure and those with >2 years' SHS exposure (< 2 years SHS: OR 1.35, 95 % CI 1.07-1.7, > 2 years SHS: OR 2.21, 95 % CI 1.9-2.57, test for trend p<0.001).

## The Integrated Respiratory Tract

Because tobacco smoke is a complex mixture, understanding its toxicology on a single toxicant-by-toxicant basis is a Sisyphian task. One approach has been to partition the smoke by filtration or the creation of extracts. Ecologic studies looking at the effects of changes in tobacco product composition provide additional information (USDHHS 1981).

The broad research question is whether the effects on the upper and lower respiratory tracts are linked. The inspired airstream travels along the respiratory tract, creating a continuum from the nose to the lower airways. The dominant histology is a pseudo-stratified ciliated columnar epithelium, but vapor uptake and particle deposition are nonuniform (Barrow 1986).

Investigators are now beginning to evaluate the larger picture of the effects of ETS on the entire respiratory system. Figure 6.8, derived from data of Hakansson et al. (2011), shows a framework for envisioning the interrelationships among tobacco smoke, asthma, and rhinitis. Other authors have developed and reviewed the idea of non-allergic pathways and respiratory system integration. Annesi-Maesano (1999) pointed out that Galen recognized the coexistence of rhinitis and asthma while Hakansson (2011) emphasized the "broad bands" of disease likely contained with the asthma and rhinitis syndromes.

### *Allergic Rhinitis and Asthma*

A sentinel synthesis (Togias 2003), published now a decade ago, summarized nearly 150 papers supporting the idea of the respiratory system as a continuous, integrated system. The author argued that allergic asthma and allergic rhinitis were manifestations of a single "chronic allergic respiratory syndrome." Rhinitis represented the "low end" of the spectrum, although evidence of lower airway inflammation could often be found. At the "high end" of the spectrum, lower airway disease was clinically evident as was rhinitis, and the two disorders tracked in parallel in terms of severity. The many interactions between the upper and lower respiratory tracts included the conditioning and filtering of inspired air by the nasal passages (and the loss of these functions when nasal congestion led to mouth breathing) and bidirectional inflammation resulting from allergen exposures.

### *Irritant Rhinitis and Asthma: Evidence for Respiratory System Integration?*

Irritant responses lack the body of evidence that exists for allergic responses, although non-allergic rhinitis and non-allergic asthma are being actively

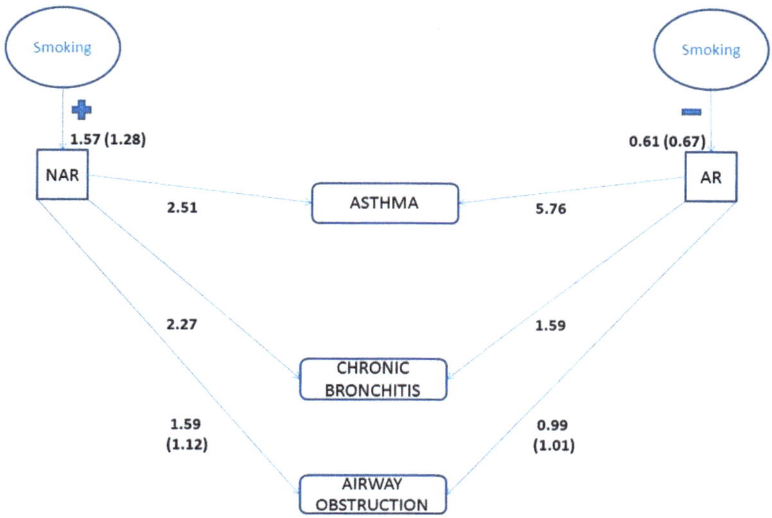


**Fig. 6.8** Associations of smoking, allergic and non-allergic rhinitis, asthma, chronic bronchitis and airway obstruction. Data used are from a population-based cross-sectional study of 7931 adults, published in Hakansson et al. 2011 "Nonallergic rhinitis and its association with smoking and lower airway disease: A general population study." Am J Rhinol Allergy 25:25–29. (no permissions)

investigated. There is heterogeneity in responses to irritants. There is interindividual variation in irritant responses, and there is variation in the effector response among irritants (Shusterman 2007).

Passive smoking is generally not associated with an increase in allergic rhinitis, but passive smoking is associated with increased wheeze apart from colds and (sometimes) increased adult asthma. This is a fascinating discrepancy with at least two possible explanations. The first is that the high baseline rate of rhinitis (nearly 60 % in NHANES) and absence of simple noninvasive biomarkers make it difficult to study risk factors. Another possibility is that there is compartmentalization of the upper and lower airway, related to the upper airway's key function of cleaning and conditioning inspired air. Data are lacking as to the similarities or the differences in effects on epithelial functions. Recently reported changes in ciliary beat frequency (CBF) effects in the nasal mucosa of passive smokers need to be evaluated in the tracheobronchial tree (Carson 2010).

Tobacco smoke-associated CRS may be more akin to the chronic bronchitis of the lower airway, related to mucous gland hyperplasia, squamous metaplasia, disordered mucociliary clearance, and susceptibility to chronic infections including biofilms.

Textbook chapters (Bascom and Ellaurie 2005; Bascom and Dolina 2007) have summarized a body of research comprising a range of irritants that demonstrate heterogeneity in the acute inflammatory response, with vascular transudation present in some but not all irritants. Shusterman proposes that atopy is an important determinant of the acute inflammatory response to STS (Shusterman 2007); additional data are needed to evaluate this hypothesis.

## Mechanisms

### *Tobacco Smoke Alters Mucosal Structure and Function*

The mechanism of tobacco smoke toxicity and its effect on the pathogenesis of asthma and allergic disease are still being elucidated. There is some evidence that smoking induces discrete changes in the airway epithelium, including an increased number of goblet cells, increased epithelial thickness, and a higher number of mast cells and a lower number of eosinophils compared to the epithelium of never smokers (Broekema et al. 2009). Smoking has also been found to affect multiple immune cell types, including eosinophils, macrophages, and neutrophils, and may potentiate the inflammatory alterations observed in asthma and rhinitis (Goncalves et al. 2011; Tamimi et al. 2012). Evaluation of bronchial biopsy specimens from the large airways of asthmatic smokers and nonsmokers demonstrated reduced number of mature CD83+ mature dendritic cells and B lymphocytes in asthmatic smokers, contributing further evidence for immune dysregulation as a mechanism of impaired asthma control among smokers (Tsoumakidou et al. 2007).

Recent work by Manoli and colleagues (2012) in a murine model of maternal cigarette smoking demonstrated abnormal alveolarization in offspring that was associated with altered retinoic acid pathway element expression, raising the possibility of altered retinoic acid signaling in lung dysfunction due to secondhand smoking.

Carson et al. (2010) demonstrated upregulation of CBF in the nasal epithelium of smokers and nonsmokers exposed to secondhand tobacco smoke. The upregulation persisted with establishing epithelial ALI in vitro cultures propagated to confluence indicating stable epigenetic modification of the ciliary cell by STS exposure.

### *Tobacco Smoke and Allergy*

Serum IgE levels are elevated in active smokers (Zetterstorm et al. 1981; Gerrard et al. 1980). A study of asthmatic probands and first-degree relatives, compared to controls, showed higher levels of IgE in current smokers compared with never smokers (controlling for gender, personal and familial history of asthma, socioeconomic class, and non-independence of subjects from the same family); the relation was independent of skin test response. The EGEA study (Epidemiological Study of the Genetics and Environment of Asthma, Bronchial Hyperresponsiveness, and Atopy) demonstrated that women who are first-degree relatives of asthmatics demonstrate elevated total IgE (103 IU/ml vs. 48 IU/ml, $p=0.02$, adjusted for asthma). The latter study suggests the presence of susceptibility factors modifying exposure–response relationships (Oryszczyn, 2000). A large multicenter European study comprising 36 centers in 16 countries (obtaining SHS exposure information through a structured interview) did not find an association between passive smoking and IgE. No sex difference was found in the association between passive smoking and total serum IgE in a secondary analysis (Janson et al. 2001).

Strachan and Cook (1998) performed a quantitative meta-analysis in 1997 of 12 studies collectively showing no adverse effect of parental smoking during pregnancy or infancy on childhood SPT positivity (pooled OR 0.87, 95 % CI 0.62–1.24). There was statistically significant heterogeneity of odds ratios relating current parental smoking to skin prick positivity.

More recent studies have examined the effect of active and SHS on serum IgE levels and SPT results in adults. The Copenhagen Allergy Study assessed 15–69-year-olds in 1990 and in 1998, performing SPT and specific IgE to common aeroallergens in 734 subjects. The risk of developing positive SPT (aOR 0.45, 95 % CI 0.21–0.98) and specific IgE positivity (aOR 0.62, 95 % CI 0.26–1.49) was lower among sustained smokers than never smokers (Linneberg 2001).

Taken together, these studies suggest that, for both children and adults, SHS exposure does not increase SPT reactivity. Active smoking, while raising total IgE, does not increase (and may decrease) incident sensitization. These studies further suggest that the positive impact of tobacco smoke on the chronic allergic respiratory syndrome occurs through an alternate, non-IgE pathway.

The epidemiologic data that tobacco smoke exposure was associated with elevated IgE levels led to the hypothesis that tobacco smoke exposure alters T cell regulation. T cells mediate the inflammatory response of asthma, with identifiable subtypes contributing to airway immune tolerance (T regulatory, or Treg, $CD4^{+}$ $CD25^{high}$ CD 127 $^{low/-}$) and airway inflammation (T effector, or Teff, $CD4^{+}$ $CD25^{neg}$). Intriguing data presented by Runyon et al. (2012) suggest that exposure to SHS (exposure within the past 5 years) alters T cell function through epigenetic modification, specifically CpG methylation within the Forkhead box P3 (FOXP3) region of Treg and the interferon gamma (IFN-$\gamma$) region of Teff cells, resulting in decreased Teff proliferation, increased IgE, and decreased tetanus titer (indicating increased TH2 and decreased TH1 functions). A unique aspect of the study design was the use of monozygotic twins discordant for asthma, thus controlling for genetic background and in utero and early childhood environmental exposures. A study of older children also found differential methylation patterns in the IFN-$\gamma$ and FOXP3 genes in T cell populations of children with asthma exposed to SHS (Kohli et al. 2012).

## *Tobacco Smoke and Epigenetic Modulation*

Recent evidence suggests that exposure to environmental tobacco smoke may lead to the development of specific asthma subtypes, particularly if this exposure occurs during the prenatal period, which has been found to represent a critical period for immune system development. Several studies have evaluated the effect of prenatal tobacco exposure on modulation of the epigenome and subsequent levels of gene expression and associations to the development of asthma and allergic phenotypes. Evaluation of 384 children participating in the Children's Health Study demonstrated differential DNA methylation patterns among children exposed to in utero smoking in eight different genes, including the previously linked GSTM1 gene (Li 2008). The methylation pattern of the TSLP gene was also found to be different among a Taiwanese cohort of children with prenatal tobacco exposure and atopic dermatitis (Wang et al. 2013). A cross-sectional study of adults from the Lovelace Smokers Cohort described differential methylation of multiple genes, including protocadherin-20 in the sputum DNA of older smokers (Sood et al. 2012).

### *Direct Effects on Bacterial Pathogens*

Research has focused primarily on the direct effects of tobacco smoke on the airway mucosa, with the increased risk of infection presumed to be related to impaired host defense. Recent studies suggest that tobacco smoke also exerts direct effects on the bacteria present on the airway surface, increasing the propensity for biofilms. Sinonasal culture taken from adults with mucoprurulent secretions of 34 patients showed that bacteria isolated from patients with tobacco smoke exposure demonstrate in vitro biofilm formation when challenged with tobacco smoke compared to those isolated from smoke-naïve patients. Bacteria from smoke-exposed patients can revert to a non-biofilm phenotype when grown in the absence of tobacco smoke (Goldstein-Daruech et al. 2011).

### *Differential Susceptibility*

Nasal inhalation challenge studies demonstrate differential effects on congestion and mucociliary clearance, providing models to explore inherited or acquired endo-phenotypes (Bascom et al. 1991, 1995). Studies of ECP genotype (GG allele) related to low $FEV_1$ and nonallergic asthma demonstrate another approach to seeking determinants of susceptibility to tobacco smoke (Jonsson 2010).

## Research Needs and Future Directions

1. How do asthma and rhinitis/CRS associated with tobacco smoke exposure differ from asthma and rhinitis/CRS unassociated with tobacco smoke exposure? Is there a distinct asthma endo/phenotype (biomarkers, gene, and protein arrays) associated with tobacco smoke exposure?

In recent years, much attention has been devoted to identifying asthma phenotypes, or endotypes, having distinct pathogenic origins and responses to medical therapy. Cluster analysis was used (Haldar et al. 2008; Moore et al. 2010) as a data-driven way to identify novel asthma endotypes. Similar methods have attempted to explore whether tobacco exposure leads to the development of a unique asthma endotype, but further work is necessary to longitudinally validate these early studies and determine whether these endotypes correspond to differential responses to medications (Howrylak et al. 2010).

Investigators originally described asthma as a disease characterized by respiratory symptoms, reversible airflow obstruction, and bronchial hyperreactivity; later definitions also emphasized the chronic airway inflammation and epithelial injury. Investigators now acknowledge that asthma is probably not a single disease but separate syndromes that overlap (Chanez and Godard 2006).

Potential phenotypic categories relate to clinical or physiologic phenotypes (severity-defined, exacerbation-prone, defined by chronic restriction, treatment resistance, and defined by age of onset); phenotype related to specific triggers (aspirin or nonsteroid anti-inflammatory drugs, environmental allergens, occupational allergens or irritants, menses, or exercise); or inflammatory phenotypes (eosinophilic, neutrophilic, or pauci-granulocytic) (Wenzel 2006). Four proposed specific endotypes are (1) hereditary, early-onset allergic asthma; (2) poorly reversible, very severe, neutrophilic asthma; (3) late-onset eosinophilic asthma; and (4) late-onset symptom-dominant obese minimal inflammation (Wenzel 2012a, b). The contribution of tobacco smoke to the latter three remains to be defined.

"Difficult asthma" was defined as "asthma, poorly controlled in terms of chronic symptoms, with episodic exacerbations, persistent and variable airway obstruction and continue requirement for short-acting β2 agonists and a reasonable dose of inhaled corticosteroids." Some investigators argue that the term severe asthma should be "reserved for those who have refractory asthma after extensive re-evaluation and an appropriate observation period of at least 6 months (Chanez and Godard 2006). The data summarized herein suggest that concomitant measurement of a biomarker of tobacco smoke exposure should be part of the evaluation of patients with "difficult asthma."

The relationship between ETS exposure and adult asthma is complex and includes consideration of persistent child-onset asthma and incident (adult-onset) asthma (Eisner and Blanc 2002). Individuals with asthma may have had in utero exposure, childhood ETS exposure, and adult ETS exposure. The child-onset asthma may or may not have been related to childhood ETS exposure. Recent studies examining the relationship between current ETS exposure and prevalent asthma do not attempt to examine this level of detail mentioned by Eisner (Eisner and Blanc 2002b).

2. What pharmacotherapy will improve asthma and rhinitis/CRS associated with tobacco smoke exposure?

Another area in which further research is necessary is in the area of drug development, specifically the development of new therapies to manage asthmatic and rhinitic patients with tobacco exposure. Given the observed modulation of corticosteroid responsiveness that occurs with tobacco exposure, developing such therapies will be important in the management of patient with asthma and tobacco exposure and resistance to corticosteroid therapy. Ongoing research has led to novel insights into the pathogenesis of obstructive lung diseases, such as asthma and COPD, and has led to the development of several new therapeutic agents targeting specific inflammatory pathways involved in these processes, including roflumilast (Fabbri et al. 2009; Calverley et al. 2009; Rabe et al. 2005) and a mitogen-activated protein kinase (MAPK) inhibitor, which is currently undergoing clinical trials for the management of COPD (Macnee et al. 2013). The inflammatory pathways targeted by these drugs have also been implicated in asthma (Gauvreau et al. 2011; Jin et al. 2010; Himes et al. 2013; Chang et al. 2012; Chung 2011) and could contribute to the growing arsenal of targeted asthma pharmacotherapies.

3. Future directions

A recent publication, "Scientific Standards for Studies on Modified Risk Tobacco Products" (Committee on Scientific Standards 2012), highlights change in tobacco health effects stakeholders: Congress has charged the Food and Drug Administration (FDA) with regulating the marketing of modified risk tobacco products—creating the unprecedented situation of bringing tobacco-related health effect research out of the shadows—and establishing criteria for measuring reduced harm. Why is this important? Because tobacco products have always been changing—but their composition has been privately held information, not reportable to any public authority. In order for a company—tobacco or pharmaceutical—to market their new products as a modified risk tobacco product, the product information will need to be submitted to and reviewed by the FDA. This creates an opportunity for biomarker development based on more precise product information.

Another landmark publication of the past decade has been the National Academy of Sciences book "Toxicity Testing in the 21st Century: A Vision and a Strategy" (Committee on Toxicity Testing 2007). This document challenges the discipline of toxicology to re-invent itself based on an understanding of pathways of toxicity, rather than an accumulation of morbidity and mortality dose–response curves for human and animal species. For the respiratory tract this presents a formidable challenge: in the human lung there are between 25 and 40+ different cells and the pathways and regulatory mechanisms for many of these cells remain poorly understood (Crapo et al. 1982).

Development of a lexicon for this effort continues. Following the conventions of pathogen-associated molecular patterns (PAMPS), Bianchi proposed conceptualizing damage-associated molecular patterns (DAMPS) and credited Joost Oppenheim with proposing the term "alarmin" for endogenous molecules that signal tissue and cell damage. Bianchi articulated that "a complete system for the detection, containment and repair of damage caused to cells in an organism requires warning signals, cells to respond to them via receptors and signaling pathways, and outputs in the form of physiologic responses" (Bianchi 2007).

Adopting this lexicon, the research agenda for tobacco smoke, asthma, and rhinitis/CRS can be summarized as a search for the DAMPS and alarmins that define these exposures and identify individuals susceptible to their effects.

## Summary

Asthma and rhinitis are prevalent conditions with significant morbidity and societal impact.

Tobacco smoke exposure, whether through active or passive smoking, remains widespread, albeit widely varying intensity across different countries and sectors of society. Shifting patterns of smoking and the emergence of modified risk tobacco products provide opportunities to understand better the impact of tobacco smoke on common diseases.

Evolving definitions focus on endo-phenotypes as both asthma and rhinitis are broad diagnoses consisting of different disease entities with different pathogenesis.

There is a critical need for understanding pathways of toxicity and deriving appropriate biomarkers. These will need to include fundamental mechanisms/pathogenesis of tobacco smoke-associated asthma and rhinitis in order to develop rational therapy. CRS associated with tobacco smoke appears more similar to bronchiectasis or chronic bronchitis.

Whether the broad bands of non-allergic rhinitis and asthma are a "common airway disease" remains to be elucidated.

The research into mechanisms of pathogenesis should include the effect of tobacco smoke on the microbiome as limited data suggest important effects.

The central pharmacologic approaches to asthma are demonstrably ineffective in asthma associated with tobacco smoke exposure. Active smokers demonstrate adverse effects related to their SHS exposure; the medical treatment of active smokers differs from nonsmokers with decreased efficacy of the main pharmacotherapeutic agents; and some effects of disease biomarkers emerging among active smokers with asthma deserve exploration in those with SHS.

## References

Annesi-Maesano I et al. Relationship of upper airway disease to tobacco smoking and allergic markers: a cohort study of men followed up for 5 years. Int Arch Allergy Immunol. 1997;114(2):193–201.

Annesi-Maesano I. Epidemiological evidence of the occurrence of rhinitis and sinusitis in asthmatics. Allergy. 1999;54:7–13.

Apseloff G et al. The importance of measuring cotinine levels to identify smokers in clinical trials. Clin Pharmacol Ther. 1994;56(4):460–2.

Arif AA et al. Prevalence and risk factors of asthma and wheezing among US adults: an analysis of the NHANES III data. Eur Respir J. 2003;21(5):827–33.

Aurrekoetxea J, et al. Determinants of self-reported smoking and misclassification during pregnancy, and analysis of optimal cut-off points for urinary cotinine: a cross-sectional study. BMJ Open. 2013; 3(1):pii.

Barnes PJ. Reduced histone deacetylase in COPD—clinical implications. Chest. 2006; 129(1):151–5.

Barrow CS. Toxicology of the nasal passages. 1986.

Bascom R et al. Upper respiratory tract environmental tobacco smoke sensitivity. Am Rev Respir Dis. 1991;143(6):1304–11.

Bascom R et al. A portable air cleaner partially reduces the upper respiratory response to sidestream tobacco smoke. Appl Occup Environ Hyg. 1996a;11(6):553–9.
Bascom R, Ellaurie M. Upper airway disorders. In: Rosenstock L, et al., editors. Textbook of clinical occupational and environmental medicine. Philadelphia:Elsevier Health Sciences; 2005.
Bascom R et al. Tobacco smoke upper respiratory response relationships in healthy nonsmokers. Fundam Appl Toxicol. 1996b;29(1):86–93.
Bascom R et al. Sidestream tobacco smoke exposure acutely alters human nasal mucociliary clearance. Environ Health Perspect. 1995;103(11):1026–30.
Bascom R, Dolina MY. Upper airway disorders. In: Rom WN, editor. Environmental and occupational medicine. Philadelphia: Lippincott Williams & Wilkins; 2007.
Bates ML et al. Longitudinal distribution of ozone absorption in the lung: comparison of cigarette smokers and nonsmokers. Toxicol Appl Pharmacol. 2009;236:270–5.
Beatty AL, Haight TJ, Redberg RF. Associations between respiratory illnesses and secondhand smoke exposure in flight attendants: a cross-sectional analysis of the Flight Attendant Medical Research Institute Survey. Environ Health. 2011;10(1):81.
Benninger MS et al. Adult chronic rhinosinusitis: definitions, diagnosis, epidemiology, and pathophysiology. Otolaryngol Head Neck Surg. 2003;129(3 Suppl):S1–32.
Biagini Myers J et al. Asking the right questions to ascertain early childhood secondhand smoke exposures. J Pediatr. 2012;160(6):1050–1.
Bianchi ME. DAMPs, PAMPs and alarmins: all we need to know about danger. J Leukoc Biol. 2007;81(1):1–5.
Bjerg A. Increased prevalence of symptoms of rhinitis but not of asthma between 1990 and 2008 in Swedish adults: comparisons of the ECRHS and GA2LEN surveys. PLoS One. 2011;6(2):e16082.
Blanc PD et al. Impact of the home indoor environment on adult asthma and rhinitis. J Occup Environ Med. 2005;47(4):362–72.
Bousquet PJ et al. Effect of smoking on symptoms of allergic rhinitis. Ann Allergy Asthma Immunol. 2009;103(3):195–200.
Bousquet J, Van Cauwenberge P, Khaltaev N. Allergic rhinitis and its impact on asthma. J Allergy Clin Immunol. 2001;108(5 suppl):S147–334.
Brody A et al. Effect of secondhand smoke on occupancy of nicotinic acetylcholine receptors in brain. Arch Gen Psychiatry. 2011;68(9):953–60.
Broekema M et al. Airway epithelial changes in smokers but not in ex-smokers with asthma. Am J Respir Crit Care Med. 2009;180(12):1170–8.
Byron K, Varigos G, Wootton A. IL-4 production is increased in cigarette smokers. Clin Exp Immunol. 1994;95(2):333–6.
California Environmental Protection Agency. Health effects of exposure to environmental tobacco smoke. Sacramento, CA: Office of Environmental Heath Hazard Assessment; 1997.
Carlsten C et al. Cotinine versus questionnaire: early-life environmental tobacco smoke exposure and incident asthma. BMC Pediatr. 2012;12:187.
Carson JL et al. Phenotypic and physiologic variability in nasal epithelium cultured from smokers and non-smokers exposed to secondhand tobacco smoke. In Vitro Cell Dev Biol Anim. 2010;46(7):606–12. doi: 10.1007/s11626-010-9310-6. Epub 2010 Apr 10.
Calverley P et al. Roflumilast in symptomatic chronic obstructive pulmonary disease: two randomised clinical trials. Lancet. 2009;374(9691):685–94.
Centers for Disease Control and Prevention. Vital signs: nonsmokers' exposure to secondhand smoke—United States, 1999–2008. Morb Mortal Wkly Rep. 2010;59(35):1141–6.
Centers for Disease Control and Prevention. Vital signs: current cigarette smoking among adults aged >= 18 years with mental illness—United States, 2009–2011. Morb Mortal Wkly Rep. 2013;62(5):81–7.
Chalmers G et al. Influence of cigarette smoking on inhaled corticosteroid treatment in mild asthma. Thorax. 2002;57(3):226–30.
Chanez P, Godard P. Is difficult asthma still clinically meaningful? Eur Respir J. 2006;28(5):897–9.

Chang P, et al. Corticosteroid insensitivity of chemokine expression in airway smooth muscle of patients with severe asthma. J Allergy Clin Immunol. 2012; 130(4).
Chaudhuri R et al. Cigarette smoking impairs the therapeutic response to oral corticosteroids in chronic asthma. Am J Respir Crit Care Med. 2003;168(11):1308–11.
Chaudhuri R et al. Role of symptoms and lung function in determining asthma control in smokers with asthma. Allergy. 2008;63(1):132–5.
Chung K. p38 mitogen-activated protein kinase pathways in asthma and COPD. Chest. 2011; 139(6).
Churg A et al. Tumor necrosis factor-alpha is central to acute cigarette smoke-induced inflammation and connective tissue breakdown. Am J Respir Crit Care Med. 2002;166(6):849–54.
Cohen R et al. In utero smoke exposure and impaired response to inhaled corticosteroids in children with asthma. J Allergy Clin Immunol. 2010;126(3):491–7.
Committee on Scientific Standards for Studies on Modified Risk Tobacco Products. Scientific standards for studies on modified risk tobacco products. Institute of Medicine of the National Academies; 2012.
Committee on Toxicity Testing and Assessment of Environmental Agents, National Research Council. Toxicity testing in the 21st century: a vision and a strategy. 2007.
Costabel U, Guzman J. Effect of smoking on bronchoalveolar lavage constituents. Eur Respir J. 1992;5(7):776–9.
Crapo JD et al. Cell number and cell characteristics of the normal human lung. Am Rev Respir Dis. 1982;126(2):332–7.
Dietz P et al. Estimates of nondisclosure of cigarette smoking among pregnant and nonpregnant women of reproductive age in the United States. Am J Epidemiol. 2010;173(3):355–9.
Dimich-Ward H. Analysis of nicotine and cotinine in the hair of hospitality workers exposed to environmental tobacco smoke. J Occup Environ Med. 1997;39(10):946–8.
Do R et al. Within- and between-person variability of exhaled breath condensate pH and NH4+ in never and current smokers. Respir Med. 2008;102(3):457–63.
Dweik RA et al. An official ATS clinical practice guideline: interpretation of exhaled nitric oxide levels (FENO) for clinical applications. Am J Respir Crit Care Med. 2011;184(5):602–15.
Ebbert JO et al. Association between respiratory tract diseases and secondhand smoke exposure among never smoking flight attendants: a cross-sectional survey. Environ Health. 2007;6:28.
Eder W, Ege MJ, von Mutius E. The asthma epidemic. N Engl J Med. 2006;355:2226–35.
Eisner MD, Blanc PD. Environmental tobacco smoke exposure during travel among adults with asthma. Chest. 2002;122(3):826–8.
Eisner MD et al. Exposure to indoor combustion and adult asthma outcomes: environmental tobacco smoke, gas stoves, and woodsmoke. Thorax. 2002a;57(11):973–8.
Eisner MD. Environmental tobacco smoke and adult asthma. Clin Chest Med. 2002b;23(4): 749–61.
EPR. Expert panel report: guidelines for the diagnosis and management of asthma (EPR 1991). Bethesda, MD: U.S. Department of Health and Human Service; National Institutes of Health; National Heart, Lung, and Blood Institute; National Asthma Education and Prevention Program; 1991.
EPR-2. Expert panel report 2: guidelines for the diagnosis and management of asthma (EPR-2 1997), 1997. Bethesda, MD: U.S. Department of Health and Human Services; National Institutes of Health; National Heart, Lung, and Blood Institute; National Asthma Education and Prevention Program; 1997.
EPR-3. Expert panel report 3: guidelines for the diagnosis and management of asthma. Full report 2007. U.S. Department of Health and Human Services, National Institutes of Health, National Heart, Lung, and Blood Institute, National Asthma Education and Prevention Program.
Fabbri L et al. Roflumilast in moderate-to-severe chronic obstructive pulmonary disease treated with longacting bronchodilators: two randomised clinical trials. Lancet. 2009;374(9691): 695–703.
Flodin U et al. An epidemiologic study of bronchial asthma and smoking. Epidemiology. 1995;6(5):503–5.

Foulds J et al. Effect of transdermal nicotine patches on cigarette smoking: a double blind crossover study. Psychopharmacology (Berl). 1992;106(3):421–7.

Gauvreau G et al. Roflumilast attenuates allergen-induced inflammation in mild asthmatic subjects. Respir Res. 2011;12:140.

Gerrard JW et al. Immunoglobulin levels in smokers and non-smokers. Ann Allergy. 1980;44(5):261–2.

Goldstein-Daruech N et al. Tobacco smoke mediated induction of sinonasal microbial biofilms. PLoS One. 2011;6(1):e15700.

Gomez M et al. Adolescent smokers are at greater risk for current asthma and rhinitis. Int J Tuberc Lung Dis. 2009;13(8):1023–8.

Goncalves R et al. Impact of smoking on inflammation: overview of molecular mechanisms. Inflamm Res. 2011;60(5):409–24.

Greer JR, Abbey DE, Burchette RJ. Asthma related to occupational and ambient air pollutants in nonsmokers. J Occup Med. 1993;35(9):909–15.

Gupta D et al. Household environmental tobacco smoke exposure, respiratory symptoms and asthma in non-smoker adults: a multicentric population study from India. Indian J Chest Dis Allied Sci. 2006;48(1):31–6.

Hakansson K et al. Nonallergic rhinitis and its association with smoking and lower airway disease: a general population study. Am J Rhinol Allergy. 2011;25(1):25–9.

Haldar P et al. Cluster analysis and clinical asthma phenotypes. Am J Respir Crit Care Med. 2008;178(3):218–24.

Harris JK et al. Demographic and geographic differences in exposure to secondhand smoke in Missouri workplaces, 2007–2008. Prev Chronic Dis. 2011;8(6):A135.

Hasday J, Dubin W, Fitzgerald T, Bascom R. Cigarettes are a rich source of bacterial endotoxin. Chest. 1996;109:63S–4.

Hersoug LG et al. Indoor exposure to environmental cigarette smoke, but not other inhaled particulates associates with respiratory symptoms and diminished lung function in adults. Respirology. 2010;15(6):993–1000.

Himes S et al. Prenatal tobacco exposure, biomarkers for tobacco in meconium, and neonatal growth outcomes. J Pediatr. 2013;162(5):970–5.

Himes BE et al. Genome-wide association analysis identifies PDE4D as an asthma-susceptibility gene. Am J Hum Genet. 2009;84(5):581–93.

Higgins MW, Keller JB, Metzner HL. Smoking, socioeconomic status, and chronic respiratory disease. Am Rev Respir Dis. 1977;116(3):403–10.

Ho SY et al. Cross-sectional and prospective associations between passive smoking and respiratory symptoms at the workplace. Ann Epidemiol. 2007;17(2):126–31.

Horváth I, Donnelly LE, Kiss A, Balint B, Kharitonov SA, Barnes PJ. Exhaled nitric oxide and hydrogen peroxide concentration in asthmatic smokers. Respiration. 2004;71:463–8.

Howrylak J, et al. Using spectral clustering of phenotypes to identify novel asthma subtypes. Am J Resp Crit Care Med. 2010; A1877.

Hu FB et al. An epidemiological study of asthma prevalence and related factors among young adults. J Asthma. 1997;34(1):67–76.

International Rhinitis Management Working Group. International consensus report on diagnosis and management of rhinitis. Allergy. 1994;49(19 suppl):1–34.

Ito K, Barnes P, Adcock I. Glucocorticoid receptor recruitment of histone deacetylase 2 inhibits interleukin-1beta-induced histone H4 acetylation on lysines 8 and 12. Mol Cell Biol. 2000;20(18):6891–903.

Janson C et al. Effect of passive smoking on respiratory symptoms, bronchial responsiveness, lung function, and total serum IgE in the European Community Respiratory Health Survey: a cross-sectional study. Lancet. 2001;358(9299):2103–9.

Janson C et al. Changes in active and passive smoking in the European Community Respiratory Health Survey. Eur Respir J. 2006;27(3):517–24.

Jatakanon A. Neutrophilic inflammation in severe persistent asthma. Am J Respir Crit Care Med. 1999;160(5):1532–9.

Jin S et al. Phosphodiesterase 4B is essential for T(H)2-cell function and development of airway hyperresponsiveness in allergic asthma. J Allergy Clin Immunol. 2010;126(6):1252–9.e12.
Juniper E. Measuring health-related quality of life in rhinitis. J Allergy Clin Immunol. 1997;99:S742–9.
Kesavan J et al. The relationship between particle deposition in the anterior nasal passage and nasal passage characteristics. J Aerosol Med. 2000;13(1):17–23.
Kesavanathan J, Bascom R, Swift DL. The effect of nasal passage characteristics on particle deposition. J Aerosol Med. 1998;11(1):27–39.
Kohli A, et al. Secondhand smoke in combination with ambient air pollution exposure is associated with increasedx CpG methylation and decreased expression of IFN-gamma in T effector cells and Foxp3 in T regulatory cells in children. Clin Epigenetics. 2012; 4(1).
Kraev T et al. Indoor concentrations of nicotine in low-income, multi-unit housing: associations with smoking behaviours and housing characteristics. Tob Control. 2009;18(6):438–44.
Kvalvik L et al. Self-reported smoking status and plasma cotinine concentrations among pregnant women in the Norwegian Mother and Child Cohort Study. Pediatr Res. 2012;72(1):101–7.
Lanza DC, Kennedy DW. Adult rhinosinusitis defined. Otolaryngol Head Neck Surg. 1997;117(3 Pt 2):S1–7.
Larsson ML et al. Environmental tobacco smoke exposure during childhood is associated with increased prevalence of asthma in adults. Chest. 2001;120(3):711–7.
Lazarus SC et al. Smoking affects response to inhaled corticosteroids or leukotriene receptor antagonists in asthma. Am J Respir Crit Care Med. 2007;175(8):783–90.
Leuenberger P et al. Passive smoking exposure in adults and chronic respiratory symptoms (SAPALDIA Study). Swiss Study on air pollution and lung diseases in adults, SAPALDIA Team. Am J Respir Crit Care Med. 1994;150(5 Pt 1):1222–8.
Li Y-F. Glutathione S-transferase P1, maternal smoking, and asthma in children: a haplotype-based analysis. Environ Health Perspect. 2008;116(3):409–15.
Lieu J, Feinstein A. Confirmations and surprises in the association of tobacco use with sinusitis. Arch Otolaryngol Head Neck Surg. 2000;126:940–6.
Levy D, Rigotti N, Winickoff J. Tobacco smoke exposure in a sample of Boston public housing residents. Am J Prev Med. 2012;44(1):63–6.
Lewis SJ et al. Cotinine levels and self-reported smoking status in patients attending a bronchoscopy clinic. Biomarkers. 2003;8(3–4):218–28.
Lin SY et al. Allergic rhinitis and secondhand tobacco smoke: a population-based study. Am J Rhinol Allergy. 2011;25(2):e66–71.
Linneberg, A., et al. Smoking and the development of allergic sensitization to aeroallergens in adults: a prospective population-based study. The Copenhagen Allergy Study. Allergy 2001; 56(4):328-332.
Lotvall J, Akdis CA, Bacharier LB, et al. Asthma endotypes: a new approach to classification of disease entities within the asthma syndrome. J Allergy Clin Immunol. 2011;127:355–60.
Lund VJ, Kennedy DW. Quantification for staging sinusitis. The Staging and Therapy Group. Ann Otol Rhinol Laryngol Suppl. 1995;167:17–21.
Manoli S et al. Maternal smoking and the retinoid pathway in the developing lung. Respir Res. 2012;13:42.
Macnee W et al. Efficacy and safety of the oral p38 inhibitor PH-797804 in chronic obstructive pulmonary disease: a randomised clinical trial. Thorax. 2013;68(8):738–45.
McSharry CP et al. Short and long-term effects of cigarette smoking independently influence exhaled nitric oxide concentration in asthma. J Allergy Clin Immunol. 2005;116(1):88–93.
McWhorter WP, Polis MA, Kaslow RA. Occurrence, predictors, and consequences of adult asthma in NHANESI and follow-up survey. Am Rev Respir Dis. 1989;139(3):721–4.
Michils A et al. Exhaled nitric oxide as a marker of asthma control in smoking patients. Eur Respir J. 2009;33(6):1295–301.
Miyake Y et al. Association of active and passive smoking with allergic disorders in pregnant Japanese women: baseline data from the Osaka Maternal and Child Health Study. Ann Allergy Asthma Immunol. 2005;94(6):644–51.

Montano-Velazquez BB et al. Rhinomanometry in young patients with perennial allergic rhinitis with/without recent exposure to tobacco smoke. Clin Otolaryngol. 2011;36(4):320–4.
Moore W et al. Identification of asthma phenotypes using cluster analysis in the Severe Asthma Research Program. Am J Respir Crit Care Med. 2010;181(4):315–23.
Muscat JE, Richie JP, Stellman SD. Mentholated cigarettes and smoking habits in whites and blacks. Tob Control. 2002;11(4):368–71.
Oryszczyn MP et al. Relationships of active and passive smoking to total IgE in adults of the Epidemiological Study of the Genetics and Environment of Asthma, Bronchial Hyperresponsiveness, and Atopy (EGEA). Am J Respir Crit Care Med. 2000;161(4 Pt 1): 1241–6.
Osborne ML et al. Assessing future need for acute care in adult asthmatics: the profile of Asthma Risk Study: a prospective health maintenance organization-based study. Chest. 2007;132(4):1151–61.
Pearce N et al. Comparison of asthma prevalence in the ISAAC and the ECRHS. Eur Respir J. 2000;16(3):420–6.
Pedersen B et al. Eosinophil and neutrophil activity in asthma in a one-year trial with inhaled budesonide. The impact of smoking. Am J Respir Crit Care Med. 1996;153(5):1519–29.
Polosa R et al. Greater severity of new onset asthma in allergic subjects who smoke: a 10-year longitudinal study. Respir Res. 2011;12(1):16.
Rabe K et al. Roflumilast–an oral anti-inflammatory treatment for chronic obstructive pulmonary disease: a randomised controlled trial. Lancet. 2005;366(9485):563–71.
Radon K et al. Passive smoking exposure: a risk factor for chronic bronchitis and asthma in adults? Chest. 2002;122(3):1086–90.
Reh DD et al. Secondhand tobacco smoke exposure and chronic rhinosinusitis: a population-based case-control study. Am J Rhinol Allergy. 2009;23(6):562–7.
Rennard SI et al. Evaluation of subclinical respiratory tract inflammation in heavy smokers who switch to a cigarette-like nicotine delivery device that primarily heats tobacco. Nicotine Tob Res. 2002;4(4):467–76.
Runyon RS et al. Asthma discordance in twins is linked to epigenetic modifications of T cells. PLoS One. 2012;7(11):e48796.
Samet JM. Adverse effects of smoke exposure on the upper airway. Tob Control. 2004;13 Suppl 1:i57–60.
Schenker MB, Samet JM, Speizer FE. Effect of cigarette tar content and smoking habits on respiratory symptoms in women. Am Rev Respir Dis. 1982;125(6):684–90.
Sebastian A, Pehrson C, Larsson L. Elevated concentrations of endotoxin in indoor air due to cigarette smoking. J Environ Monit. 2006;8(5):519–22.
Shipton D et al. Reliability of self reported smoking status by pregnant women for estimating smoking prevalence: a retrospective, cross sectional study. BMJ. 2009;339:b4347.
Shusterman D. Environmental nonallergic rhinitis. Clin Allergy Immunol. 2007;19:249–66.
Silverman RA et al. Cigarette smoking among asthmatic adults presenting to 64 emergency departments. Chest. 2003;123(5):1472–9.
Simoni M et al. Respiratory symptoms/diseases and environmental tobacco smoke (ETS) in never smoker Italian women. Respir Med. 2007;101(3):531–8.
Sippel JM et al. Associations of smoking with hospital-based care and quality of life in patients with obstructive airway disease. Chest. 1999;115(3):691–6.
Siroux V et al. Relationships of active smoking to asthma and asthma severity in the EGEA study. Epidemiological study on the Genetics and Environment of Asthma. Eur Respir J. 2000;15(3):470–7.
Smith J, et al. Estimating cotinine associations and a saliva cotinine level to identify active cigarette smoking in Alaska native pregnant women. 2013.
Sood A et al. Methylated genes in Sputum among older smokers with asthma. Chest. 2012;142(2):425–31.
Spanier A et al. Comparison of biomarkers and parent report of tobacco exposure to predict wheeze. J Pediatr. 2011;159(5):776–82.

Spencer K, Cowans N. Accuracy of self-reported smoking status in first trimester aneuploidy screening. Prenat Diagn. 2013;33(3):245–50.

Strachan DP, Cook DG. Health effects of passive smoking. 5. Parental smoking and allergic sensitisation in children. Thorax. 1998;53(2):117–23.

Strickland I et al. High constitutive glucocorticoid receptor beta in human neutrophils enables them to reduce their spontaneous rate of cell death in response to corticosteroids. J Exp Med. 2001;193(5):585–93.

Sunyer J. Smoking and bronchial responsiveness in nonatopic and atopic young adults. Spanish Group of the European Study of Asthma. Thorax. 1997;52(3):235–8.

Tamimi A, Serdarevic D, Hanania N. The effects of cigarette smoke on airway inflammation in asthma and COPD: therapeutic implications. Respir Med. 2012;106(3):319–28.

Tammemagi CM et al. Secondhand smoke as a potential cause of chronic rhinosinusitis: a case-control study. Arch Otolaryngol Head Neck Surg. 2010;136(4):327–34.

Tanou K et al. Inflammatory and oxidative stress biomarkers in allergic rhinitis: the effect of smoking. Clin Exp Allergy. 2009;39(3):345–53.

Taylor D et al. Exhaled nitric oxide measurements: clinical application and interpretation. Thorax. 2006;61(9):817–27.

Thorn J, Brisman J, Toren K. Adult-onset asthma is associated with self-reported mold or environmental tobacco smoke exposures in the home. Allergy. 2001;56(4):287–92.

Togias A. Rhinitis and asthma: evidence for respiratory system integration. J Allergy Clin Immunol. 2003;111(6):1171–83. quiz 1184.

Topp R et al. The effect of environmental tobacco smoke exposure on allergic sensitization and allergic rhinitis in adults. Indoor Air. 2005;15(4):222–7.

Troisi RJ et al. Cigarette smoking and incidence of chronic bronchitis and asthma in women. Chest. 1995;108(6):1557–61.

Tsoumakidou M et al. Cigarette smoking alters bronchial mucosal immunity in asthma. Am J Respir Crit Care Med. 2007;175(9):919–25.

U.S. Department of Health, Education, and Welfare. Smoking and health: report of the advisory committee to the surgeon general of the public health service. Washington: U.S. Department of Health, Education, and Welfare, Public Health Service, Center for Disease Control; 1964.

U.S. Department of Health and Human Services Public Health Service Office on Smoking and Health. The changing cigarette: a report of the surgeon general. 1981.

U.S. Department of Health and Human Services. The health consequences of involuntary smoking. a report of the surgeon general. Rockville, MD: U.S. Department of Health and Human Services, Public Health Service, Centers for Disease Control, Center for Health Promotion and Education, Office on Smoking and Health; 1986. DHHS publication no. (CDC) 87-8398.

U.S. Department of Health and Human Services. The health benefits of smoking cessation, 1990. U.S. Department of Health and Human Services. Public Health Service. Centers for Disease Control. Center for Chronic Disease Prevention and Health Promotion. Office on Smoking and Health; 1990.

U.S. Department of Health and Human Services, editor. The health consequences of smoking: a report of the surgeon general. Atlanta, GA: U.S. Department of Health and Human Services, Centers for Disease Control and Prevention, National Center for Chronic Disease Prevention and Health Promotion, Office on Smoking and Health; 2004.

U.S. Department of Health and Human Services, editor. The health consequences of involuntary exposure to tobacco smoke: a report of the surgeon general. Atlanta, GA: U.S. Department of Health and Human Services, Centers for Disease Control and Prevention, Coordinating Center for Health Promotion, National Center for Chronic Disease Prevention and Health Promotion, Office on Smoking and Health; 2006.

van Eeden S, Hogg J. The response of human bone marrow to chronic cigarette smoking. Eur Respir J. 2000;15(5):915–21.

Van Hoydonck PGA et al. Quantitative analysis of 8-isoprostane and hydrogen peroxide in exhaled breath condensate. Eur Respir J. 2004;23(2):189–92.

Verleden GM, Dupont LJ, Verpeut AC, Demedts MG. The effect of cigarette smoking on exhaled nitric oxide in mild steroid–naive asthmatics. Chest. 1999;116:59–64.

Vesterinen E, Kaprio J, Koskenvuo M. Prospective study of asthma in relation to smoking habits among 14,729 adults. Thorax. 1988;43:534–9.

Wang J, et al. Differential activation of killer cells in the circulation and the lung: a study of current smoking status and chronic obstructive pulmonary disease (COPD). PLoS One. 2013; 8(3).

Webster J et al. Proinflammatory cytokines regulate human glucocorticoid receptor gene expression and lead to the accumulation of the dominant negative beta isoform: a mechanism for the generation of glucocorticoid resistance. Proc Natl Acad Sci USA. 2001;98(12):6865–70.

Wenzel S. Severe asthma: from characteristics to phenotypes to endotypes. Clin Exp Allergy. 2012a;42(5):650–8.

Wenzel SE. Asthma: defining of the persistent adult phenotypes. Lancet. 2006;368(9537): 804–13.

Wenzel S. Asthma phenotypes: the evolution from clinical to molecular approaches. Nat Med. 2012b;18(5):716–25.

Wieslander G et al. Changes in the ocular and nasal signs and symptoms of aircrews in relation to the ban on smoking on intercontinental flights. Scand J Work Environ Health. 2000;26(6):514–22.

Wilson K et al. Tobacco-smoke exposure in children who live in multiunit housing. Pediatrics. 2010;127(1):85–92.

Wright T, Collier A. Agreement of umbilical cord drug and cotinine levels with maternal self-report of drug use and smoking during pregnancy. J Perinatol. 2012; 32(2).

Wright T et al. Agreement of umbilical cord drug and cotinine levels with maternal self-report of drug use and smoking during pregnancy. J Perinatol. 2011;31(5):324–9.

Zetterstrom O et al. Another smoking hazard: raised serum IgE concentration and increased risk of occupational allergy. Br Med J (Clin Res Ed). 1981;283(6301):1215–7.

Zhu A et al. The ability of plasma cotinine to predict nicotine and carcinogen exposure is altered by differences in CYP2A6: the influence of genetics, race, and sex. Cancer Epidemiol Biomarkers Prev. 2013;22(4):708–18.

# Chapter 7
# Irritant and Airborne Contact Dermatitis

**Payton A. Kuhlenbeck and Tanner J. Parrent**

**Abstract** Understanding and recognizing contact dermatitis is a vital tool in any healthcare provider's armamentarium. Making the correct diagnosis will not only lead to the appropriate treatment of your patient but also save the healthcare system excessive, unnecessary costs. Contact dermatitis is an eczematous reaction that encompasses two major forms: irritant and allergic. While clinical appearance can often be indistinguishable, the pathophysiology, etiology, and history are often very different. Irritant contact dermatitis (ICD) can be thought of as a direct toxic effect on the skin by an irritant while allergic contact dermatitis (ACD) is a hypersensitivity reaction to an allergen.

Airborne contact dermatitis can be caused by various substances that come into contact with the skin via an aerosolized or an airborne form. Both ICD and ACD are included in this category. Together, irritant and airborne contact dermatitis comprise a majority of the diseases that have been labeled as occupational contact dermatitis (OCD). Each year, OCD leads to the indirect and direct costs of nearly a billion dollars in lost wages and medical expenses.

**Keywords** Contact • Dermatitis • Airborne • Allergic • Irritant • Occupational skin diseases

P.A. Kuhlenbeck, B.S. • T.J. Parrent, M.D. (✉)
Division of Dermatology, Department of Medicine, Brody School of Medicine at East Carolina University, Greenville, NC, USA
e-mail: parent@ecu.edu

W.J. Meggs (ed.), *The Toxicant Induction of Irritant Asthma, Rhinitis, and Related Conditions*, DOI 10.1007/978-1-4614-9044-9_7,

## Introduction

Contact dermatitis is an eczematous reaction that encompasses two major forms: irritant and allergic. While clinical appearance can often be indistinguishable, the pathophysiology, etiology, and history are often very different. Irritant contact dermatitis (ICD) is an inflammatory reaction triggered by activation of the innate immune system by direct contact with a cytotoxic substance. Allergic contact dermatitis (ACD) is a type IV delayed-type hypersensitivity reaction mediated by T-cells (Kanerva 1999).

Airborne contact dermatitis is caused by various toxic substances and allergens that come into contact with the skin via an aerosolized or an airborne form. Both ICD and ACD causes compose this category (Handa et al. 2011). Together, irritant and airborne contact dermatitis comprise a majority of the diseases that have been labeled as occupational contact dermatitis (OCD). OCD is of immense importance as it has led to the indirect and direct costs of nearly a billion dollars in lost wages and medical expenses (McCall et al. 2005).

## Irritant Versus Allergic Contact Dermatitis

Understanding the difference between irritant and allergic contact dermatitis is often difficult from appearance, but several key differences can help elucidate the etiology. Table 7.1 summarizes these differences (Fyhrquist-Vanni et al. 2007).

**Table 7.1** Differences between irritant and allergic contact dermatitis

| | Irritant | Allergic |
|---|---|---|
| Substance | Water, solvents, acids/alkalis, soaps | Low-molecular-weight allergen |
| Concentration | Often high amounts at lengthy exposure | Can be very low |
| Mechanism | Nonimmunologic, cytotoxic effect to epidermis | Type IV delayed-type hypersensitivity reaction |
| Onset | Immediate (hours) | Delayed (days) |
| Symptom | Pain and burning | Itch |
| Distribution | Often indistinct borders | Corresponds well to exposed skin (leather sandals, nickel jewelry, rubber material in underwear) |
| Immunology | No activated T-cells present | Activated T-cells present |
| Patch testing | Negative | Positive |
| Therapy | Avoidance and protection from prolonged exposure | Absolute avoidance |

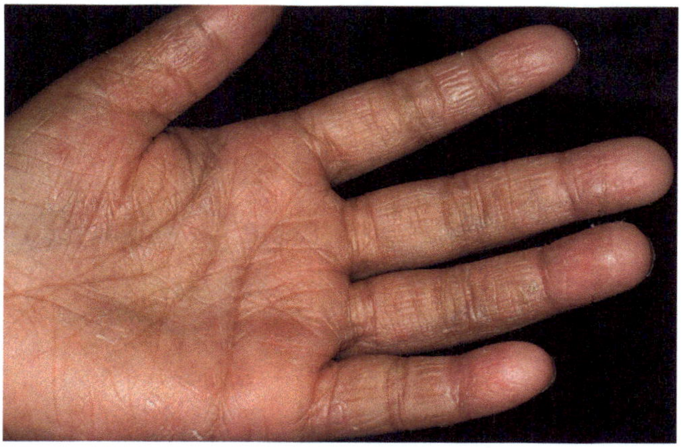

**Fig. 7.1** An example of irritant hand dermatitis

## Irritant Contact Dermatitis

### *Epidemiology*

ICD comprises about 70–80 % of contact dermatitis cases. Most of the causes of ICD are due to the direct toxic effect of a substance on the epidermal keratinocytes. The array of expression of ICD varies greatly from dryness of the skin to actual burns. Often it is the nature of the substance, concentration, and length of exposure that determine the severity of the reaction (Fyhrquist-Vanni et al. 2007). Many cases can be attributed to one's occupation. The classic example is housewife's hand eczema, which is caused from repeated exposure to water (handwashing, dishwashing, child bathing, etc.). Often the patient does not realize that a substance as mild as water is causing their painful, dry, and cracked hand eczema. Figure 7.1 contrasts irritant hand dermatitis with Fig. 7.2 allergic hand dermatitis.

### *Pathophysiology*

The exact cellular mechanisms of ICD are still largely unknown. Three basic steps can be thought of when trying to understand the pathogenesis of an ICD reaction. (1) Cytotoxic or direct injury to the epidermal keratinocytes leads to necrosis, apoptosis, and activation of the innate immune response. This can occur in both acute and chronic phases. The more toxic substances that cause direct keratinocyte damage lead to the acute ICD. The substances, like solvents and detergents, degrade the lipid barrier of the epidermis leading to a slower destruction of the keratinocytes and a chronic ICD picture. (2) The cellular necrosis and apoptosis lead to the release of

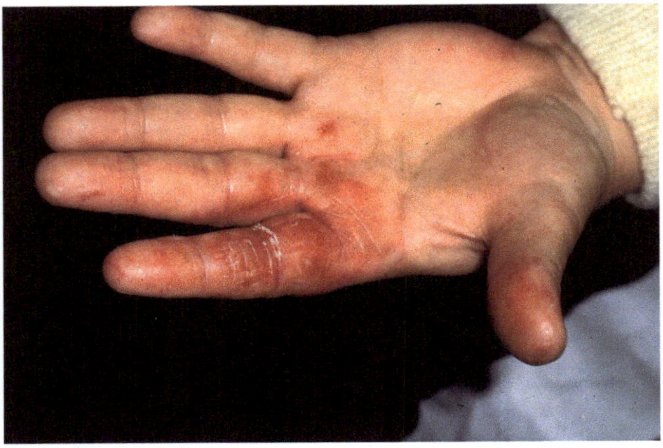

**Fig. 7.2** An example of allergic contact dermatitis of the hand

inflammatory chemokines and cytokines which in turn causes leukocyte recruitment. (3) The inflammatory infiltrate that responds to the irritant causes the local inflammation which is clinically portrayed as spongiotic dermatitis, also known as eczema (Nosbaum et al. 2009).

## *Features and Causes*

As mentioned above, the spectrum of ICD can range from xerotic, dry skin to burns depending on the nature and exposure of the irritant. Commonly, ICDs present as dry, scaly, fissured skin that is often painful and occasionally bleeding. Below, we discuss several of the common causes of ICD.

## *Acids*

Acids are corrosive substances that can be separated into inorganic and organic categories. Acids cause damage to the epidermis both through direct toxicity and denaturation of proteins. The inorganic acids are often used in industrial work and include nitric acid, sulfuric acid, hydrochloric acid, hydrofluoric acid, and phosphoric acid among others. The reactions of each are different but all cause a general redness, vesiculation, and cell necrosis. Sulfuric acid is often used by iron, brass, bronze, and copper workers and can cause a brownish charring of the skin (Flammiger and Maibach 2006). Hydrofluoric acid is one of the strongest inorganic acids and is used as a rust remover as well as in plastics and glass etching. Exposure to it can cause severe ICD resulting in ulceration (Stuke et al. 2008).

Organic acids include acetic, formic, benzoic, glycolic, and salicylic acids and often tend to be less irritating. Several of these acids are used in the cosmetic industry in chemical peels and facewash for acne treatment. Prolonged exposure to certain individuals can cause redness, dryness, and fissuring of the skin.

## *Alkalis*

Alkalis are caustic substances such as lye soaps, detergents, bleach, ammonia, oven cleaner, and drain pipe cleaner, amongst others that tend to be more irritating to the skin than acids. They are capable of degrading the lipid barrier and denaturing epidermal proteins. This often leaves the skin unprotected, hard, dry, and cracked. Occupational exposures occur in workers linked to the industries which provide the products listed above (Baxter et al. 2004).

## *Solvents*

Solvents are often organic molecules used in industry for purposes such as chemical synthesis, degreasing, paint removal, as well as personal use such as nail polish remover. Solvents cause ICD by degrading the epidermal lipid barrier producing dry, painful, and fissured skin. Hexane is a component of gasoline as well as a common solvent used in chemical synthesis. Absorption by either inhalation or direct contact with skin can lead to paresthesias and paresis. Other solvents include trichloroethylene, benzene, methylene chloride, xylene, toluene, and turpentine. Xylene is a common irritant in histopathology laboratories, while turpentine is both a known cause of ICD and ACD (Baxter et al. 2004).

## *Unsuspected Causes*

Outside of the industrial causes of ICD, for which there is a countless list, many causes of ICD are common to the entire population. Water is one of the most common causes of ICD as listed above with housewife's hand eczema. Other occupations at risk for water-induced ICD include hairdressers, bartenders, food handlers, and healthcare workers. Often, simple reduction to the exposure to water can aid in relief to these individuals' disease.

Irritant diaper dermatitis is one of the most common, if not the most, causes of ICD. Urine, feces, and occlusive diapers are notorious for causing redness and irritation to exposed skin. Often, skin folds and concave surfaces are spared in these areas. One needs to remember that this can present both in babies and the elderly. Lip-licker's dermatitis is another common cause of ICD. In this case, salvia causes a repeated wetting and drying cycle that leads to production of chronically dry, red, chapped lips.

Food-induced ICD is not only caused from the wet work of preparation and handling but also from innate chemicals within the food itself. Broccoli, cabbage, and cauliflower amongst other vegetables contain isothiocyanate which can cause an ICD in some who handle these products when wet. Pineapple, which contains bromelain, is another example of a food with the ability to cause ICD (Bolognia et al. 2008).

## *Miscellaneous*

The list for causes of ICD is extensive and endless. A literature search of occupational ICD will lead to pages of case reports of various causes for this condition. Other broad categories include metal salts, hydrocarbons, fiberglass, airbags, capsaicin, disinfectants, plastics, as well as many others (Bolognia et al. 2008).

## *Diagnosis*

Unfortunately, patch testing does not elucidate causes of ICD. Patch testing is used for ACD and has limitations in this area. History and physical are critical for making an accurate diagnosis. Once etiology is apparent, confirmation can be found when the patient improves with avoidance of irritant.

## *Management*

The simplest resolution to ICD is avoidance of triggers. This is often easier said than done for many patients. In the case of water-induced ICD, one can limit exposure by less water usage or by protection with gloves. Restoration of the epidermal barrier is crucial to management of ICD, and several steps can be taken to assist with this measure. First, shielding and protection from the trigger are of utmost importance. This can be accomplished by protective clothing, gloves, and face shields. Remember that ICD is related to concentration of irritant and exposure. Limiting the exposure through a protective barrier can resolve the issue for many patients. Second, restoring the epidermal barrier through the use of emollients and ointments can innately protect the skin from the irritant. This is easily accomplished with the use of petrolatum products. These can be applied several times a day, including at night with the use of cotton gloves in the case of irritant hand eczema. Lastly, the use of topical steroids in an ointment base helps to reduce local inflammation as well as provides a lipid barrier from the ointment base. Together, these three steps are useful techniques to help resolve the majority of ICD. In the case these therapies do not help, one should refer to dermatology for use of systemic therapies.

## Airborne Contact Dermatitis

### *Epidemiology*

Airborne contact dermatitis (ABCD) represents a subset of contact dermatitis caused from pollen, dust, spray, fumes, or volatile chemicals without the direct handling of the substance. It is represented by both allergic and irritant causes and commonly affects exposed areas such as the face, neck, upper chest, and forearms (Kumar et al. 2012). It is often this distribution which leads clinicians to suspect an airborne cause of contact dermatitis. Persons affected by ABCD can be categorized into occupational and non-occupational subsets. It is often the allergic form of ABCD that is often reported, but various irritant ABCD exist as well. Allergic ABCD patients are often sensitized through direct or indirect contact, inhalation, or ingestion in herbal teas and supplements (Handa et al. 2011).

### *Pathophysiology*

As stated above, ABCD can be both irritant and allergic. The pathogenesis for ICD has been described earlier in the chapter. Allergic ABCD falls into the ACD category. In order for ACD to occur, one must be sensitized to the allergen. The allergen initially comes into contact with the skin or the mucosa and penetrates the epidermal barrier. It then binds to epidermal proteins where it is phagocytized by antigen-presenting cells (APCs). The allergen and protein are processed and presented on the APCs which migrate to the draining lymph nodes where they stimulate naïve T-cells. This leads to the formation of activated T-cells, both effector and memory types, which are released into circulation. Re-exposure to the specific allergen activates these T-cells stimulating the type IV delayed-type hypersensitivity reaction (Handa et al. 2011; Kumar et al. 2012). Cytokine profiles for patients often show increased amounts of Th1 pro-inflammatory cytokines like IL-6, IL-8, IL-17, and TNF-a as well as decreased levels of Th2 anti-inflammatory cytokines IL-4 and IL-10 (Akhtar et al. 2010). This immunologic response can take at times several days when patients are exposed to low levels of allergen, which is why ACD is referred to as delayed-type contact dermatitis.

### *Features and Causes*

The classic example of ACD is rhus dermatitis, or poison ivy dermatitis. When a person is exposed to this allergen initially, there is no response noted in most cases. This is because by the time the cell-mediated response occurs, the allergic hapten has been degraded. In cases where there is massive exposure to the allergen, ACD

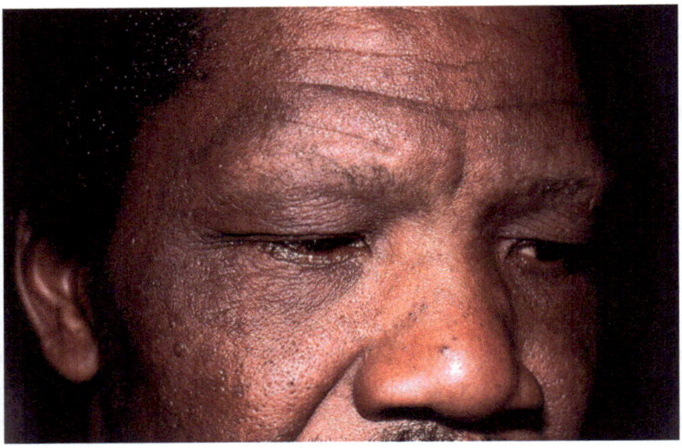

**Fig. 7.3** An example of the 'V' shaped distribution about the neck and chest of classical airbourne contact dermatitis

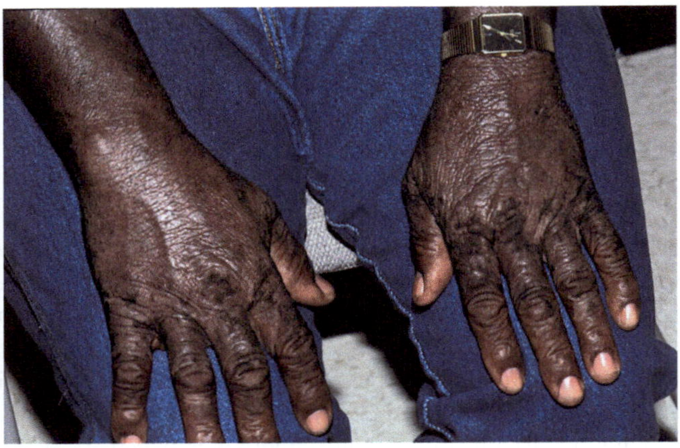

**Fig. 7.4** An example of involvement of the hands and arms in classical airbourne contact dermatitis

can occur on first exposure. Classically, rhus dermatitis occurs on second exposure and is characterized by acute erythema, linear vesiculation, and intense itching. ABCD has numerous causes, several of which are discussed below. Clinical manifestations include acneiform eruptions, lichenoid eruptions, exfoliative dermatitis, fixed drug eruptions, and erythema multiforme, amongst others. It is not uncommon for one allergen to present with different manifestations (Handa et al. 2011). Classic ABCD involves the exposed face, the "V" of neck and upper chest, hands, and forearms (Figs. 7.3 and 7.4).

## *Parthenium Dermatitis*

Perhaps the classic example of ABCD is parthenium dermatitis caused by *Parthenium hysterophorus* which belongs to the family of Compositae. This particular dermatitis is quite common in India and was likely introduced to the country through import of wheat (Handa et al. 2011). The pollen from this plant is responsible for approximately 40 % of patients in contact dermatitis clinics. The component within this group of allergens is sesquiterpene lactone, which is located in the lipophilic oleoresin portion of the plant. Parthenin, a type of sesquiterpene lactone, is the major allergen in parthenium dermatitis. *P. hysterophorus* produces an allergic ABCD as well as photocontact dermatitis. A third of patients in India with atopic dermatitis can have a type I hypersensitivity reaction to *P. hysterophorus* as evidenced by a Th2 cytokine profile of increased IL-4 and IL-10 (Akhtar et al. 2010).

## *Dusts*

Several different aerosolized dusts can lead to ABCD. Cement dust in masons can lead to both irritant and allergic ABCD. The chromates and cobalt in the cement are notorious causes of ACD, and the alkaline properties of the material can cause ICD. Dust from work in this area can lead to a dry, lichenified dermatitis. Sawdust from various trees including teak, mahogany, and redwood can cause ABCD from both the aerosolized dust and smoke when burnt. They tend to cause a dry dermatitis on the face and groin of workers in this industry (Handa et al. 2011). Coal dust has been reported as a cause of ABCD in a power plant employee (Monzon et al. 2007).

## *Sprays*

Spray cleaners, insecticides, and pesticides are causes of ABCD which lead to eyelid dermatitis in patients (Rietschel and Fowler 2008).

## *Latex*

Latex is both a cause of immediate type I hypersensitivity and delayed type IV hypersensitivity. As an airborne cause, it can occur through aerosolized powders from latex gloves. Components within the latex gloves that can cause allergic ABCD include the latex as well as benzothiazoles, thiurams, paraphenylenediamines, thioureas, and dithiocarbamates. Classic clinical manifestations have been reported. The move in healthcare to non-latex, non-powdered gloves has drastically reduced these reactions (Page et al. 2000).

## *Miscellaneous*

Other culprits known to cause airborne dermatitis are turpentine, plastics, rubber, glues, pesticides, solvents, metal salts, fiberglass, sewage sludge, animal feed, acids, alkalis, and others. Benzoyl peroxide has been implicated as both a cause of allergic and irritant ABCD, including a case caused from burning candle wax in which benzoyl peroxide was found in the candle (Bonnekoh and Merk 1991). Table 7.2 contains several examples of both allergic and irritant ABCD (Ghosh 2011; Haustein et al. 1985; Lensen et al. 2006; Nethercott 1981; Patiwael et al. 2005; Santos and Goossens 2007).

## *Diagnosis*

Determining the etiology of a patient's ABCD is a challenge for the practitioner. Recognizing the pattern of ABCD is the first step in making a correct diagnosis. History and physical examination are critical. Questions should be asked about occupation, hobbies, recent travels, and exposures as well as other relevant questions pertaining to the location of the patient and time of year. Patch testing can be used in cases of allergic ABCD.

## *Management*

As with most contact dermatitis, prevention through avoidance of irritant and allergen is key to managing the disease. With ABCD this can be extremely difficult for some. Simple measures like avoiding the outdoors when pollen count is high; showering after outdoor exposure; frequent changing into clean clothes; and use of barrier creams and ointments can help limit exposure to allergen or irritant. Even when under the strictest measures, some patients have been forced to change professions due to their ABCD.

As with other dermatitis, topical steroids are the therapy of choice for most. Ointments tend to be preferred by most practitioners as they are more occlusive and do not contain preservatives like creams which can cause a compounded ACD in some cases. Oral prednisone may be used in some patients who do not respond to topical therapy, but duration should be tapered over at least 3 weeks to avoid a rebound reaction. Dosing at 1 mg/kg/day of prednisone is generally sufficient. Still, some patients are unable to avoid exposure to their trigger and must be placed on systemic immunosuppressive agents.

**Table 7.2** Examples of allergic and irritant airbourne contact dermatitis. Adapted from Santos and Goossens (2007)

| *Allergic ABCD* | *Source* |
|---|---|
| Metals | |
| • Cobalt | Dickel et al. (2001) |
| • Mercury | Bartolome et al. (2000) |
| • Nickel | Candura et al. (2001) |
| Hydrocarbons | |
| • Benzoyl peroxide | Forschner et al. (2002) |
| • Epoxy resin | Sasseville et al. (2000) |
| • Formaldehyde | Ezughah et al. (2001) |
| • Isocyanates | Goossens et al. (2002) |
| • Acrylates | Bong and English (2000) |
| Plants | |
| • Ambrosia | Schumacher and Silvis (2003) |
| • Cashew nut | Criado et al. (2002) |
| • Chamomilla | Rycroft (2003) |
| • Chrysanthemum | Groenewoud et al. (2002) |
| • Compositae | Fortina et al. (2005) |
| • Garlic | Bassioukas et al. (2004) |
| • Latex | Nettis et al. (2001) |
| • Thyme | Spiewak et al. (2001) |
| Chemicals | |
| • Azathioprine | Lauerma et al. (2001) |
| • Azithromycin | Milković-Kraus and Kanceljak-Macan (2001) |
| • Budesonide | Pontén (2006) |
| • Diacetylmorphine | Coenraads et al. (2001) |
| • Cinnamic aldehyde | Decapite and Anderson (2004) |
| • Lansoprazole | Vilaplana and Romaguera (2001) |
| • Methotrexate | Dastychová (2003) |
| • Mesna | Kiec-Swierczynska and Krecisz (2003) |
| • Oxycodone | MacFarlane et al. (2003) |
| • Paraphenylenediamine | Dyche and Goldsmith (2003) |
| • Simvastatin | Peramiquel et al. (2005) |
| • Ranitidine | Ryan et al. (2003) |
| *Irritant ABCD* | |
| • Air-conditioning filter fibers | Patiwael et al. (2005) |
| • Chlorothalonil | Lensen et al. (2006) |
| • Particleboard | Saary et al. (2001) |
| • Phosphates | Lazarov et al. (2002) |

## Summary

Irritant and airborne contact dermatitis are common causes of both occupational and non-occupational disease. As a practitioner, recognizing these manifestations and asking the appropriate answer will often lead to the diagnosis. An eczematous dermatitis is caused in both cases, and avoidance of irritant and allergen is key to improvement in patients. Topical steroids and barrier protection from causes aid in the resolution of symptoms and restoration of epidermal barrier.

## References


Akhtar N, Verma KK, Sharma A. Study of pro- and anti-inflammatory cytokine profile in the patients with parthenium dermatitis. Contact Dermatitis. 2010;63:203–8.

Bartolome B, Cordoba S, Sanchez-Perez J, Fernandez-Herrera J, Garcia-Diez A. Baboon syndrome of unusual origin. Contact Dermatitis. 2000;43:113.

Bassioukas K, Orton D, Cerio R. Occupational airborne allergic contact dermatitis from garlic with concurrent type I allergy. Contact Dermatitis. 2004;50:39–41.

Baxter P, Adams P, Aw T, et al. Hunter's diseases of occupations. 9th ed. London: Arnold; 2004. p. 307–14.

Bolognia J, Jorizzo J, Rapini R. Dermatology. 2nd ed. St. Louis: Mosby; 2008.

Bong JL, English JSC. Allergic contact dermatitis from airborne exposure to acrylates. Contact Dermatitis. 2000;43:242.

Bonnekoh B, Merk HF. Airborne allergic contact dermatitis from benzoyl peroxide as a bleaching agent of candle wax. Contact Dermatitis. 1991;24(5):367–8.

Candura SM, Locatelli C, Butera R, Gatti A, Fasola D, Manzo L. Widespread nickel dermatitis from inhalation. Contact Dermatitis. 2001;45:174–5.

Coenraads PJ, Hogen Esch AJ, Prevoo RLMA. Occupational contact dermatitis from diacetylmorphine (heroin). Contact Dermatitis. 2001;45:114.

Criado RF, Criado PR, Malaman F, Ensina LF, Vasconcellos C, Aun WT, et al. Nonoccupational allergic contact dermatitis to cashew nut simulating photosensitivity eczema. Am J Contact Dermat. 2002;13:85–6.

Dastychová E. Allergic contact dermatitis in methotrexate manufacture. Contact Dermatitis. 2003;48:226.

Decapite TJ, Anderson BE. Allergic contact dermatitis from cinnamic aldehyde found in an industrial odour-masking agent. Contact Dermatitis. 2004;51:312–3.

Dickel H, Radulescu M, Weyher I, Diepgen TL. Occupationally-induced "isolated cobalt sensitization". Contact Dermatitis. 2001;45:246–7.

Dyche JA, Goldsmith PC. Case report of occupational sensitization to p-phenylenediamine in a microbiology laboratory. Br J Dermatol. 2003;149:96.

Ezughah FI, Murdoch SR, Finch TM. Occupational airborne allergic contact dermatitis from medium-density fibreboard containing phenol-formaldehyde resin-2 (PFR-2). Contact Dermatitis. 2001;45:242.

Flammiger A, Maibach H. Sulfuric acid burns (corrosion and acute irritation): evidence-based overview to management. Cutan Ocul Toxicol. 2006;25(1):55–61.

Forschner K, Zuberbier T, Worm M. Benzoyl peroxide as a cause of airborne contact dermatitis in an orthopaedic technician. Contact Dermatitis. 2002;47:241.

Fortina AB, Romano I, Peserico A. Contact sensitization to Compositae mix in children. J Am Acad Dermatol. 2005;53:877–80.

Fyhrquist-Vanni N, Alenius H, Alenius H, Lauerma A. Contact dermatitis. Dermatol Clin. 2007;25:613–23.

Ghosh S. Airborne-contact dermatitis of non-plant origin: an overview. Indian J Dermatol. 2011;56(6):711–4.

Goossens A, Detienne T, Bruze M. Occupational allergic contact dermatitis caused by isocyanates. Contact Dermatitis. 2002;47:304–8.

Groenewoud GCM, Jong NW, Burdorf A, De Groot H, Gerth van Wÿk R. Prevalence of occupational allergy to Chrysanthemum pollen in greenhouses in the Netherlands. Allergy. 2002;57:835–40.

Handa S, De D, Mahajan H. Airborne contact dermatitis—current perspectives in etiopathgenesis and management. Indian J Dermatol. 2011;56:700–6.

Haustein U, Tegetmeyer L, Ziegler V. Allergic and irritant potential of benzoyl peroxide. Contact Dermatitis. 1985;13(4):252–7.

Kanerva L, Elsner P, Wahlberg JE, et al. Handbook of occupational dermatology. Berlin: Springer; 2000.

Kiec-Swierczynska M, Krecisz B. Occupational airborne allergic contact dermatitis from mesna. Contact Dermatitis. 2003;48:171.

Kumar S, Khandpu S, Rao D, Wahaab S, Khanna N. Immunological response to Parthenium hysterophorus in India patients with Partheium sensitive atopic dermatitis. Immunol Invest. 2012;41(1):75–86.

Lauerma AI, Koivuluhta M, Alenius H. Recalcitrant allergic contact dermatitis from azathioprine tablets. Contact Dermatitis. 2001;44:129.

Lazarov A, Yair M, Lael E, Baitelman L. Airborne irritant contact dermatitis from phosphates in a fertilizer factory. Contact Dermatitis. 2002;46:53–4.

Lensen GJ, Jungbauer FHW, Goncalo M, Coenraads PJ. Chlorothalonil: outbreak of airborne occupational irritant facial contact dermatitis. Contact Dermatitis. 2006;55:17.

McCall B, Horwitz I, Feldman S, et al. Incidence rates, costs, severity, and work-related factors of occupational dermatitis. Arch Dermatol. 2005;141:713–8.

MacFarlane CS, Charman C, Fertig A, English JSC. An outbreak of contact dermatitis in an opiate manufacturing plant. Br J Dermatol. 2003;149:95.

Milković-Kraus S, Kanceljak-Macan B. Occupational airborne allergic contact dermatitis from azithromycin. Contact Dermatitis. 2001;45:184.

Monzon S, Morales A, Perez-Camo I, et al. Airborne occupational allergic contact dermatitis from coal dust. Allergy. 2007;62:1346.

Nethercott J. Airborne irritant contact dermatitis due to sewage sludge. J Occup Med. 1981;23(11):771–4.

Nettis E, Colanardi MC, Ferrannini A, Tursi A. Airborne allergic contact dermatitis. Allergy. 2001;56:583–4.

Nosbaum A, Voscanson M, Rozieres A, et al. Allergic and irritant contact dermatitis. Eur J Dermatol. 2009;19:325–32.

Page E, Esswein E, Petersen M, Lewis D, Bledsoe R. Natural rubber latex: glove use, sensitization, and airborne and latent dust concentrations at a Denver hospital. J Occup Environ Med. 2000;6:613–20.

Patiwael JA, Wintzen M, Rustemeyer T, Bruynzeel DP. Airborne irritant contact dermatitis due to synthetic fibres from an air-conditioning filter. Contact Dermatitis. 2005;52:126–9.

Peramiquel L, Serra E, Dalmau J, Vila AT, Mascaró JM, Alomar A. Occupational contact dermatitis from simvastatin. Contact Dermatitis. 2005;52:286–7.

Pontén A. Airborne occupational contact dermatitis caused by extremely low concentrations of budesonide. Contact Dermatitis. 2006;55:121–4.

Rietschel RL, Fowler JF. Fisher's contact dermatitis. Hamilton: BC Decker Inc; 2008. p. 69–101.

Ryan PJJ, Rycroft RJG, Aston IR. Allergic contact dermatitis from occupational exposure to ranitidine hydrochloride. Contact Dermatitis. 2003;48:67–8.

Rycroft RJG. Recurrent facial dermatitis from chamomile tea. Contact Dermatitis. 2003;48:229.

Saary MJ, House RA, Holness DL. Dermatitis in a particleboard manufacturing facility. Contact Dermatitis. 2001;44:325–30.

Santos R, Goossens A. An update on airborne contact dermatitis: 2001–2006. Contact Dermatitis. 2007;57:353–60.

Sasseville D, Moreau L, Brassard J, Leclerc G. Allergic contact dermatitis to epoxy resin in microscopy immersion oil: cases from Canada. Am J Contact Dermat. 2000;11:99–103.

Schumacher MJ, Silvis NG. Airborne contact dermatitis from Ambrosia deltoidea (triangle-leaf bursage). Contact Dermatitis. 2003;48:212–6.

Spiewak R, Skorska C, Dutkiewicz J. Occupational airborne contact dermatitis caused by thyme dust. Contact Dermatitis. 2001;44:235–9.

Stuke LE, Arnoldo BD, Hunt JL, Purdue GF. Hydrofluoric acid burns: a 15-year experience. J Burn Care Res. 2008;29(6):893–6.

Vilaplana J, Romaguera C. Allergic contact dermatitis due to lansoprazole, a proton pump inhibitor. Contact Dermatitis. 2001;44:39–40.

# Chapter 8
# Exposure Limits

**Grace Ziem**

*If you give an employer some poison repeatedly, it is called a crime.*
*If your employer does this to you, it is called an exposure limit.*

Dr. James Keogh, Occupational Medicine Physician.

**Abstract** Exposure limits are concentrations in air of potentially harmful chemicals that should not be exceeded in the workplace. Regional and national exposure limits are arrived at by private and governmental groups by considering available data which may be limited. The intent is to protect the majority of workers from harmful effects of occupational chemicals. Some but not all have the force of law. Exposure limits are often modified as new data becomes available. Difficulties with exposure limits include lack of applicability to mixtures of chemicals with synergistic toxicities and inability to protect sensitivity populations such as asthmatics and those with impaired detoxification abilities.

**Keywords** Exposure limits • Threshold limit values • Permissible exposure limits • Chemical exposures

## Introduction

Exposures to harmful chemicals, the majority being respiratory irritants, are common and occur in homes, schools, offices, factories, and outdoors. Working with hazardous chemicals occurs in many occupations. Inhalational exposures are common to

G. Ziem, M.D., M.P.H., D.P.H. (✉)
Occupational and Environmental Health, 16926 Eyler's Valley Road, Emmitsburg, MD 21727-9729, USA

W.J. Meggs (ed.), *The Toxicant Induction of Irritant Asthma, Rhinitis, and Related Conditions*, DOI 10.1007/978-1-4614-9044-9_8,

airborne gases, vapors, fumes, and particles. Exposure limits are concentrations in air that should not be exceeded unless workers use properly selected personal protection equipment with detailed training. Many countries have developed exposure limits. In addition, cities, states, and provinces may also have exposure limits. In some cases, exposure limits have the force of law, while in others they are guidelines or recommendations that are not mandatory. Serious problems affecting the validity of exposure limits are discussed below.

When health complaints occur in an occupational setting, often managers/decision makers are interested in creating healthy conditions before measuring exposure. This can be done by increasing ventilation; removing hazardous chemicals, procedures, and equipment; replacing mold-contaminated areas; improving protective equipment and training; and eliminating other problems. While these approaches can improve health for future persons, *measurements and inspections would then NOT represent the original conditions* under which the illness began. It is important for clinicians and others to understand and ask affected patient(s) about original exposure conditions because they often have helpful information about such changes.

It is also common for there to have been NO measurements performed, even when multiple persons have developed health problems. Concerns about budget, neglected responsibility, liability, etc. can affect exposure evaluation decisions significantly.

Although many exposures are untested, when testing is done, threshold limit values (TLVs) are often mentioned. These seldom updated (Castleman 2006) values are published in the United States by the American Conference of Governmental Industrial Hygienists (ACGIH), a nongovernmental organization. Their website at www.acgih.org can be consulted for methods used to determine TLVs and recommendations for their use.

Since it is reasonable that a longer duration of exposure to a given concentration is more dangerous than a short-term exposure, exposure limits vary with durations of exposures and are defined as follows:

Time-weighted average (TWA) exposure limit—the maximum average concentration of a chemical in air for a normal 8-h working day and 40-h week.

Short-term exposure limit (STEL)—the maximum average concentration to which workers can be exposed for a short period (usually 15 min).

Ceiling value—the concentration that should not be exceeded at any time.

Exposure limits are given with modifiers: TLV-TWA, TLV-STEL, PEL-TWA, etc. where PEL refers to the National Institute of Occupational Safety and Health (NIOSH) Permissible Exposure Limits (PEL), which are only recommendations without enforcement. Exposure limits vary among jurisdictions and can be modified over time, as more data becomes available, if funds are provided. Exposure limits are in general not determined by controlled studies but are set by committees that consider epidemiological data, when available, controlled studies in laboratory animals with extrapolation to humans, and limited human exposure data.

In the United States, NIOSH develops and periodically but seldom revises specific PELs. The Occupational Safety and Health Administration (OSHA) is tasked with workplace safety using these limits, but economics greatly limit enforcement status. PELs are published in the US Code of Federal Regulations, Occupational Safety and Health Standards on Toxic and Hazardous Substances, 29CFR 1910.10000.

The NIOSH Pocket Guides to Chemical Hazards are available at the NIOSH website, www.cdc.gov/niosh. These cards give PELs for a number of chemicals as well as hazards associated with exposures and recommendations for personal protective equipment. TLVs and PELs are only applicable to the workplace and do not apply to exposure in homes and outdoor exposures.

Many states have guidelines that can differ from federal guidelines and can be enforced under state laws. Some states have exposure limits for outdoor air. The website of the International Labor Organization (www.ilo.org) provides a convenient listing of international and state jurisdictions that have exposure limits, with links to online databases maintained by each jurisdiction.

## Early Problems with Validity

The US occupational exposure limits, the majority involving respiratory irritants, have been largely developed with scant scientific documentation. The process of their development was poorly understood for decades after their first annual listing in 1946. They were issued by a nongovernmental body with the perhaps misleading name of the American Conference of Governmental Industrial Hygienists (ACGIH). The exposure limits were referred to by 1948 as TLVs, despite early corporate influence (Castleman 1997) and internal acknowledgement that they were "industry's values" (Stokinger 1969).

When the Occupational Safety and Health Act was passed in 1970, industry "liaison" members from various chemical companies (e.g., Dow, DuPont) began to play a major but publicly unacknowledged role in both the writing of official TLV documentation as well as proposing the actual levels for TLV exposure limits (Castleman and Ziem 1988).

The published documentation of TLVs continued to withhold this fact and refuses to allow public access to their minutes (Castleman and Ziem 1994). Despite their widespread use, the TLVs have been criticized by NIOSH, OSHA, and others (Castleman and Ziem 1994). The majority of criticized TLVs are respiratory irritants.

Toxicologist Herbert Stokinger (1969) early on critiqued the lack of adequate human and even chronic animal data but tried to coax such data from the industries that manufactured the respiratory irritants and toxins. Dr. Hector Blejer resigned from the TLV committee in 1980 after 10 years of service because of the increasingly strong pro-industry bias and conflicts with scientific approaches among government scientists at NIOSH and OSHA (Blejer 1999).

## Lack of Scientific Basis

A medical review was done of articles evaluating human health effects at specific exposure levels (Ziem 1989). Significant health effects were documented at or below the TLVs for 23 chemicals. The majority were respiratory irritants. This is despite limiting the review to 33 months from only four occupational medicine journals.

Another study (Roach and Rappaport 1990) compared the TLV levels to both the levels described in the ACGIH TLV Documentation literature as causing health effects and also with the levels reported as prevailing measurements in industry. No statistical correlation was found with health effects, but a strong correlation was found between TLV published levels and industry prevailing exposure levels. This disparity was found for respiratory and eye irritation effects, for neurologic/brain effects (Roach and Rappaport 1990) and for other types of illness.

## Why Are TLVs Important?

Without knowing the history of flaws in TLV formation, OSHA adopted the TLVs as the legally enforced workplace PELs and use the TLVs at worksite inspections to determine whether a health risk or a current problem exists. (Most worksites are seldom inspected.) Other countries in Europe and Asia also adopted these levels. Further, TLVs have been misused for environmental (non-workplace) standards (Castleman and Ziem 1989).

*The result is a worldwide lack of protection for many workers.* If measurements are done, the need for corrective measures is often minimized. Workers who seek medical care with measurements below the TLV level are likely to be misdiagnosed. With inadequate exposure controls and lack of medical recognition, the illness can more readily become disabling.

Also, many workplace measuring instruments are designed to only detect exposure near or above the TLV. These often miss (recording as zero or undetectable) lower but significant exposure levels. Further, ventilation system design is often based on the TLVs and thus more likely to allow significant exposures that could cause harmful health effects.

When workers become disabled from exposure, the TLVs are often used to deny compensation. This deprives people with respiratory and other illnesses the resources for health-improving measures. It prevents adequate preventive measures from being developed, so co-workers continue to be exposed. New hires continue to be assured that exposure measurements indicated a safe work environment, creating a form of toxic "musical chairs."

TLVs are often misused in evaluation of risk in schools and health facilities despite increased vulnerability of children, elderly, and ill or injured persons. They are also misused to evaluate home environments, despite much longer duration of exposure, contamination of food-contact surfaces, and often more vulnerable inhabitants.

This author (Ziem 1989) has seen, both as a clinical treating physician for decades and as a medical worksite inspector with Maryland OSHA (1978–1980), many persons with obvious respiratory illness of irritant origin below the legally used exposure limits called TLVs. The author (Ziem 1989) visited the national office where official TLV "documenting" files were then kept and was astounded to see lack of literature searches. In many cases there was obvious reliance on industry letters or even a phone call with scant data lacking scientific rigor.

## Chemical Mixtures

Workplace and other environmental monitoring, if chemicals are monitored at all, often measure a very limited number of chemicals (rather than all or even most chemicals used and released). Often a review of monitoring results focuses on whether one or possibly a few measurements exceed the TLVs. At best, effects are considered to be merely additive for those which can be measured by TLV-based monitoring equipment.

However, mixtures of chemicals create harm in a synergistic (much more than additive) manner (Hempel-Jorgensen et al. 1999). As chemical mixtures become more complex, containing more chemicals, the effects become more hyperadditive (Cometto-Muniz et al. 1997). This would cause further risk of harm even when individual chemical levels are below TLVs.

Mixtures including both water-soluble and fat-soluble or "lipophilic" chemicals (a common situation) more readily penetrate the respiratory tract and can trigger and exacerbate irritant asthma/reactive airways (both upper and lower) at far lower exposure levels (Zeliger 2003).

Chemical mixtures can interact with each other either as gases/vapors or particles to create tissue-damaging free radicals (Weschler et al. 2006) which increase respiratory inflammation when breathed in. Even a 4-h exposure of humans in newly built or remodeled buildings can increase inflammatory immune cells in the respiratory system (Koren et al. 1992). Exposure to chemical mixtures, e.g., VOCs, even at levels below legal guidelines increases irritant-related asthma (Rumchev et al. 2004).

When one thinks about any workplace or other environmental setting, there is virtually always a complex chemical mixture and thus for irritants a synergistic effect on respiratory inflammation.

## Indoor Respiratory Hazards

Solvents, glues, coating agents, welding/soldering materials, and other chemicals/substances introduced are almost always an irritant mixture in even one container. Often multiple types of mixtures are used. Mixing, heating, or otherwise treating mixtures often creates more irritants.

Add to this the respiratory irritant chemical mixtures introduced by each of many products. These include commercial cleaning agents, "air fresheners," pesticide residues, and VOC off-gassing from renovations, carpet and other furnishings, HVAC contaminants, molds, etc. The airborne mixture can readily contain hundreds of chemicals, often a mixture of water- and fat-soluble chemicals.

Air fresheners, using gas chromatography-mass spectrometry, are VOC complex chemical mixtures that are respiratory irritants (Potera 2011). Indeed, 19 % of the US adults report health symptoms from exposure to "air fresheners" (Caress and Steinemann 2009).

Reduced building ventilation for energy conservation has led to reduced circulation of fresh air (Ashford and Miller 1998). This can include increased caulking, sealing, tight windows, and further insulation. An EPA study of four building (Wallace 1985) found 800 VOCs as indoor air pollutants. Levels measured were typically 2–5 times greater than outdoor levels and not uncommonly ten times or more. Within the buildings, measured levels could vary by 3–4 orders of magnitude, indicating intense indoor sources (Wallace 1985). This clearly indicates that persons in some areas of the building were at much higher risk than others and that indoor VOC mixtures are a significant respiratory hazard.

Virtually all airborne exposures occur in mixtures because of multiple substances creating off-gassing indoors and even many outdoor environments. These include VOCs from molds (Schleibinger 1999), scented products (Potera 2011), pesticide residues (Cox and Surgan 2006; Rohrer et al. 2003), cleaning products (Nazaroff et al. 2006), renovation and repair products (Koren et al. 1992), and combustion products (Brooks et al. 1985; Kilburn 2000; Sharman et al. 2002). Each of these is in fact often a complex chemical mixture. There are many indoor environments with many of these products, each containing chemical mixtures. The result is a very complex chemical mixture.

## Synergistic Risk from Chemical Mixtures

Mixtures of VOCs (most of which are airborne irritants) interact much more than additively even at subthreshold (below detection) levels (Hudnell et al. 1992). Respiratory irritation shows no signs of adaptation (Hudnell et al. 1992). Such exposure causes an inflammatory effect in the respiratory track (Hudnell et al. 1992).

When mixtures are more complex (obviously common in many indoor environments), the effects become more hyperadditive (Cometto-Muniz et al. 1997; Hempel-Jorgensen et al. 1999) and effects can be seen far below the TLV (Hempel-Jorgensen et al. 1999). Eye irritation effect of mixtures is similar to upper and lower respiratory irritation (Hempel-Jorgensen et al. 1999). This makes eye irritation a valuable warning symptom to help prevent respiratory damage from airborne irritants: controlling exposure rather than just steroid eye drops, for example.

Mixtures of lipid (fat)-soluble chemicals (e.g., VOC mixtures) penetrate the respiratory tract far more easily (Zeliger 2003). Chemical mixtures can interact with each other and/or airborne particle surfaces, creating tissue-damaging free radicals (Weschler et al. 2006).

Thus chemical mixtures can cause respiratory inflammation even at "low exposure" levels (Koren et al. 1992). Repeated low-dose chemical mixture airborne exposure over time increases the potential for sensitization (Hudnell 1993).

Chemical mixtures involving indoor pesticides are common given lack of a national practice of least toxic pest control. Chemical mixtures are found in many pesticides. Pesticides very often have a higher toxicity compared to their odor detection level. These pesticide chemical mixtures even at modest levels can produce dramatic increase in damage to many body organs (Hayes et al. 2006).

## Genetic Diversity and Other Vulnerability

Exposure limits have not given significant consideration to genetic diversity in the population regarding the ability to detoxify (clear foreign substances from the body).

Prior to the last century, there was much less genetic need for detoxification ability due to dramatically less prevalent exposure to both pollutants and drugs. Thus genetic impairment in detoxification ability would be unlikely to have affected survival and reproduction. Natural selection would be more likely to include healthy persons with genetic detoxification limitations.

For example: *Methylation* is important for detoxification, neurotransmitters, and other functions. Epinephrine and norepinephrine metabolism, which affect the airways and other body functions, require methylation. Yet at least *half of the population has genetic impairment in methylation* (Engbersen et al. 1995).

*Glutathione* is a very *major detoxifying agent* and also "neutralizes" inflammatory free radicals (Parkinson 2001) that would otherwise cause respiratory inflammation when inhaled. Glutathione reduces lung inflammation (Bishop et al. 2005). *Over half of the population has genetic impairment in glutathione function* (Board et al. 1990).

*Acetylation* is important for the *ability of the respiratory tract to cope with many toxins* (Parkinson 2001). Yet *acetylation impairment is also commonly found* in the general population (Hein et al. 2000).

There are other lung airway defense mechanisms (Kobzik 2007; Lippmann and Chen 2007), including bronchial fluid lining, airway shape and size, mucociliary clearance, and numerous immune defenses. Genetic or other diversity in exposed persons can significantly affect respiratory response to inhaled irritants and particulate (Kobzik 2007; Lippmann and Chen 2007). Genetic diversity is common in many of these factors.

Adding together genetic diversity in the above respiratory response mechanisms, it is clear that one exposure limit for all is as unscientific as one sulfite or pollen limit for all.

## Human Exposure and Other Vulnerabilities

There are other factors that make exposure limits not valid. These include the following:

1. Length of exposure
   Longer duration of exposure increases harmful effects of toxins and irritants (Eaton and Klaassen 2001). Workers on longer shifts and residents in homes or institutions all have longer exposures and less time away from exposure for recovery or improvement.
2. Age
   Infants and children are more susceptible because of more body need for cell growth, a more rapid respiratory rate, and developing but still immature respira-

tory tracts, immune systems, and defense mechanisms. The smaller Eustachian tube when exposed to irritants is more susceptible to swelling that can lead to recurring, respiratory infections with irritant exposure.

3. Other vulnerabilities and problems
   Pregnant women needing to also detoxify for a fetus can be at greater risk. Significant vital organ development can occur before a woman is aware of her pregnancy.

Persons with inflammation from allergies, previous irritant exposure (Hudnell et al. 1992), or other respiratory diseases have greater risk with irritant/toxic exposure.

## Lack of Research

Respiratory effects of long-term repeated exposures over months and years have received minimal scientific study related to exposure limits. All the above-listed factors which have major respiratory safety implications have very serious research gaps and some receive minimal scientific study.

Obviously therefore, threshold exposure limits and many other exposure limits lack scientific validity. Documentation of respiratory safety in the many complex circumstances described above is so faulty that it cannot be relied upon for protection of either healthy or ill humans.

This leads to a much greater need for scientific clinical acumen in observation and documentation. It requires the use of clinical criteria that are protective of health and that document illness. Documentation is essential to prevent further deterioration of affected person(s) to avoid disability and to avoid placing another healthier person in a hazardous environment.

### *Diagnostic Criteria for Evaluating Exposure-Related Effects*

When there is a change in respiratory symptoms, such as increased inflammation, without a documented infection, irritant exposure should be considered in the differential diagnosis. When symptoms include burning, the likelihood of an irritant cause becomes much greater, because this symptom is often associated with the pathologic changes seen in airway inflammation after irritant exposure (Meggs et al. 1996).

Mucous membrane irritant burning symptoms can be easily evaluated by asking "Have you had a burning-like feeling in the eyes, nose, throat, and/or chest? If yes, when did this first occur?"

Respiratory symptoms of irritant origin can also include headache in the area of the sinuses or ear(s), or other ear symptoms (if there is Eustachian tube involvement), irritation of tongue, mouth, throat, larynx, voice changes/hoarseness, chest irritation, coughing, chest tightness, and sometimes wheezing. Patients may have a few of these symptoms but often do not have them all.

To avoid missing an irritant situation, one should apply accepted medical criteria to evaluate an exposure relationship to airborne irritants (Landrigan and Baker 1991).

1. The relationship in time between the onset of illness symptoms and exposure.
   In the case of airborne irritants, some persons will experience symptoms with initial or the first few exposures, but others may not develop symptom onset until weeks, months, or even years of first irritant exposure. However, it is typical that the irritant symptoms begin within 2–3 days of the most recent irritant exposure. It is very important to ask when the first symptoms started, as patients often focus on when they could no longer work or function. Asking when they were last well or without symptom(s) can be very helpful.
2. Improvement of symptoms during times away from exposure.
   Once symptoms become chronic, variation is much less obvious to the person. Thus it is essential to focus on when they first noticed symptoms and did symptoms change in specific locations. This avoids a questioning bias. Some patients may not recall the first days or even weeks, when changes may have been better during an 8–12-h period. Thus it is important to ask whether the symptoms changed if they were in different location for a few days or longer. For those with longer chronic changes, longer time away from exposure is often needed to evaluate a change such as during vacations or longer times away from suspected sources.
3. Recurrence or worsening of symptoms after re-exposure.
   This can be evaluated by similar questioning as above. A trial removal of a few weeks or more away from a suspected environment is helpful, asking about the severity of specific symptoms before and then later after return. Longer removal is needed for more severity and/or more chronic effects.

If lower airway changes are suspected, a portable peak flow meter can be used. Since combustion products during travel or commute may exacerbate already inflamed airways, readings should be done and recorded:

- At home before commute/travel
- After commute/travel and prior to entry into area of suspected exposure
- Then periodic readings in areas of suspected exposure

Recording date, time, circumstances, location, and symptoms along with peak flow readings is often useful.

For patients with primarily reactive upper airways (since irritants deposit differently depending on many factors) peak flow readings may yield less information than a symptom log.

All patients should be advised to leave an area when adversely affected: the supervisor should have a medical note to ensure that further harm does not occur.

## Summary

It is tragic but true that there are no known safe irritant exposure levels that will protect all individuals. Any symptomatic exposure poses a risk. For pesticides and certain other chemicals, one exposure may be sufficient to induce chronic effects. Repeated symptomatic exposures further increase the risk of chronic disabling respiratory inflammation. Under these circumstances, there is no safe exposure level if that exposure exacerbates symptoms.

## References

Ashford NA, Miller CS. Chemical exposures: low levels and high stakes. 2nd ed. New York, NY: Wiley; 1998. p. 10–3.

Bishop C, Hudson VM, Hilton SC, Wilde C. A pilot study of the effect of inhaled buffered reduced glutathione on the clinical status of patients with cystic fibrosis. Chest. 2005;127:308–17.

Blejer HP. Letter to Col. V. L. Carter Chairman of the TLV committee dated 5 June 1980.

Board P, Coggan M, Johnston P, Ross V, Suzuki T, Webb G. Genetic heterogeneity of the human glutathione transferases: a complex of gene families. Pharmacol Ther. 1990;48:357–69.

Brooks SM, Weiss MA, Bernstein IL. Reactive airways dysfunction syndrome. Case reports of persistent airways hyperreactivity following high-level irritant exposures. J Occup Med. 1985;27:473–6.

Caress SM, Steinemann AC. Prevalence of fragrance sensitivity in the American population. J Environ Health. 2009;71:46–50.

Castleman BI, Ziem GE. American Conference of Governmental Industrial Hygienists: low threshold of credibility. Am J Ind Med. 1994;26:133–43.

Castleman BI, Ziem GE. Corporate influence on threshold limit values. Am J Ind Med. 1988;13:531–59.

Castleman B. How threshold limits for lead were established in the 1950s. Am J Ind Med. 1997;32:702–3.

Castleman BI. Legacy of corporate influence on threshold limit values and European response. Re: Am J Ind Med 44: 204–213, 2003. Am J Ind Med. 2006;49:307–9.

Castleman BI, Ziem GE. Toxic pollutants, science, and corporate influence. Arch Environ Health. 1989;44:68–127.

Cometto-Muniz JE, Cain WS, Hudnell HK. Agonistic sensory effects of airborne chemicals in mixtures: odor, nasal pungency, and eye irritation. Percept Psychophys. 1997;59:665–74.

Cox C, Surgan M. Unidentified inert ingredients in pesticides: implications for human and environmental health. Environ Health Perspect. 2006;114:1803–6.

Eaton DL, Klaassen CD. Principles of toxicology. In: Klaassen CD, editor. Casarett & doull's toxicology: the basic science of poisons. 6th ed. New York, NY: McGraw-Hill; 2001. p. 14–31.

Engbersen AM, Franken DG, Boers GH, Stevens EM, Trijbels FJ, Blom HJ. Thermolabile 5,10-methylenetetrahydrofolate reductase as a cause of mild hyperhomocysteinemia. Am J Hum Genet. 1995;56:142–50.

Hayes TB, Case P, Chui S, Chung D, Haeffele C, Haston K, et al. Pesticide mixtures, endocrine disruption, and amphibian declines: are we underestimating the impact? Environ Health Perspect. 2006;114 Suppl 1:40–50.
Hein DW, Doll MA, Fretland AJ, Leff MA, Webb SJ, Xiao GH, et al. Molecular genetics and epidemiology of the NAT1 and NAT2 acetylation polymorphisms. Cancer Epidemiol Biomarkers Prev. 2000;9:29–42.
Hempel-Jorgensen A, Kjaergaard SK, Molhave L, Hudnell KH. Sensory eye irritation in humans exposed to mixtures of volatile organic compounds. Arch Environ Health. 1999;54:416–24.
Hudnell H. Time course of odor and irritation effects in humans exposed to a mixture of 22 volatile organic compounds. In: Agency USEP, editor; 1993
Hudnell HK, Otto DA, House DE, Molhave L. Exposure of humans to a volatile organic mixture. II. Sensory. Arch Environ Health. 1992;47:31–8.
Kilburn KH. Effects of diesel exhaust on neurobehavioral and pulmonary functions. Arch Environ Health. 2000;55:11–7.
Kobzik L. Lung immune defenses against environmental agents. In: Rom WN, editor. Environmental and occupational medicine. 4th ed. New York, NY: Lippincott Williams & Wilkins; 2007. p. 189–99.
Koren HS, Graham DE, Devlin RB. Exposure of humans to a volatile organic mixture. III. Inflammatory response. Arch Environ Health. 1992;47:39–44.
Landrigan PJ, Baker DB. The recognition and control of occupational disease. JAMA. 1991;266:676–80.
Lippmann M, Chen L. Particle deposition and pulmonary defense mechanisms. In: Rom WM, editor. Environmental and occupational medicine. 4th ed. New York, NY: Lippincott Williams & Wilkins; 2007. p. 168–86.
Meggs WJ, Elsheik T, Metzger WJ, Albernaz M, Bloch RM. Nasal pathology and ultrastructure in patients with chronic airway inflammation (RADS and RUDS) following an irritant exposure. J Toxicol Clin Toxicol. 1996;34:383–96.
Nazaroff WW, Coleman BK, Destaillats H, Hodgson DL, Lunden MM, Singer BC et al. Indoor air chemistry: cleaning agents, ozone and toxic air contaminants. California Air Resources Board California Environmental Protection Agency; 2006.
Parkinson A. Biotransformation of xenobiotics. In: Klaassen CD, editor. Casarett & doull's toxicology: the basic science of poisons. 6th ed. New York, NY: McGraw-Hill; 2001. p. 213–8.
Potera C. Scented products emit a bouquet of VOCs. Environ Health Perspect. 2011;119:A16.
Roach SA, Rappaport SM. But they are not thresholds: a critical analysis of the documentation of threshold limit values. Am J Ind Med. 1990;17:727–53.
Rohrer CA, Hieber TE, Melnyk LJ, Berry MR. Transfer efficiencies of pesticides from household flooring surfaces to foods. J Expo Anal Environ Epidemiol. 2003;13:454–64.
Rumchev K, Spickett J, Bulsara M, Phillips M, Stick S. Association of domestic exposure to volatile organic compounds with asthma in young children. Thorax. 2004;59:746–51.
Schleibinger H. Occurrence of microbiologically produced aldehydes and ketones from filter materials of HVAC systems field and laboratory experiments. In: Practical Engineering for IAQ. Oct 22–24 edn. Denver CO: American Society oof Heating, Refrigeration and Air Conditioning Engineers, Inc. Proceedings jointly published with US EPA and DOE; 1995.
Sharman JE, Coombes JS, Geraghty DP, Fraser DI. Exposure to automotive pollution increases plasma susceptibility to oxidation. Arch Environ Health. 2002;57:536–40.
Stokinger HE. Current problems of setting occupational exposure standards. Arch Environ Health. 1969;19:277–81.
Wallace LA. Organics:overview. In: Gammage RB, Kaye SV, editors. Indoor air and human health. 2nd ed. Chelsea, MI: Lewis Publishers, Inc.; 1985. p. 331–3.
Weschler CJ, Wells JR, Poppendieck D, Hubbard H, Pearce TA. Workgroup report: Indoor chemistry and health. Environ Health Perspect. 2006;114:442–6.
Zeliger HI. Toxic effects of chemical mixtures. Arch Environ Health. 2003;58:23–9.
Ziem G. Physical symptoms after neurotoxic exposure. J Occup Med. 1989;31:410–1.

# Chapter 9
# Occupational Issues Related to Respiratory Irritants

**Ricky Langley and David Lipton**

**Abstract** Numerous substances in the workplace can cause irritation of the mucus membranes and respiratory tract. Both physical characteristics and chemical composition of the irritant may influence the effects seen on the airways. Particle size determines the location of deposition in the airways. Water solubility, pH, electric charge, hygroscopicity, and propensity to bind with tissue proteins influence the uptake, deposition, and degree of damage from inhaled respiratory irritants. Health effects of inhaled irritants include rhinitis, vocal cord dysfunction, asthma, emphysema, chronic bronchitis, and reactive airways dysfunction syndrome. In addition inhaled irritants can cause annoyance reactions, irritation, and corrosive changes and even increase the risk of infection. In evaluating complaints from irritant exposure both the worker and worksite should be evaluated. Worker evaluation should include a thorough medical and occupational history, a physical exam focusing on the skin and upper and lower respiratory tract, and appropriate laboratory test which may include pulse oximetry, complete blood count, spirometry, and allergy skin testing. Radiographic scans of the affected organ may give an indication of localized or widespread involvement of that organ. Peak flow monitoring may be useful to determine where exposure may be occurring.

**Keywords** Chemical • Irritants • Asthma • RADS • RUDS • Vocal cord dysfunction

R. Langley, M.D., M.P.H. (✉) • D. Lipton, M.S.P.H., C.I.H.
Occupational and Environmental Epidemiology Branch, North Carolina Division of Public Health, Raleigh, NC 276-1912, USA
e-mail: rick.langley@dhhs.nc.gov

W.J. Meggs (ed.), *The Toxicant Induction of Irritant Asthma, Rhinitis, and Related Conditions*, DOI 10.1007/978-1-4614-9044-9_9,

## Introduction

A wide variety of airborne substances in the workplace can cause irritation of the respiratory system. One definition of irritation is nonspecific, reversible, direct, acute inflammatory response with injury to epithelial cells without an immune response. Irritant symptoms usually begin immediately or within minutes to hours after the exposure. Irritants can affect any part of the respiratory system. In addition to short-term acute effects, long-term chronic effects are increasingly recognized as consequence from single high-level exposure and chronic low-level irritant exposures in the workplace (Taylor 1996).

Chemical and physical characteristics of the inhaled agent have an important role in determining where in the respiratory tract the agent has its main impact. The effect of an irritant on the respiratory tract is influenced by whether the agent is a solid, liquid, or gas.

In addition, there are host factors that affect the body's response to inhalation of an irritant. Anatomical and physiological factors, lung defense mechanisms, and immunological state of the host all have a role in protecting the host from the inhaled agent. Airway geometry, breathing rates and patterns, ciliary action, clearance rates, macrophage function, allergic diathesis, atopy, and tissue type, are factors that influence the effects of inhaled agents (Morgan 1995).

This chapter reviews chemical and physical properties, epidemiology of illnesses, and host factors in the physiological response to occupational exposure to respiratory irritants. It also provides practical guidance for evaluation of potential risks from irritants in the workplace.

## Factors Influencing the Effects of an Inhaled Irritant

### *Physical and Chemical Factors Influencing the Effects of Inhaled Irritants*

The effect of an irritant on the respiratory tract is influenced by the physical characteristics and chemical composition of the contaminant. They influence the site of deposition or uptake, absorption into tissue, elimination, metabolism, or neutralization of the contaminant. Physical characteristics that are important include the physical state of the agent, whether particle, mist, vapor, fume, or gas; size and density of the agent; shape and penetrability; solubility; hygroscopicity; and electric charge. Chemical properties of importance include pH of the agent, fibrogenicity, antigenicity, and propensity to bind with substances in the tissues (Morgan 1995).

An important physical characteristic is the particle size. Particles with an aerodynamic diameter of greater than 5 μm are deposited in the upper respiratory tract and proximal airways. Particles with an aerodynamic diameter between 0.5 and 5 μm penetrate and deposit in the bronchioles and alveoli, the airway exchange region of

**Table 9.1** EPA particle size and description

| EPA description | Aerodynamic diameter |
|---|---|
| Super coarse | >10 μm |
| Coarse | 2.5–10 μm |
| Fine | 0.1–2.5 μm |
| Ultrafine | <0.1 μm |

the lungs. Particles with a diameter smaller than 0.5 μm act like gases and are more readily exhaled.

The American Conference of Governmental Industrial Hygienists Threshold Limit Values for Chemical Substances and Physical Agents categorizes the potential hazard of inhaled particles by size. Particle size-selective threshold limit values are expressed in three forms. Inhalable particulate matter (IPM) is hazardous when deposited anywhere in the respiratory tract. IPM replaces the term total dust. Samplers for IPM have a collection efficiency of 50 % for particles with an aerodynamic diameter of 100 μm. Collection efficiency increases with decreasing particle size; essentially all particulate matter (100 %) less than 1 μm is collected by the device. Thoracic particulate matter (TPM) is hazardous when deposited anywhere in the airways and gas-exchange region. TMP samplers have a collection efficiency of 50 % for a particle with an aerodynamic diameter of 10 μm. Respirable particles (RP) are hazardous when deposited in the gas-exchange regions of the lungs. RP samplers have a collection efficiency of 50 % for a particle with an aerodynamic diameter of 4 μm (ACGIH 2012).

For air pollution control, the Environmental Protection Agency (EPA) terminology for airborne particles is presented in Table 9.1.

EPA also uses terms such as Total Suspended Particles for aerosols with aerodynamic diameter between 0.1 and about 30 μm. EPA defines $PM_{10}$ as particles with and aerodynamic diameter between 2.5 and 10 μm and $PM_{2.5}$ as aerodynamic diameter of less than or equal to 2.5 μm. Both $PM_{10}$ and $PM_{2.5}$ are regulated as criteria pollutants under the National Ambient Air Quality Standards (NAAQS). The NAAQS includes primary and secondary standards. Primary standards provide public health protection, including protecting the health of "sensitive" populations such as asthmatics, children, and the elderly. The secondary standards protect public welfare including decreased visibility and damage to animals, crops, and vegetation. $PM_{2.5}$ are important for air pollution control because these particles settle slowly compared to larger particles and can be transported long distances. In addition $PM_{2.5}$ often contains sulfates, nitrates, organic compounds, and ammonium compounds.

Fine and ultrafine particles can represent a significant fraction of particulate emissions from certain types of combustion, waste incineration, and metallurgical sources and are hard to collect in field sampling (EPA 2010).

In addition to submicrometer or ultrafine particles incidental to processes, engineered particles with one, two, or three external dimensions between 1 and 100 nm (0.001–0.1 μm) are increasingly being used in optoelectronic, electronic, magnetic, medical imaging, drug delivery, cosmetic, catalytic, and other applications. Although beyond the scope of this review, a growing body of evidence indicates that exposure to some of these engineered nanomaterials can cause adverse health effects that may be different from the parent materials (NIOSH 2012).

Particle size is important for biological availability of particles. Geometry dictates that for spherical particles, the ratio of surface area to volume varies inversely with the radius of the sphere. In other words, a large number of small particles will have a greater surface area compared to a few larger particles. The greater surface area may impact bioavailability of an inhaled dose.

Geometry also dictates that for spherical particles, the ratio of volume to the radius varies with the cube of the radius. In other words, a few large particles may dominate the total mass in an air sample of an aerosol with a homogenous density but a highly variable particle size distribution. Therefore, it is crucial that the sampling method has accurate particle size selection capabilities to provide an accurate estimation of the inhaled dose.

Another important characteristic is the physical state of the substance. Solids, mists, fumes, and gases behave differently when inhaled. Fumes are sometimes called condensable particulate matter because the material is not a particle under process conditions. The particle forms within seconds or less by condensation or reaction upon cooling and dilution with ambient air. Most fume particles are agglomerations usually less than 2.5 μm in diameter. Fumes are produced when a solid material is heated beyond the point of vaporization and quickly condense and are common in metal working processes such as welding and thermal cutting.

The shape of the particle whether round or fibrous influences the hazards associated with inhaled particles. Fibers are long thin particles. In the NIOSH Criteria for a Recommended Standard: Occupational Exposure to Fibrous Glass, fibers are defined as particles with a diameter less than or equal to 3.5 μm and a length of greater than or equal to 10 μm (NIOSH 1977). For chrysotile asbestos a fiber with an aerodynamic diameter of 10 μm roughly corresponds to a physical diameter of 3 μm.

Some evidence suggests that long fibers are more hazardous than short fibers of the same material. One hypothesis is that fibers shorter than the diameter of a macrophage are more easily engulfed and removed from the lungs than longer fibers of the same diameter. Animal and in vitro studies also suggest that long fibers (greater than 5 μm) are associated with increased lung disease and are more capable of transport to the pleura and peritoneum (NIOSH 1999; ATSDR 2002).

A major chemical characteristic that influences the site of deposition and uptake of chemical irritants is the solubility in water. Water-soluble gases, vapors, and droplets tend to deposit and affect the upper airways while water-insoluble agents tend to deposit in the lower airways. The pH, electric charge, hygroscopicity, and propensity to bind with substances in tissues also influence the uptake, deposition, and degree of damage from inhaled respiratory irritants.

Although the effects of exposure to individual irritants have been well characterized, less is known about the irritating effects of complex mixtures such as smoke. Smoke is a complex mixture resulting from incomplete combustion containing gases, fine particles, and condensation nuclei. The individual components and concentration of contaminants in smoke are determined by specific circumstances.

### *Host-Related Factors*

A number of host factors influence a person's sensitivity and susceptibility to inhaled irritants. Anatomical and physiological factors such as airway geometry, breathing rates and patterns, effectiveness of the mucociliary clearance mechanisms, and macrophage function are important considerations. The immunological state of the host as well as the potential for allergic diathesis, atopy, and tissue type all have a role in influencing the effects of inhaled agents (Morgan 1995).

In addition to somatic changes to cells exposed to an irritant, people can experience chemically stimulated feelings known as chemesthesis. The appreciation of irritation (i.e., chemesthesis) affecting the eyes, nose, and throat is principally mediated by the trigeminal nerve (cranial nerve V). Pulmonary irritation is mainly under vagal (cranial nerve X) nerve control. Odors are detected by the olfactory nerve, but strength of odor does not always equate to toxicity.

## Health Effects of Inhaled Irritants

Irritants can affect any portion of the respiratory system from the upper airways (nasal cavity, sinuses, larynx, and trachea) to the lower respiratory tract (bronchi, bronchioles, and alveoli). Irritation of the nasal passages and sinuses is associated with rhinitis. Irritation of the larynx and the vocal cords is associated with vocal cord dysfunction, a set of symptoms that can mimic asthma because of similar clinical presentations (Shamon 2009). Asthma is an obstructive and inflammatory disease of the lower airways. Other health effects of irritation of the lower airways and air exchange regions of the lungs include chronic obstructive pulmonary disease (COPD) (emphysema and chronic bronchitis) and reactive airways dysfunction syndrome (RADS). In addition inhaled irritants can cause annoyance reactions, irritational effects, sensitization, corrosive changes, and even increase the risk of infections (Bardana 2008).

## Epidemiology

Respiratory diseases associated with workplace exposures are responsible for approximately 70 % of occupational disease mortality (Weston 2011). Occupational respiratory diseases can be described as three basic types: interstitial lung diseases, airway diseases, and pleural diseases. Interstitial lung diseases include asbestosis, byssinosis, chronic beryllium disease, silicosis, coal worker pneumoconiosis, and farmer's lung disease. Examples of airway diseases are work-related or exacerbated asthma, chronic obstructive lung disease, and bronchiolitis obliterans. Pleural diseases include mesothelioma and pleural plaques. Work-related exposures associated with respiratory disorders are numerous as evidenced in Table 9.2 (CDC 2008).

**Table 9.2** Work-related respiratory conditions: most frequent associated hazards (excluding asbestos), 1994–2004. From NIOSH No. 2008-143a p 297

| Respiratory hazards | Number | Percent |
|---|---|---|
| Indoor air pollutants | 431 | 19.8 |
| Crystalline silica | 186 | 8.5 |
| Solvents n.o.s. | 92 | 4.2 |
| Smoke n.o.s. | 83 | 3.8 |
| Coal (incl. coal dust) | 75 | 3.4 |
| Dust n.o.s. | 75 | 3.4 |
| Chemicals n.o.s. | 73 | 3.3 |
| Mold | 63 | 2.9 |
| Isocyanates n.o.s. | 58 | 2.7 |
| Paint (incl. epoxy, latex, oil based) | 50 | 2.3 |
| Cutting oils | 44 | 2.0 |
| Latex, natural rubber | 41 | 1.9 |
| Tuberculosis | 41 | 1.9 |
| Welding n.o.s. (incl. fumes) | 40 | 1.8 |
| Hydrocarbons n.o.s. | 27 | 1.2 |
| Formaldehyde | 24 | 1.1 |
| Cleaning materials n.o.s. (incl. disinfectants) | 22 | 1.0 |
| Glutaraldehyde | 22 | 1.0 |
| Wood dust n.o.s. | 18 | 0.8 |
| Diesel exhaust | 17 | 0.8 |
| Glues n.o.s. | 17 | 0.8 |
| Carbon monoxide | 16 | 0.7 |
| Lubricants n.o.s. | 15 | 0.7 |
| Metal fumes n.o.s. | 15 | 0.7 |
| Acids, bases, oxidizers n.o.s. | 14 | 0.6 |
| Epoxy resins | 13 | 0.6 |
| Photo-developing chemicals n.o.s. | 10 | 0.5 |
| Toluene | 10 | 0.5 |
| Flour n.o.s. | 9 | 0.4 |
| Methyl ethyl ketone | 9 | 0.4 |
| Acrylates n.o.s. | 8 | 0.4 |
| Asphalt | 8 | 0.4 |
| Bleach | 8 | 0.4 |
| Freon® | 8 | 0.4 |
| Odors | 8 | 0.4 |
| Pesticides n.o.s. | 8 | 0.4 |
| Polymers n.o.s. | 8 | 0.4 |
| Sulfuric acid | 8 | 0.4 |
| Ammonia solution n.o.s. | 7 | 0.3 |
| Ethylene oxide | 7 | 0.3 |
| Hydrochloric acid | 7 | 0.3 |
| Plastic smoke | 7 | 0.3 |
| Acrolein | 6 | 0.3 |
| Cement dust | 6 | 0.3 |
| Hydrogen sulfide | 6 | 0.3 |
| Irritant gases n.o.s. | 6 | 0.3 |
| Man-made mineral fibers | 6 | 0.3 |
| Plant material n.o.s. | 6 | 0.3 |
| Polyvinyl chloride | 6 | 0.3 |
| All others | 435 | 20.0 |
| Total | 2,179 | 100.0 |

**Table 9.3** Allergic asthmagens

| Work activity | Agent |
|---|---|
| *High-molecular-weight substances* | |
| Bakers, farmers, flour mill workers, grain elevator workers | Flour, grain dust |
| Silk-processing workers, research laboratory workers, insect-raising facility workers | Insects |
| Prawn, snow-crab, and fish processors | Seafood, other marine organisms |
| Laboratory workers, animal handlers | Animal dander |
| Detergent producers, food industry workers, blood-processing laboratory workers | Enzymes |
| Carpet manufacturing workers, pharmaceutical industry workers, latex glove-manufacturing workers, health care workers | Gums, latex |
| *Low-molecular-weight substances* | |
| Plastic, rubber, or foam-manufacturing workers, spray painters, foam insulation installers | Diisocyanates (toluene, diphenylmethane, hexamethylene) |
| Solderers, electronic industry workers | Colophony (abietic acid) |
| Woodworkers, foresters, artisans | Plicatic acid (Western red cedar wood dust) |
| Refinery workers | Metals (chromium, platinum, nickel) |
| Textile workers | Dyes |
| Plastic and epoxy resin workers | Anhydrides (trimellitic, phthalic) |
| Adhesive handlers | Acrylates |
| Health care workers | Glutaraldehyde, formaldehyde |
| Pharmaceutical industry workers | Pharmaceuticals |

Work-related asthma can be differentiated as asthma caused by work, (occupational asthma) or asthma exacerbated by work. It has been estimated that 10–16 % of asthma cases in adults are attributable to occupational exposures (Bardana 2008; CDC 2012; Scherer et al. 2012). Occupational asthma (OA) can be allergic or non-allergic in origin. The allergic variant can be further divided into the classic IgE-mediated form and polyimmunologic form. Allergic cases are usually caused by high-molecular-weight allergens such as animal proteins in hair or saliva or grain dusts, pollens, and molds. Some lower molecular weight compounds, such as the isocyanates, can also cause asthma. There is often a latency period from initial exposure of days or months before a person develops typical asthmatic symptoms, especially for allergic cases.

Table 9.3 provides examples of occupations and associated agents known to cause allergic occupational asthma (Youakim 2001).

Non-allergic occupational asthma can be divided into RADS, pharmacologic bronchoconstriction, and reflex bronchospasm. RADS is a sudden onset of asthma-like symptoms following a high-level irritant gas, vapor, or fume exposure. The diagnosis of RADS requires that asthma-like symptoms begin within 24 h of an exposure that is characteristically single, high level, and brief (Brooks et al. 1998). Exposures associated with RADS are sometimes repetitive and occur throughout the work cycle. Table 9.4 provides examples of exposures associated with RADS.

**Table 9.4** Chemicals associated with RADS

| Irritants | Sensitizers |
|---|---|
| Pesticide spraying | Diphenylmethane diisocyanate |
| Cement sealant | Hexamethylene diisocyanate |
| Mixed solvent vapors and mist | Toluene diisocyanate |
| Household bleach vapor | Flour dust |
| Spray paint | Acrylates, methacrylate, and cyanoacrylate ester |
| Sulfur dioxide gas | |
| Titanium tetrachloride mist | |
| Ammonia vapors | |
| Muriatic (hydrochloric) acid spill | |
| Welding fume | |
| Chlorine gas | |
| Burned Freon fumes | |
| Sodium hydroxide exposure | |

Work-related rhinitis may be differentiated as occupational rhinitis due to an exposure at a workplace or work-exacerbated rhinitis that is preexisting or concurrent rhinitis exacerbated by workplace exposures. Occupational rhinitis (OR) is an inflammatory disease of the nose characterized by symptoms such as nasal congestion, sneezing, rhinorrhea, itching, and/or nasal airflow limitation and/or hypersecretions due to a workplace exposure (Endre 2010; Moscato and Siracusa 2009; Moscato et al. 2009). Occupational rhinitis is two to four times more common than OA. The majority of patients with work-related asthma also suffer from occupational rhinitis. OR often precedes the development of OA, especially if high molecular agents are involved. As with OA, occupational rhinitis symptoms may be caused by IgE- or non-IgE-mediated immunological hypersensitivity reactions. Non-allergic occupational rhinitis can be caused through irritant, non-immunologic mechanisms. Single or multiple high-dose exposures to irritants can cause transient or permanent symptoms of rhinitis and have been referred to as reactive upper airway dysfunction syndrome or RUDS (Meggs 1994).

Laryngeal dysfunction can be associated with workplace exposures (Hoy 2012). Vocal cord dysfunction (VCD) is a syndrome characterized by the intermittent, abnormal paradoxical adduction of the true vocal cords during respiration resulting in variable upper airway obstruction. It is also commonly referred to as paradoxical vocal fold motion disorder. Patients with VCD usually present with intermittent shortness of breath of varying intensity, wheezing, stridor, choking, throat tightness, voice changes, or cough, and these symptoms often resolve quickly after relaxation or cessation of activity (de la Hoz et al. 2008). Episodic dyspnea, dysphonia, cough, and sensation of tingling in the throat have been described from workplace exposures to fumes, perfumes, and cleaning agents. Situations of high psychological distress may be associated with recurrent symptoms of vocal cord dysfunction (Hoy 2012).

## Worksite Evaluation

The worksite evaluation should begin with obtaining background information about processes, chemical usage, environmental control measures, personal protective equipment, and employee education/training. Material Safety Data Sheets can provide information about chemical hazards. Any measurements of worker exposure should be reviewed. Logs of first-aid cases and any records the employer maintains on occupational injuries and illnesses should be reviewed. Many employers are required to maintain the OSHA form 300 and supplemental form 301 to record work-related injuries and illnesses. All occupational illnesses are recordable. A review of worker's compensation claims should also be conducted.

The number of workers exposed and the physical and chemical characteristics and patterns of exposure can be estimated from a careful walkthrough with interviews of potentially affected employees. The use, effectiveness, and maintenance of engineering controls such as exhaust ventilation enclosure of aerosol-producing processes should be reviewed.

## Worker Evaluation

A thorough medical and occupational history should be performed for individuals presenting with respiratory symptoms. Is there any cough, shortness of breath, or sputum production? Does the patient note any decrease in physical activity due to dyspnea on exertion or chest pain? Details of smoking including exposure to secondhand smoke are important. The person should be asked about indoor pet and pest problems. Any history of water damage inside the home should be discussed as indoor mold may be causing symptoms. Does the person have allergies to tree, weed, or grass pollens?

The occupational history should include questions on general cleanliness/dustiness of the work environment. Does the job involve exposure to dust or dirt/rocks? Does the person work directly with chemicals? If not, does he/she walk through areas where chemicals may be used? Does his/her work involve exposure to animals/animal feed of any type? Is the person aware of water damage to the worksite such as backed-up sewer line or a leaking roof? Does anyone wear respirators at the worksite and why?

If the employee is required to wear a respirator, the medical evaluation to determine if the individual can tolerate the physiological burden associated with respirator use without serious medical consequences should be reviewed. The Occupational Safety And Health Respiratory Protection Standard 29CFR 1910-134 requires medical evaluations performed by a physician or other licensed health care professional following a standard medical questionnaire or equivalent to be performed for every employee required to wear a respirator at work. There should be a written medical opinion for each employee required to wear a respirator which should be maintained by the employer. If respirators such as dust masks (filtering face piece respirators) are available for voluntary use certain elements of the respirator standard are relaxed as long as the respirator itself does not present a hazard (U.S. Department of Labor 1998).

In addition in the OSHA Permissible Exposure Limits listed in 29CFR 1910-1000, there are approximately 30 substance-specific health-related standards for substances such as asbestos, coal tar pitch volatiles, inorganic arsenic, lead, formaldehyde, chromium (VI) cadmium, ethylene oxide, and vinyl chloride. These substance-specific or expanded standards will have additional medical surveillance requirements (U.S. Department of Labor 1993).

Next a physical exam is performed focusing on the skin and upper and lower respiratory tract. Is there evidence of any contact dermatitis? Are the nasal passages patent? Is there nasal discharge? Are the sinuses tender to palpation/percussion? Is there any redness of the throat of evidence of lymphadenopathy? Is there any evidence of hoarseness? What is the respiratory rate? Are there any rales/rhonchi/wheezing noted on exam? Is there evidence of cyanosis or clubbing?

Several guidance documents from the Agency for Toxic Substances and Disease Registry (U.S Department of Health and Human Services 2008), the American Academy of Clinical Toxicology (2010), and others (Lax et al. 2008) have been published detailing obtaining an exposure history and a symptom history and performing a clinical examination.

Depending on the findings additional laboratory procedures are often indicated. Pulse oximetry or arterial blood gas measurements may provide useful information. Office spirometry or full pulmonary function testing may indicate obstructive or restrictive changes. A complete blood count may show evidence of eosinophilia in persons that are suspected of having an allergic component to their symptoms. Allergy skin testing may be useful if one suspects environmental allergens such as pollen or molds. In certain cases antibodies against specific chemicals, e.g., isocyanates, can be sought, but the absence of antibodies does not necessarily mean that the suspected agent is not the cause of the symptoms due to the frequent low sensitivity/specificity qualities of many of these tests. Methacholine challenge testing can be used to evaluate bronchial reactivity. Exhaled nitrous oxide levels may suggest inflammation in the lungs (Murugan et al. 2009). Sputum eosinophils may suggest an inflammatory component (Snell and Newbold 2008). For certain agents, specific inhalation challenge test may be useful to aid in diagnosis. Other tests may include bronchoalveolar lavage and microscopy of the washings. Laryngoscopy may be useful to diagnose VCD. If infection is suspected, culture of sputum and bronchial washings may identify the infectious agent. Biopsy of the involved tissue with special staining and spectroscopy may indicate the etiology. Peak flow monitoring at work can provide useful information and may indicate areas of the worksite that deserve closer industrial hygiene assessment. Radiological studies such as CXR and CT scans may give an indication of localized or widespread involvement of the particular organ.

## References


Agency for Toxic Substances and Disease Registry. Technical briefing paper: health effects from exposure to fibrous glass, rock wool, or slag wool. 2002. http://www.atsdr.cdc.gov/DT/fibrous-glass.html#appendix-a

American Academy of Clinical Toxicology Exposure History Form. 2010. http://www.clintox.org/documents/AACTExposureHistoryForm.pdf.

American Conference of Governmental Industrial Hygienists Threshold limit values for chemical substances, physical agents and biological exposure indices. 2012.

Bardana Jr EJ. Occupational asthma. J Allergy Clin Immunol. 2008;121(2 suppl):408–11.

Brooks SM et al. The spectrum of irritant-induced asthma: sudden and not-so-sudden onset and the role of allergy. Chest. 1998;113:1.

Centers for Disease Control and Prevention. Work-related lung disease surveillance report 2007. Morganton: NIOSH; 2008, W.V. No 2008-143a.

Centers for Disease Control and Prevention. Work-related asthma—38 states and District of Columbia, 2006–2009. Morb Mortal Wkly Rep. 2012;61(20):375–8.

de la Hoz RE, Shohet MR, Bienenfeld LA, Afilaka AA, Levin SM, Herbert R. Vocal cord dysfunction in former World Trade Center (WTC) rescue and recovery workers and volunteers. Am J Ind Med. 2008;51(3):161–5.

Endre L. Occupational rhinitis. Orv Hetil. 2010;151(23):941–5.

Environmental Protection Agency, Air Pollution Training Institute. Basic concepts in environmental sciences, module 3, characteristics of particles—particle size categories 2010. http://www.epa.gov/apti/bces/module3/category/category.htm.

Hoy R. Work related laryngeal syndromes. Curr Opin Allergy Clin Immunol. 2012;12(2): 95–101.

Lax MB, Grant WD, Manetti FA, Klein R. Recognizing occupational disease—taking an effective occupational history. Am Fam Physician. 2008; 58(4):935–44. http://www.aafp.org/afp/1998/0915/p935.html.

Meggs WJ. RADS and RUDS-the toxic induction of asthma and rhinitis. J Toxicol Clin Toxicol. 1994;32(5):487–501.

Moscato G, Siracusa A. Rhinitis guidelines and implications for occupational rhinitis. Curr Opin Allergy Clin Immunol. 2009;4(2):110–5.

Moscato G, Vandenplas O, Van Wijk RG, Malo JL, Perfetti L, et al. EAACI position paper on occupational rhinitis. Respir Res. 2009. doi:10.1186/1465-9921-10-16.

Morgan WKC. The deposition and clearance of dust from the lungs-their role in the etiology of occupational lung diseases. In: Morgan WKC, Seaton A, editors. Occupational lung disease. Philadelphia: W.B. Saunders Company; 1995. p. 111–6.

Murugan A, Prys-Picard C, Calhoun WJ. Biomarkers in asthma. Curr Opin Pulm Med. 2009; 15(1):12–8.

National Institute for Occupational Safety and Health. Criteria for a recommended standard: occupational exposure to fibrous glass. DHHS (NIOSH) publication number 77-152. 1977.

National Institute for Occupational Safety and Health. Interdivisional fiber subcommittee, final report. March 17, 1999.

National Institute for Occupational Safety and Health. General safe practices for working with engineered nanomaterials in research laboratories. DHHS (NIOSH) publication no. 2012-147, 2012.

Scherer HK, Bircher A, Tamm M, Miedinger D. Occupational rhinitis and asthma. Ther Umsch. 2012;69(4):261–7.

Shamon S. Vocal cord dysfunction: current understanding and approach to disease. UBC Med J. 2009;1(1):2009.

Snell N, Newbold P. The clinical utility of biomarkers in asthma and COPD. Curr Opin Pharmacol. 2008;8(3):222–35.

Taylor AJN. Respiratory Irritants encountered at work. Thorax. 1996;51(5):541–5.
United States Department of Labor, Occupational Safety and Health Administration, 29 Code of Federal Regulations, 1910.134. 1998 http://www.osha.gov/pls/oshaweb/owadisp.show_document?p_id=12716&p_table=standards (see appendix C for OSHA respirator medical evaluation questionnaire and appendix D for employees using respirators when not required under the standard).
United States Department of Labor, Occupational Safety and Health Administration. 29 code of federal regulations, subpart Z, toxic and hazardous substances. 1993 http://www.osha.gov/pls/oshaweb/owadisp.show_document?p_table=STANDARDS&p_id=1014.
U.S. Department of Health and Human Services. Agency for Toxic Substances and Disease Registry (ATSDR), Case Studies in Environmental Medicine. Taking an Exposure History 2008 http://www.atsdr.cdc.gov/csem/csem.html.
Weir NA, Gulati M, Radlich CA. Approach to the patient/diagnostic methods. In: Rosenstock L, Cullen MR, Brodkin CA, Radlich CA, editors. Textbook of clinical occupational and environmental medicine. Philadelphia: Elsevier Saunders; 2005. p. 285–92.
Weston A. Work-related lung diseases. IARC Sci Publ. 2011;163:387–405.
Youakim S. Work related asthma. Am Fam Physician. 2001;64(11):1839–49.

# Chapter 10
# The Brain as a Target Organ for Allergic and Irritant Sensitivity: A Review and Suggestions for Research

**William J. Meggs, Richard M. Bloch, and Kori L. Brewer**

**Abstract** Objective: Clinical descriptions of behavioral and neurological manifestations of allergy and irritant sensitivity are described. Public health implications and mechanisms are discussed, with recommendations for further research. Data sources: MedLine searches of articles combining the terms allergy, asthma, rhinitis, irritant rhinitis, irritant asthma, chemical sensitivity, and multiple chemical sensitivity syndrome were combined with searches on fatigue, chronic fatigue syndrome, depression, anxiety, and insomnia. Textbooks of allergy and books on irritant sensitivity were reviewed.

Data extraction and synthesis: Quantitative evidence on the neurological and psychiatric manifestations of asthma and chemical sensitivity is limited, though a few controlled studies exist. Irritant sensitivity is generally self-reported in studies, though objective parameters exist for diagnosis of allergy. Clinical descriptions and controlled studies are analyzed for their support for the hypothesis that the brain is a target organ for allergic and irritant sensitivity.

Conclusions: This literature review supports the hypothesis that the brain is a target organ for allergic and irritant reactions with neuropsychological manifestations. Technology exists to conduct controlled challenge studies using real-time

W.J. Meggs, M.D., Ph.D., F.A.C.M.T., F.A.C.E.P. (✉)
Department of Emergency Medicine, Brody School of Medicine
at East Carolina University, Greenville, NC, USA
e-mail: meggsw@ecu.edu

R.M. Bloch, Ph.D.
Department of Psychiatry, Brody School of Medicine
at East Carolina University, Greenville, NC, USA

K.L. Brewer, Ph.D.
Department of Emergency Medicine, Brody School of Medicine
at East Carolina University, Greenville, NC, USA

W.J. Meggs (ed.), *The Toxicant Induction of Irritant Asthma, Rhinitis, and Related Conditions*, DOI 10.1007/978-1-4614-9044-9_10,

monitoring of cerebral function with state-of-the-art imagining modalities, correlating neuropsychological manifestations, and serum biomarkers. This research could have implications for treatment and prevention of some forms of neuropsychological illnesses.

**Keywords** Allergy • Respiratory irritants • Fatigue • Depression • Sleep disorders • Attention-deficit disorder

## Introduction

Illnesses related to exposures to allergens or irritants involve a two-step process. There has to be an initiating mechanism followed by a responsive organ. In the case of allergy, the initiating mechanism is the binding of a substance to IgE antibodies. For irritant reactions, the initiating mechanism is binding of a substance to nociceptors on sensory nerves. The second step is reactivity in a target organ producing a clinical manifestation. This chapter discusses the evidence that the brain can be a target organ, that is manifest cerebral dysfunction, in susceptible individuals encountering an allergen or an irritant.

The Joint Task Force on Practice Parameters, representing the American Academy of Allergy, Asthma & Immunology; the American College of Allergy, Asthma and Immunology; and the Joint Council of Allergy, Asthma and Immunology, states (Wallace et al. 2008): "Although sometimes mistakenly viewed as a trivial disease, symptoms of allergic and non-allergic rhinitis may significantly affect a patient's quality of life and can be associated with conditions such as *fatigue, headache, cognitive impairment, and sleep disturbance*." (Italics added). How does inflammation of the upper airway, whether induced by allergens, irritants, or other factors, become associated with neurological symptoms?

Allergens and irritants affect susceptible individuals at lower levels than tolerated by the population at large. Primary target organs in these individuals can be the upper airway, lower airway, conjunctiva, or skin, although other organs less commonly can have hyper-reactivity to exposures. A wealth of clinical descriptions from earlier eras suggests that the brain may be a target organ for allergic and irritant exposures in susceptible individuals. These clinical descriptions have largely been ignored in our scientific era of evidence-based medicine due in part to an inability to objectively assess cerebral function. The development of technologies for the objective analysis of changes in cerebral function over brief time periods now gives the ability to study cerebral function in challenge studies to allergens and irritants. Just as a patient with asthma can have pulmonary function tests, bronchoalveolar washings, and other objective parameters of disease analyzed pre- and post-allergen and irritant challenges, an individual with changes in cognition, mood, alertness, or other cerebral manifestations can undergo objective challenges with allergens and irritants with real-time monitoring of cerebral function.

This review article defines allergic sensitivity, irritant sensitivity, and target organs. The clinical descriptions that suggest that the brain may be a target organ for allergens and irritants are reviewed. Studies supporting such as association are discussed. In the final section, research directions and methodological confounders are outlined, with discussion of modalities for objectively monitoring cerebral reactivity on a real-time basis.

## Allergy, Irritant Sensitivity, and Target Organs

Voluminous scientific data has led to universal acceptance of the existence and nature of allergy. Allergic individuals make specific antibodies of the IgE class to antigens that are either environmental proteins or adducts of environmental chemicals with indigenous proteins. IgE is bound to high-affinity receptors on mast cells and basophils. Cross-linking of IgE molecules by antigens triggers mast cell and basophil degranulation with release of histamine, cytokines, chemotactic factors, and other mediators that trigger an inflammatory response.

The target organs of allergy are most commonly the site of inoculation with antigen. Allergic rhinitis and allergic asthma represent airway inflammation triggered by inhaled proteins to which the individual is producing specific IgE antibody molecules. Urticaria occurs with inoculation of the skin with antigen; examples are insect stings or iatrogenic urticaria induced by skin testing. The target organ is not always the site of inoculation. For example, some individuals with pollen allergy develop urticaria during pollen seasons (Anuradha et al. 2006; Hesselmar et al. 2007). Dogs with pollen allergy commonly develop dermatitis during the pollen season (Chanthick et al. 2008). A small percentage of individuals with asthma have attacks triggered by food antigens (Yazicioglu et al. 1999). Systemic anaphylaxis occurs when there is immediate reactivity of multiple target organs—including respiratory, skin, and cardiovascular with manifestations of bronchospasm, bronchorrhea, rhinorrhea, urticaria, hypotension, and tachycardia. One hypothesis for responsiveness in an organ different from the inoculated organ is neurogenic switching (Meggs 1995), in which activation of sensory nerve fibers at the site of inoculation sends a message that is rerouted to other sites.

The chemicals given in Table 1.1 in Chap. 1 are ubiquitous in developed and many developing societies. Virtually everyone is exposed daily to some of these chemicals at concentrations that are tolerated by the majority of individuals. Many clinical descriptions and case definitions have been advanced to describe populations with reactivity to these substances, such as multiple chemical sensitivity (MCS) syndrome (Cullen 1987), chemical sensitivity (Rea 1994), environmental illness (Randolph 1962), idiopathic environmental intolerances (International Programme on Chemical Safety 1996), and toxicant-induced loss of tolerance (TILT) syndrome (Miller 1999, 2001). Population studies suggest that self-reported sensitivity to these agents is common (Meggs 1996; Kreutzer et al. 1999; Voorhees

1998; Caress and Steinemann 2004a, b; Hausteiner et al. 2005) and can range as high as 30 % when survey questions are designed to include individuals with symptoms limited to airway inflammation associated with substances in Table 1.1 in Chap. 1 (Meggs 1996). Opinions concerning the nature of chemical sensitivity vary from a psychosomatic disorder (Terr 1986; Staudenmayer et al. 2003), hyperventilation syndrome (Leznoff 1997), and a disorder of nasal mucosa (Bascom 1992; Meggs 1992; Meggs and Cleveland 1993) to attributing a broad range of diseases to low-level chemical exposures (Randolph 1962).

It is now scientifically established and universally accepted that chemicals such as those given in Table 1.1 in Chap. 1 can induce airway inflammation in susceptible individuals (Brooks et al. 1998; Elberling et al. 2007; Qian et al. 2007). The mechanism is known to be neurogenic inflammation, with irritant chemicals binding chemoreceptors on sensory nerve fibers and triggering an inflammatory cascade by the release of neurokinens (Nielsen 1991; Groneberg et al. 2004; Lacroix and Landis 2008). In addition, increased levels of nerve growth factor are found in the airways of allergic and irritant rhinitis patients relative to controls (Sanico et al. 1999, 2000; Millqvist et al. 2005; Sarin et al. 2006).

Asthma and rhinitis triggered by irritants are generally accepted and known as irritant rhinitis and irritant asthma. A PubMed search of irritant rhinitis and irritant asthma yielded 235 and 820 articles, respectively (November 2009). For the purpose of this chapter, we will use the term *irritant sensitivity* to make it clear that we are referring specifically to responsiveness to irritant chemicals at levels tolerated by the population at large, with objective markers of airway inflammation, mediated via neurogenic inflammation. That said, most of the data discussed on chemical sensitivity in the remainder of this chapter include individuals with self-reported chemical sensitivity without screening for airway inflammation.

Challenge studies in humans document that chemical exposures can provoke signs and symptoms of airway inflammation in susceptible individuals (Doty et al. 1988; Millqvist and Lowhagen 1996; Willes et al. 1992, 1998; Baur et al. 1999; Jorres et al. 2000; Nordenhall et al. 2001; Elberling et al. 2004, 2007). Animal studies too numerous to review here document associations between chemical irritant exposures and airway inflammation. A study of MCS patients found increases in nasal airway resistance after chemical challenge (Doty et al. 1988). Millqvist and her collaborators have performed a number of elegant challenge studies in patients with chemical sensitivities that simultaneously prove sensory hyper-reactivity in these patients while supporting neurogenic inflammation and the concept of neurogenic switching (Millqvist and Lowhagen 1996; Millqvist et al. 1999, 2005, 2008). Inoculation of the conjunctiva with perfume in subjects breathing through a mask designed to avoid detection of odor was demonstrated to produce symptoms of airway inflammation in controlled blinded challenge studies of chemically sensitive individuals but not controls, even though no perfume reached the airway (Millqvist and Lowhagen 1996). A study of MCS patients found increased levels of nerve growth factor and substance P in plasma of patients but not control groups that increased with chemical challenge (Kimata 2004).

Irritant exposures can induce asthma and rhinitis that can persist, with heightened sensitivity to irritants. These syndromes are called reactive airways dysfunction syndrome (RADS) (Brooks et al. 1985, 1998) and reactive upper-airways dysfunction syndrome (RUDS) (Meggs and Cleveland 1993; Meggs 1994; Meggs et al. 1996a, b). Further, irritant exposures can act as environmental adjuvants and lead to allergy to proteins when there are concomitant exposures to irritants and allergens. Though most of the work has been done in experimental models, diesel exhaust particles is a notable example that has been verified as an environmental adjuvant in humans (Diaz-Sanchez et al. 1997, 1999).

To summarize, allergic diseases result from a combination of having specific IgE antibodies to antigens in the environment having one or more responsive target organs that can be objectively assessed. Irritant sensitivity is a hyper-responsiveness to environmental chemicals via neurogenic inflammation triggered by the interaction of chemicals with sensory nerve fibers with responsive target organs that can be objectively assessed. A target organ is an organ that undergoes pathophysiological and clinical changes when activated by allergens or irritants.

## Descriptions of the Brain as Target Organ for Allergy and Irritancy

There are abundant descriptions of the brain reactions to allergens and irritants (Speer 1972), dating back at least to 1923 (Duke 1923). Descriptions include asthenia, delirium, confusion, depression, psychosis, and even seizures. The Davison-Campbell Descriptive Classification is given in Table 12.2 in Chap. 12. Campbell comments: "Since our present knowledge does not well explain the origin and pathogenesis of allergic reactions in the nervous system, we are obliged to classify them on a descriptive basis." (Campbell 1972). At the current time, knowledge has not yet advanced to the point of explaining these reactions. Contemporary medical practice has not embraced the concept that some behavioral disorders arise from reactivity to allergens and irritants. At the same time, behavioral disorders including depression and attention-deficit disorder are increasing, particularly among the young who have unprecedented exposures to environmental chemicals (CDC 2005).

Association between depression, anxiety, allergy, and irritant sensitivity are suggested by a number of studies. Allergy skin tests performed on all depressed individuals referred for a psychiatric evaluation during a 1-year period were positive in 93 of 109 subjects (Ossofsky 1976), though only 50 % reported allergy symptoms. 33 % of psychiatric patients with depression had documented allergy but only 6 % of patients with schizophrenia (Nasr et al. 1981). Individuals in a large insurance database with allergic rhinitis were more likely to file claims for anxiety and depression than those making insurance claims without allergic rhinitis (Cuffel et al. 1999). A study found that, of those reporting depression, 71 % reported allergy and 64 % had a health professional diagnosis of allergy (Bell et al. 1991). A history of asthma, hay fever, urticaria, or eczema was found in 26 % of those with monopolar depression, versus 17 % in a nondepressed control group (Matussek et al. 1983). Marshall reviewed the literature relating allergy and depression and hypothesized that autonomic reactions to allergens in allergic people who also tend to be depressed can be sufficient to induce depression (Marshall 1993). Ragweed allergy season brings greater sadness and fatigue among allergy sufferers than when ragweed allergens are out of season (Marshall et al. 2002).

Anxiety is also associated with allergy and in particular a subtype of anxiety disorder, panic disorder. A study found allergies in 72 % of patients with panic disorder (Kennedy et al. 2002). A strong association was found between panic disorder and allergy in children (Kovalenko et al. 2001). Children with panic disorder were five times more likely to utilize allergy services than children with other anxiety disorders or without anxiety disorders. A large health care insurance database study found that patients with allergic rhinitus have high rates of comorbid anxiety disorders (Cuffel et al. 1999). Addolarato et al. compared the state and trait anxiety of patients with food allergies to those of patients with irritable bowel syndrome, of patients with lactose intolerance, and of healthy controls. Both food allergy and irritable bowel patients showed higher levels of both state and trait anxiety than the other two groups (Addolarato et al. 1998).

Simon reviewed psychological studies of chemically sensitive patients and found that the percentage with depression and anxiety is higher in the chemically sensitive group than in control groups (Simon 1994). A study comparing patients with chemical sensitivity to chronic back pain and repetitive motion syndrome patients found that 44 % of the patients with chemical sensitivity suffered from anxiety or depression compared to 15 % of the comparison groups (Simon et al. 1993). Current depressive disorders were found in 50 % of a cohort of patients presenting to an occupational medicine clinic for treatment of symptoms related to chemical exposure (Fiedler et al. 1992). Using a structured interview, depressive disorders were found in 40 % of chemically sensitive patients recruited from the community but only 13 % of nonsensitive controls (Black et al. 1990). Current symptoms of depression or anxiety where found in approximately 75 % of patients developing chemical sensitivity associated with occupational exposure to solvents (Simon et al. 1990). A study found that after adjusting for age, gender, and education, patients with multiple chemical sensitivities scored higher than normal workers on both the depression and anxiety subscales of the SCL-90, although only the depression difference reached significance (Osterberg et al. 2002).

A study comparing subjects with self-reported allergy and chemical sensitivity, with instruments designed to detect anxiety and depression, found significant increases in both anxiety and depression in those reporting allergy and those reporting chemical sensitivity. There was no significant difference, however, in those reporting allergy from those reporting chemical sensitivity (Bloch and Meggs 2007). This study suggests a common feature relating allergy and chemical sensitivity that leads to anxiety and depression. That feature may be upper airway inflammation.

Seizures described as induced by foods include grand mal seizures, petit mal seizures, and brief focal seizures. Attempts to correlate electroencephalogram studies and allergy skin tests with seizure activity have had variable results (Campbell 1968). Fatigue in association with allergy and irritant exposures is a recurring theme in descriptions of neurological allergy. Ragweed allergic patients reported increased general and mental fatigue, reduced motivation, increased sadness, and reduced pleasure but not increased anxiety or emotional distress during the ragweed pollen season (Marshall et al. 2002). A study of chronic fatigue syndrome patients found that 24 % had no significant rhinitis complaints, 30 % had positive skin tests suggesting the potential for allergic rhinitis complaints, and 46 % had nonallergic rhinitis (Baraniuk et al. 1998). One interpretation of this study is that in a significant subset of patients with chronic fatigue, allergic and/or irritant rhinitis is the cause of the fatigue. Chronic fatigue syndrome patients were found to report increased levels of chemical sensitivity relative to healthy controls (Nawab 2000). Ill Gulf War veterans reporting chemical sensitivity and exposed to diesel vapors and acetaldehyde suffered increased malaise relative to controls (Fiedler et al. 2004). Listlessness/fatigue and long-term fatigue were among the five most common symptoms in a population with self-reported chemical sensitivity (Gibson and Vogel 2009).

Cognitive function was found to be impaired in children suffering from seasonal allergic rhinitis using a didactic computer simulation in a realistic classroom situation. Impairment was exacerbated by treatments with sedating antihistamines and partially but not totally reversed by treatment with nonsedating antihistamine (Vuurman et al. 1993). This research concluded that allergic rhinitis can lead to impairment cognition and that sedating histamines can exacerbate that impairment. A study comparing symptoms in individuals who developed chemical sensitivity in association with pesticide exposure versus remodeling found that cognitive symptoms were most severe in both groups, with no statistically significant difference between the two groups (Miller and Mitzel 1995). Difficulty concentrating and memory difficulties were among the five most common symptoms in a population with self-reported chemical sensitivity (Gibson and Vogel 2009).

Randolph described behavioral disorders and other neurological symptoms arising from exposures to environmental chemicals (Randolph 1962). He described paired stimulatory symptoms triggered by exposures and withdrawal symptoms that occur after removal from the exposure, whether iatrogenic for testing purpose or from random exposures to chemicals in the diet, air, and water in daily life. For example, manic behavior is described as triggered by exposure, while depression is a withdrawal symptom after the exposure is removed. Grand mal seizures are described as occurring from stimulation, while coma is described as a withdrawal symptom.

Some authors, while recognizing relationships between depression, fatigue, anxiety, and cognitive dysfunction, consider these associations as comorbid disorders with allergic rhinitis and/or chemical sensitivity (Black 1990, Bloch 2007) rather than the mental issues being caused or as a consequence of allergic and irritant exposures.

Sick building syndrome (World Health Organization 1983) is described as illnesses occurring in occupants of tightly sealed buildings with poor air exchange. The two organ systems most commonly affected are respiratory (cough, nasal congestion, ...) and the nervous system (confusion, cognitive dysfunction, difficulty with concentration, headache, difficulty with memory) (Robertson et al. 1985; Seppänen and Fisk 2004). Irritants in buildings include volatile organic chemicals out-gassing from paints, carpets, wall board, adhesives, and office machinery.

Insecticides, perfumes, fragrances, and cleaning products contribute to the mix. Volatile mycotoxins from mold growth are found in water-damaged buildings (Jarvis 2002; Fog Nielsen 2003; Rios et al. 2009), though their impact on human health is at this time controversial (Hardin et al. 2003). Occupants of poorly ventilated buildings have an increased risk of asthma (Hoffman et al. 1993). The brain as a target organ for irritant reactions could explain the neurological symptoms that accompany respiratory complaints in poorly ventilated buildings.

One of the most perplexing features of chemical sensitivity is that some individuals are highly disabled by their sensitivities and undertake remarkable lifestyle changes to avoid chemicals (Kipen et al. 1995; Fiedler et al. 1992; Gibson & Vogel 2009). Perhaps the reason that some are so disabled is that they suffer from irritant sensitivity with the brain as a target organ.

Autonomic dysfunction has been observed in children with allergic rhinitis by studies of heart rate variability (Tascilar et al. 2009). In a controlled study subjects with non-arteriosclerotic cardiac arrhythmias and/or chest pain refractory to medication and having symptoms related to smooth muscle sensitization were studied in a rigidly controlled, relatively fume- and particle-free environment. Symptoms and arrhythmias abated while in the controlled environment and were induced by re-exposure to irritants (Rea 1978). The observation that some subjects with self-reported chemical sensitivity develop respiratory alkalosis (Leznoff 1997; Fiedler et al. 2004) when challenged has been interpreted as evidence that chemical sensitivity is an anxiety disorder; an alternative interpretation is that the brain is a target organ for irritant sensitivity with central dysregulation of autonomic responses in some individuals.

In summary, there is literature supporting the hypothesis that the brain is a target organ for allergic and irritant sensitivity. Rigorous scientific demonstration of pathophysiology to support the association is lacking. With the burdensome prevalence of allergy, depression, anxiety, attention-deficit disorder, fatigue, and sleep disturbances in our society, scientific study of the brain as a target organ for allergic and irritant sensitivity has the potential to impact both prevention and treatment of a spectrum of neurological disorders.

## Possible Mechanisms

Discussion about the mechanisms in the brain that could lead to symptoms such as fatigue, depression, anxiety, hyperactivity, cognitive dysfunction, disordered attention, and sleep disturbances may be speculative at this time. Based on the physiological mechanisms underlying allergic and irritant reactivity in other organs, vasomotor phenomena, edema, capillary leak, cytokines, neurokinens, chemotaxis, and cellular migrations could all play a role. Microglia cells are involved in host defense in the brain and could play a role. Clinical descriptions and limited controlled studies suggest that individuals with allergic and/or irritant sensitivity have variable cerebral manifestations, ranging from none to depression, anxiety, cognitive dysfunction, sleep disturbances, and fatigue. A possible explanation of this variability is that different regions of the brain are involved in different individuals, just as different regions of the airway can be involved in the different individuals, ranging from sinusitis, rhinitis and pharyngitis to asthma. Individuals with urticaria and dermatitis can have involvement of variable regions of the dermis that is sometimes fixed with recurrences in a given individual.

That allergic and irritant sensitivity may exacerbate psychiatric illnesses becomes more plausible as data accumulates about the role of inflammation in these disorders. To quote from Beumer et al., "There is accumulating evidence for activation of microglia (histopathology and PET scans) and circulating monocytes (enhanced gene expression of immune genes, an overproduction of monocyte/macxrophage-related cytokines) in patients with bipolar disorder, major depressive disorder, and schizophrenia." (Beumer et al. 2012). Postmortem studies of individuals with schizophrenia who committed suicide have found increases in microglia numbers.

It is now established that systemic inflammation can excite microglia in the brain. The mechanisms have been elucidated in experimental studies (Perry 2004, 2010; Perry et al. 2003; Teeling and Perry 2009). It follows that inflammation induced by allergens and irritants potentially activate central nervous system inflammation. Immunoglobulins (Menachem et al. 2013) and cytokines impact central nervous system function and can affect function (Larson and Dunn 2001). Down regulation of neurogenesis in the hippocampus by microglial activation is another potential mechanism for systemic inflammation, including allergy and irritant exposures, to impact neuropsychological behaviors (Di Filippo et al. 2013; Kohman and Rhodes 2013).

## Research Needs

The scientific study of seasonal allergic asthma is a valid model that can guide the study of the brain as a possible target organ for allergic and irritant sensitivity. Individuals with allergic asthma who are asymptomatic outside of a pollen season can undergo double-blinded placebo-controlled inhalational challenges to pollen with objective markers of a physiological response to pollen but not placebo challenges such as pulmonary function tests. We now have new tools for studying changes in brain function that can be monitored over the time frames necessary for challenge studies. These include functional magnetic resonance imagining (fMRI), magnetoencephalography (MEG), electroencephalography (EEG), optical imaging, and PET scans (Bandettini 2009). Studies of imagining in allergic rhinitis patients concentrate on sinus pathology. A PET scan study of MCS patients determined that the patient group activated odor-processing brain regions less than controls and showed an odorant-related increase in activation of the anterior cingulate cortex and cuneus-precuneus (Hillert et al. 2007). A PET scan study of 12 patients meeting the criteria for IEI found six patients with deficits in verbal learning and memory, three of whom had reduced information processing speed. A group analysis of the patients found no areas with significantly reduced glucose metabolism

(Bornschein et al. 2007). Studies pre- and post-challenge with chemical irritants were not performed in this study.

Pupillography offers a technique to measure subtle changes in autonomic responses (Shirakawa et al. 1990) as does heart rate variability though proper attention to methodology is required (Tak et al. 2009). Serum factors such as cytokines and other mediators of inflammation could be monitored simultaneously. These objective parameters could be correlated with symptom scores, neuropsychological instruments, and blinded assessments of behavior.

It must be recognized that not all individuals with allergic and irritant sensitivity have behavioral manifestations. Just as only a subset of individuals with allergic rhinitis get urticaria during pollen seasons, it may be that only a subset have the brain as target organ for allergic and irritant sensitivity.

There are recognized confounders for studying irritant sensitivity. Most irritants have odors which make blinding difficult. A technique worthy of investigation is sleep studies, in which subjects with irritant sensitivity are challenged during sleep. Adverse reactions to odors could coexist with irritant sensitivity, making odor masking with stronger odors problematic. Since olfactory-linked responses are easily conditioned, it has been hypothesized that irritant reactivity to odorous substances could condition irritant responses to odor at levels below the irritancy threshold (Meggs 1999).

Patient selection can be problematic, particularly in the case of irritant sensitivity in which there are no validated objective markers such as the presence of specific IgE antibody in allergy to validate self-reported claims of sensitivity. The presence of upper airway inflammation, whether symptomatic or not, may be important in choosing a population for initial study. A characteristic finding of blotchy yellow-to-white discoloration of the nasal mucosal surrounding visible blood vessels has been observed in patients who meet a case definition for the multiple chemical sensitivity syndrome and have upper airway inflammation.

Not all allergic and irritant sensitive subjects have associated neuropsychological illnesses. In one study 65 % of subjects with chemical sensitivity were found to meet the criteria for a current or a past mood, anxiety, or somatoform disorder by an unblinded structured interview, versus 28 % of controls. Hence 35 % of the chemically sensitive subjects in this study may not have had cerebral manifestations (Black et al. 1990). Studying those without cerebral manifestations would be analogous to including food allergy patients who do not develop urticaria upon food challenges in a skin biopsy study and could dilute results in a statistical analysis, unless they were included as a control group.

Similarly, not all patients with depression, anxiety, and other neuropsychological difficulties necessarily have reactions to allergens or to chemical irritants. Since depression, anxiety, allergy, and self-described sensitivity to odors or irritants all have relatively high prevalence, there can be substantial overlap without any relationship between the mediating processes. In studying the relationship between irritants and brain pathophysiology, care must be taken to insure that depression and anxiety do not act as confounders. Groups being compared in challenge tests should have comparable levels of irritant sensitivity, allergy, depression, and anxiety.

Since pollen levels fall to zero during certain seasons, it is easy to perform challenges outside of the pollen season in subjects with isolated seasonal allergies. The ubiquitous nature of irritants in our society makes it difficult to perform challenges without isolating subjects from irritants. One proposed solution is to house subjects in residential environmental control units which are designed to minimize exposures to irritants and allergens.

Use of environmental control units to study irritant/chemical sensitivity has been recommended (National Research Council 1992a, b). These residential units would be constructed and maintained to minimize exposure to chemical irritants. A national environmental control unit could be constructed that would be available to investigators to perform challenge studies to allergens and irritants in a controlled environment. Investigators would apply on a competitive basis for access to the facility for specific studies. A residential unit would be necessary to allow adequate washout periods between challenges and to isolate subjects from aeroallergens and chemical irritants. Such a facility would need appropriate analytical capabilities, imagining modalities, and laboratory support to precisely monitor exposures and physiological responses. State-of-the-art neuroimagning. capability would be necessary. While such a facility would be expensive to construct and maintain, the burden of neuropsychiatric illnesses in our society mandates that we explore causes of epidemics. There is sufficient support for the notion that the brain is a target organ for allergic and irritant sensitivity with important clinical implications to justify study.

## Conclusion

There is an extensive literature suggesting that exposure to allergens and irritants is associated with clinical manifestations of altered cerebral function ranging from depression and anxiety to fatigue and cognitive effects. Scientific verification of this association could impact public health and lead to new approaches to treatment and prevention of a subset of patients with neuropsychiatric illnesses.

**Acknowledgments** The authors recognize that the contributions to this field are so numerous that many references to many relevant articles are not possible within the limits of this review. We apologize to those whose important work is not discussed or referenced.

## References

Addolarato G, Marsigli L, Capristo E, Caputo F, Dall'Aglio C, Baudanza P. Anxiety and depression: a common feature of health care seeking patients with irritable bowel syndrome and food allergy. Hepatogastroenterology. 1998;45:1559–64.

Anuradha B, Vijayalakshmi V, Suman Latha G, Hari Sai Priya V, Murthy KJR. Profile of pollen allergies in patients with asthma, allergic rhinitis and urticaria in Hyderabad. Indian J Chest Dis Allied Sci. 2006;48:221–2.

Bandettini PA. What's new in neuroimaging methods? Ann N Y Acad Sci. 2009;1156:260–93.

Baraniuk JN, Clauw DJ, Gaumond E. Rhinitis symptoms in chronic fatigue syndrome. Ann Allergy Asthma Immunol. 1998;81:359–65.

Bascom R. Multiple chemical sensitivity: a respiratory disorder. Toxicol Ind Health. 1992; 8:221–8.

Baur X, Schneider EM, Wieners D, Czuppon A. Occupational asthma to perfume. Allergy. 1999;54:1334–5.

Bell IR, Jasnoski ML, Katgan J, King DS. Depression and allergies: survey of a nonclinical population. Psychother Psychosom. 1991;55:24–31.

Beumer W, Gibney SM, Drexhage RC, Pont-Lezica L, Doorduin J, Klein HC, et al. The immune theory of psychiatric diseases: a key role for activated microglia and circulating monocytes. J Leukoc Biol. 2012;92:959–75.

Black D, Rathe A, Goldstein RB. Environmental illness: a controlled study of 26 subjects with 20th century disease. JAMA. 1990;264:3166–70.

Bloch RM, Meggs WJ. Co-morbidity patterns of self-reported chemical sensitivity, allergy, and other medical illnesses with anxiety and depression. J Nut Environ Med. 2007;16:136–48.

Bornschein S, Hausteiner C, Drzezga A, Theml T, Heldmann B, Grimmer T, Perneczky R, Jahn T, Schwaiger M, Zilker T, Förstl H. Neuropsychological and positron emission tomography correlates in idiopathic environmental intolerances. Scand J Work Environ Health. 2007 Dec; 33(6):447–53.

Brooks SM, Weiss MA, Bernstein IL. Reactive airways dysfunction syndrome (RADS). Persistent asthma syndrome after high level irritant exposures. Chest. 1985;88:376–84.

Brooks SM, Hammad Y, Richards I, Giovinco-Barbas J, Jenkins K. The spectrum of irritant-induced asthma: sudden and not-so-sudden onset and the role of allergy. Chest. 1998;113: 42–9.

Campbell MB. Allergy is not epilepsy. Electroencephalogr Clin Neurophysiol. 1968;24:398.

Campbell MB. Allergy and epilepsy, chapter 5. In: Speer F, editor. Allergy of the nervous system. Springfield: CC Thomas; 1972. p. 59–78.

Caress SM, Steinemann AC. Prevalence of multiple chemical sensitivities: a population-based study in the southeastern United States. Am J Public Health. 2004a;94:746–7.

Caress SM, Steinemann AC. A national population study of the prevalence of multiple chemical sensitivity. Arch Environ Health. 2004b;59:300–5.

Centers for Disease Control and Prevention (CDC). Mental health in the United States. Prevalence of diagnosis and medication treatment for attention-deficit/hyperactivity disorder–United States, 2003. MMWR Morb Mortal Wkly Rep. 2005;54:842–7.

Chanthick C, Anaman S, Buathet K. The prevalence of positive intradermal allergy tests in 114 dogs with atopic dermatitis in the Bangkok metropolis, Thailand. Vet Immunol Immunopathol. 2008;126:256–62. Epub 2008 Aug 3.

Cuffel B, Wamboldt M, Borish L, Kennedy S, Crystal-Peters J. Economic consequences of comorbid depression, anxiety, and allergic rhinitis. Psychosomatics. 1999;40:491–6.

Cullen MR. The worker with multiple chemical sensitivities. Occup Med State Art Rev. 1987;2:655–62.

Di Filippo M, Chiasserini D, Gardoni F, Viviani B, Tozzi A, Giampà C, et al. Effects of central and peripheral inflammation on hippocampal synaptic plasticity. Neurobiol Dis. 2013;52:229–36.

Diaz-Sanchez D, Tsien A, Fleming J, Saxon A. Combined diesel exhaust particulate and ragweed allergen challenge markedly enhances human in vivo nasal ragweed-specific IgE and skews cytokine production to a T helper cell 2-type pattern. J Immunol. 1997;158:2406–13.

Diaz-Sanchez D, Garcia MP, Wang M, Jyrala M, Saxon A. Nasal challenge with diesel exhaust particles can induce sensitization to a neoallergen in the human mucosa. J Allergy Clin Immunol. 1999;104:1183–8.

Doty RL, Deems DA, Frye RE, Pelberg R, Shapiro A. Olfactory sensitivity, nasal resistance, and autonomic function in patients with multiple chemical sensitivities. Arch Otolaryngol Head Neck Surg. 1988;114(12):1422–7.

Duke WW. Food allergy as a cause of illness. JAMA. 1923;81:886.
Elberling J, Linneberg A, Mosbech H, Dirksen A, Frolund L, Madsen F, et al. A link between skin and airways regarding sensitivity to fragrance products? Br J Dermatol. 2004;151:1197–203.
Elberling J, Skov PS, Mosbech H, Holst H, Dirksen A, Johansen JD. Increased release of histamine in patients with respiratory symptoms related to perfume. Clin Exp Allergy. 2007;37:1676–80.
Fiedler N, Maccia C, Kipen H. Evaluation of chemically sensitive patients. J Occup Med. 1992;34:529–38.
Fiedler N, Giardino N, Natelson B, Ottenweller JE, Weisel C, Lioy P, et al. Responses to controlled diesel vapor exposure among chemically sensitive Gulf War veterans. Psychosom Med. 2004;66:588–98.
Fog Nielsen K. Mycotoxin production by indoor molds. Fungal Genet Biol. 2003;39:103–17.
Gibson PR, Vogel VM. Sickness-related dysfunction in persons with self-reported multiple chemical sensitivity at four levels of severity. J Clin Nurs. 2009;18:72–81.
Groneberg DA, Quarcoo D, Frossard N, Fischer A. Neurogenic mechanisms in bronchial inflammatory diseases. Allergy. 2004;59:1139–52.
Hardin BD, Kelman BJ, Saxon A. Adverse human health effects associated with molds in the indoor environment. J Occup Environ Med. 2003;45:470–8.
Hausteiner C, Bornschein S, Hansen J, Zilker T, Forstl H. Self-reported chemical sensitivity in Germany: a population-based survey. Int J Hyg Environ Health. 2005;208:271–8.
Hesselmar B, Eriksson B, Aberg N. Urticaria is associated with birch-pollen sensitization. Pediatr Allergy Immunol. 2007;18:692–5.
Hillert L, Musabasic V, Berglund H, Ciumas C, Savic I. Odor processing in multiple chemical sensitivity. Hum Brain Mapp. 2007;28:172–82.
Hoffman RE, Wood RC, Kreiss K. Building-related asthma in Denver office workers. Am J Public Health. 1993;83:89–93.
International Programme on Chemical Safety. Conclusions and recommendations of a workshop on multiple chemical sensitivities (MCS). Regul Toxicol Pharmacol. 1996;24:S188–9.
Jarvis BB. Chemistry and toxicology of molds isolated from water-damaged buildings. Adv Exp Med Biol. 2002;504:43–52.
Jorres RA, Holz O, Zachgo W, Timm P, Koschyk S, Muller B, et al. The effect of repeated ozone exposures on inflammatory markers in bronchoalveolar lavage fluid and mucosal biopsies. Am J Respir Crit Care Med. 2000;161:1855–61.
Kennedy BL, Morris RL, Schwab JJ. Allergy in panic disorder patients: a preliminary report. Gen Hosp Psychiatry. 2002;24:265–8.
Kimata H. Effect of exposure to volatile organic compounds on plasma levels of neuropeptides, nerve growth factor and histamine in patients with self-reported multiple chemical sensitivity. Int J Hyg Environ Health. 2004;207:159–63.
Kipen HM, Hallman W, Kelly-McNeil K, Fiedler N. Measuring chemical sensitivity prevalence: a questionnaire for population studies. Am J Public Health. 1995;85:574–7.
Kohman RA, Rhodes JS. Neurogenesis, inflammation and behavior. Brain Behav Immun. 2013;27:22–32.
Kovalenko PA, Hoven CW, Wu P, Wicks J, Mandell DJ, Tiet Q. Association between allergy and anxiety disorders in youth. Aust N Z J Psychiatry. 2001;35:815–21.
Kreutzer R, Neutra RR, Lashuay N. Prevalence of people reporting sensitivities to chemicals in a population-based survey. Am J Epidemiol. 1999;150:1–12.
Lacroix JS, Landis BN. Neurogenic inflammation of the upper airway mucosa. Rhinology. 2008;46:163–5.
Larson SJ, Dunn AJ. Behavioral effects of cytokines. Brain Behav Immun. 2001;15:371–87.
Leznoff A. Provocative challenges in patients with multiple chemical sensitivity. J Allergy Clin Immunol. 1997;99:438–42.
Marshall PS. Allergy and depression: a neurochemical threshold model of the relation between the illnesses. Psychol Bull. 1993;113:23–43.

Marshall PS, O'Hara C, Steinberg P. Effects of seasonal allergic rhinitis on fatigue levels and mood. Psychosom Med. 2002;64:684–91.

Matussek P, Agerer D, Seibt G. Allergic disorders in depressive patients. Compr Psychiatry. 1983;24:25–34.

Meggs WJ. Multiple chemical sensitivities and the immune system. Toxicol Ind Health. 1992;8:203–14.

Meggs WJ. RADS and RUDS: toxic induction of asthma and rhinitis. J Toxicol Clin Toxicol. 1994;32:487–501.

Meggs WJ. Mechanisms of allergy and chemical sensitivity. Toxicol Ind Health. 1999;15:331–8.

Meggs WJ, Cleveland Jr CH. Rhinolaryngoscopy findings in patients with the multiple chemical sensitivity syndrome. Arch Environ Health. 1993;48:14–8.

Meggs WJ, Dunn KA, Goodman PE, Bloch RM, Davidoff AL. Prevalence of allergy and chemical sensitivity in a general population. Arch Environ Health. 1996a;51:275–82.

Meggs WJ, Elsheik T, Metzger WJ, Albernaz M, Bloch RM. Nasal pathology and ultrastructure in patients with chronic airway inflammation (RADS and RUDS) following an irritant exposure. Clin Toxicol. 1996b;334:383–96.

Meggs WJ. Neurogenic switching: a hypothesis for a mechanism for shifting the site of inflammation in allergy and chemical sensitivity. Environ Health Perspect 1995;103:2–4.

Meggs WJ, Dunn KA, Bloch RM, Goodman PE, and Davidoff AL. Prevalence and nature of allergy and chemical sensitivity in a general population. Arch Environ Health 1996;51: 275–282.

Menachem A, Chapman J, Deri Y, Pick CG, Katzav A. Immunoglobulin-mediated neurocognitive impairment: new data and a comprehensive review. Clin Rev Allergy Immunol. 2013;45: 248–55.

Miller CS. Are we on the threshold of a new theory of disease? Toxicant-induced loss of tolerance and its relationship to addiction and abdiction. Toxicol Ind Health. 1999;15:284–94.

Miller CS. Toxicant-induced loss of tolerance. Addiction. 2001;96:115–37.

Miller CS, Mitzel HC. Chemical sensitivity attributed to pesticide exposure versus remodeling. Arch Environ Health. 1995;50:119–29.

Millqvist E, Lowhagen O. Placebo-controlled challenges with perfume in patients with asthma-like symptoms. Allergy. 1996;51:434–9.

Millqvist E, Bengtsson U, LoÈwhagen O. Provocations with perfume in the eyes induce airway symptoms in patients with sensory hyperreactivity. Allergy. 1999;54:495–9.

Millqvist E, Ternesten-Hasséus E, Ståhl A, Bende M. Changes in levels of nerve growth factor in nasal secretions after capsaicin inhalation in patients with airway symptoms from scents and chemicals. Environ Health Perspect. 2005;113:849–52.

Millqvist E, Ternesten-Hasse'us E, Bende M. Inhaled ethanol potentiates the cough response to capsaicin in patients with airway sensory hyperreactivity. Pulm Pharmacol Ther. 2008;21:794–7.

Nasr S, Altman EB, Meltzer HY. Concordance of atopic and affective disorders. J Affect Disord. 1981;3:291–6.

National Research Council. Biological markers in immunotoxicology. Washington, DC: National Academy Press; 1992a. p. 43. 138.

National Research Council. Multiple chemical sensitivities: addendum to biological markers in immunotoxicology. Washington, DC: National Academy Press; 1992b. p. 43. 138.

Nawab SS, Miller CS, Dale JK, Greenberg BD, Friedman TC, Chrousos GP, Straus SE, Rosenthal NE. Self-reported sensitivity to chemical exposures in five clinical populations and healthy controls. Psychiatry Res. 2000 Jul 24;95(1):67–74.

Nielsen GD. Mechanisms of activation of the sensory irritant receptor by airborne chemicals. Crit Rev Toxicol. 1991;21:183–208.

Nordenhall C, Pourazar J, Ledin MC, Levin JO, Sandstrom T, Adelroth E. Diesel exhaust enhances airway responsiveness in asthmatic subjects. Eur Respir J. 2001;17:909–15.

Ossofsky HJ. Affective and atopic disorders and cyclic AMP. Compr Psychiatry. 1976;17: 335–46.

Osterberg K, Karlson B, Orbaek P. Personality, mental distress, and risk perception in subjects with multiple chemical sensitivity and toxic encephalopathy. Scand J Psychol. 2002;43:169–75.
Perry VH. The influence of systemic inflammation on inflammation in the brain: implications for chronic neurodegenerative disease. Brain Behav Immun. 2004;18:407–13.
Perry VH. Contribution of systemic inflammation to chronic neurodegeneration. Acta Neuropathol. 2010;120:277–86.
Perry VH, Newman TA, Cunningham C. The impact of systemic infection on the progression of neurodegenerative disease. Nat Rev Neurosci. 2003;4:103–12.
Qian Z, He Q, Kong L, Xu F, Wei F, Chapman RS, et al. Respiratory responses to diverse indoor combustion air pollution sources. Indoor Air. 2007;17:135–42.
Randolph T. Human ecology and susceptibility to the chemical environment. Springfield: C.C. Thomas; 1962.
Rea WJ. Environmentally triggered cardiac disease. Ann Allergy. 1978;40:243–51.
Rea WJ. Chemical sensitivity, vol. 1. Boca Raton: CRC Press; 1994.
Rios JL, Boechat JL, Gioda A, dos Santos CY, de Aquino Neto FR, Lapa e Silva JR. Symptoms prevalence among office workers of a sealed versus a non-sealed building: associations to indoor air quality. Environ Int. 2009;35:1136–41.
Robertson AS, Burge PS, Hedge A, Sims J, Gill FS, Finnegan M, et al. Comparison of health problems related to work and environmental measurements in two office buildings with different ventilation systems. Br Med J (Clin Res Ed). 1985;291(6492):373–6.
Sanico AM, Koliatsos VE, Stanisz AM, Bienenstock J, Togias A. Neural hyperresponsiveness and nerve growth factor in allergic rhinitis. Int Arch Allergy Immunol. 1999;118:154–8.
Sanico AM, Stanisz AM, Gleeson TD, Bora S, Proud D, Bienenstock J, et al. Nerve growth factor expression and release in allergic inflammatory disease of the upper airways. Am J Respir Crit Care Med. 2000;161:1631–5.
Sarin S, Undem B, Sanico A, Togias A. The role of the nervous system in rhinitis. J Allergy Clin Immunol. 2006;118:999–1016.
Seppänen OA, Fisk WJ. Summary of human responses to ventilation. Indoor Air. 2004;14 Suppl 7:102–18.
Shirakawa S, Ishikawa S, Miyata M, Rea WJ, Johnson AR. A pupillographical study on the presence of organochlorine pesticides in autonomic nerve disturbance. Nippon Ganka Gakkai Zasshi. 1990;94:418–23.
Simon GE. Psychiatric symptoms in multiple chemical sensitivity. Toxicol Ind Health. 1994;10:487–96.
Simon GE, Daniell W, Stockbridge H, Claypoole K, Rosenstock L. Immunologic, psychological, and neuropsychological factors in multiple chemical sensitivity: a controlled study. Ann Intern Med. 1993;119:97–103.
Simon GE, Katon WJ, Sparks PJ. Allergic to life: psychological factors in environmental illness. Am J Psychiatry. 1990;147:901–6.
Speer F. Allergy of the nervous system. Springfield: CC Thomas; 1972.
Staudenmayer H, Binkley KE, Leznoff A, Phillips S. Idiopathic environmental intolerance: part 2: a causation analysis applying Bradford Hill's criteria to the psychogenic theory. Toxicol Rev. 2003;22:247–61.
Tak LM, Riese H, de Bock GH, Manoharan A, Kok IC, Rosmalen JG. As good as it gets? A meta-analysis and systematic review of methodological quality of heart rate variability studies in functional somatic disorders. Biol Psychol. 2009;82:101–10.
Tascilar E, Yokusoglu M, Dundaroz R, Baysan O, Ozturk S, Yozgat Y, et al. Cardiac autonomic imbalance in children with allergic rhinitis. Tohoku J Exp Med. 2009;219:187–91.
Teeling JL, Perry VH. Systemic infection and inflammation in acute CNS injury and chronic neurodegeneration: underlying mechanisms. Neuroscience. 2009;158:1062–73.
Terr AI. Environmental illness. A clinical review of 50 cases. Arch Intern Med. 1986;146:145–9.
Voorhees RM. Memorandum from New Mexico Deputy State Epidemiologist to Joe Thompson, Special Council, Office of the Governor. 1998.

Vuurman EF, van Veggel LM, Uiterwijk MM, Leutner D, O'Hanlon JF. Seasonal allergic rhinitis and antihistamine effects on children's learning. Ann Allergy. 1993;71:121–6.

Wallace DV, Dykewicz MS, Bernstein DI, Blessing-Moore J, Cox L, Khan DA, et al. The diagnosis and management of rhinitis: an updated practice parameter. J Allergy Clin Immunol. 2008;122:S1–84.

Willes SR, Fitzgerald TK, Bascom R. Nasal inhalation challenge studies with sidestream tobacco smoke. Arch Environ Health. 1992;47:223–30.

Willes SR, Fitzgerald TK, Permutt T, Proud D, Haley NJ, Bascom R. Acute respiratory response to prolonged, moderate levels of sidestream tobacco smoke. J Toxicol Environ Health A. 1998;53:193–209.

World Health Organization. The "sick" building syndrome. Indoor air pollutants exposure and health effects. EURO report and studies 78. Copenhagen: World Health Organization; 1983. p. 23–7.

Yazicioglu M, Baspinar I, Ones U, Pala O, Kiziler U. Egg and milk allergy in asthmatic children: assessment by immulite allergy food panel, skin prick tests and double-blind placebo-controlled food challenges. Allergol Immunopathol. 1999;27:287–93.

# Chapter 11
# An Approach to Treating Irritant Airway Inflammation

**Grace Ziem**

**Abstract** Treatment of irritant-induced airway inflammation can be difficult. Standard pharmaceutical therapies are often ineffective or only provide limited relief. Based on the current understanding of inflammation biochemistry, a treatment approach has been developed that combines avoidance of noxious exposures with supplements that reduce oxidative damage to the airway and scavenge nitric oxide. Scientific basis and practical guidelines for exposure reduction to reduce exacerbations in affected persons are described, including easy-to-use accommodations.

**Keywords** Reactive airways treatment • Reactive airway disease • Treatment of asthma and rhinosinusitis • Treatment of occupational asthma

## Introduction

Physicians also use the term reactive airways for this condition.

As a physician, I have specialized in reactive airway treatment for several decades. My discussion includes that experience and provides scientific documentation. The introduction highlights concepts to be discussed in greater detail in the chapter. The chapter also seeks to provide useful clinical tools for accurate treatment and efficient evaluation aides.

---

The author has never had any financial relationship or reward structure with any laboratory; pharmacy; and drug, substance, or equipment supplier.

G. Ziem, M.D., M.P.H., D.P.H. (✉)
Occupational and Environmental Health, 16926 Eyler's Valley Road, Emmitsburg, MD 21727-9729, USA

W.J. Meggs (ed.), *The Toxicant Induction of Irritant Asthma, Rhinitis, and Related Conditions*, DOI 10.1007/978-1-4614-9044-9_11,

I am cautious about dosing and I describe that approach. I have never had a reactive airway patient die under my care and rarely had more than brief, minor symptoms, never requiring ER or hospital attention. Patients should not "tough out" symptoms. A healing approach helps the patient feel better. It is wise for the patient to introduce one treatment at a time. Side effects mean slow down and dilute/use smaller dose. If symptoms still occur, defer or omit suspect substance.

Presenting symptoms often include a *burning sensation in upper and/or lower airways*. This usually accompanies acquired exacerbations with irritant and particulate exposures at intensities and durations that were previously not symptomatic.

Environmental controls are essential for clinical success. These need to be adequate to avoid any symptomatic exacerbation. Evaluation of where symptoms are worse and what circumstances seem to exacerbate them is critical. Comparing peak flow and/or symptom log in different situations can help identify problems. Samples are given of patient resources and physician support for irritant control.

Symptom-masking drugs are often poorly tolerated: inhalants because of irritants (Hudnell et al. 1992) and systemic because of impaired detoxification (Ziem 1999). Drugs do not address cause: either biochemical mechanisms or environmental factors. Drugs can mask adverse responses and mislead both patient and clinician to miss exacerbating exposures at home, school, or work. A healing approach is initially more complex than drugs: I was also initially trained to use the latter. However, it is exciting for doctor and patient to watch healing progress and to observe patients act physiologically younger when the focus is on healing.

Medical treatment that down regulates the self-perpetuating biochemical nitric oxide/peroxynitrite cycle can result in major clinical improvement. This chapter attempts to help clinicians do this without a degree in biochemistry. To be most effective, treatment should be test based because patients differ widely in which healing substances are needed for repair. Total "cure" may not occur because the body tends to retain a sufficient warning system to help prevent further harm.

Nutrition plays an important role in speeding repair. To help patient and clinician and correct serious nutritional misinformation, the author has attached a nutritional fact sheet, which has worked well. Beware that dieticians and even some clinical nutritionists may not be aware of the nutritional needs of these patients.

## Evaluation of Progress

Many diagnostic approaches are discussed elsewhere. To avoid confusing or missing the diagnosis, the author has also found the following tools to be useful. They are largely derived from epidemiologic research and have further demonstrated their value in use on over a thousand patients.

Letting the patient complete various written questions saves provider time. Questions are listed by type here for discussion but can easily be combined by the provider for a single, more complete patient questionnaire: which the provider can review in 2–3 min.

For *baseline comparison*, the following questions greatly help distinguish irritant-related respiratory effects from allergies, infections, smoking, pneumoconioses, etc.:

## Intake Patient Questions

*Have you had a burning-like feeling in eyes, nose, sinuses, throat, lungs, and other areas? Check:* □ *No* □ *Yes CIRCLE AFFECTED AREAS.*

*If yes, when did this first occur?*

---

*Location/circumstances where symptoms* first *noticed?*

---

---

*Location/circumstances where symptoms* first *felt better?*

---

---

*Where and when are symptoms currently worse?*

---

If desired, more space can allow the patient to describe circumstances.

*Baseline and follow-up* can use an abbreviated version of epidemiologic research first done at Johns Hopkins, with question wording later published (Ziem and McTamney 1997). This standardized, epidemiologic, and validated question wording did distinguish between affected groups and controls. The items below focus on respiratory airways.

## Intake and Follow-Up Patient Questions

*For the symptoms and health problems listed below:* ***Circle*** *the number that best describes how often the symptom occurs. Also* ***circle specific symptoms when several are listed.***

| *Symptom* | *Almost daily* | *Several times a week* | *Once a week* | *Several times a month* | *Once a month or less* | *Rarely if ever* | *Not sure* |
|---|---|---|---|---|---|---|---|
| *Sinus, nose, throat irritation/burning* | 1 | 2 | 3 | 4 | 5 | 6 | 7 |
| *Ear congestion or discomfort* | 1 | 2 | 3 | 4 | 5 | 6 | 7 |
| *Weak voice, hoarseness* | 1 | 2 | 3 | 4 | 5 | 6 | 7 |
| *Chest tightness, irritation, or burning* | 1 | 2 | 3 | 4 | 5 | 6 | 7 |
| *Coughing, wheezing* | 1 | 2 | 3 | 4 | 5 | 6 | 7 |

To evaluate and compare *intensity of exacerbations in a dose–response manner*, the author selected the Johns Hopkins questions that are useful screening items to spare patient and clinician a longer questionnaire. Obviously, other irritants can be a problem also.

## *Exacerbation Patient Questions*

*For each situation described below, answer the questions at the top of each column. By "sick" we mean anything YOU consider to be either a major or a minor health problem. Put a check in the appropriate box.*

| *Would you be sick if you had to spend 4 h …?* | | | | | |
|---|---|---|---|---|---|
| Exposures | *No* | *A little* | *Moderate* | *A lot* | *Don't know* |
| *Next to a person smoking cigarettes outside* | | | | | |
| *Driving in heavy traffic with windows open* | | | | | |
| *In a room sprayed with pesticides 4 h ago* | | | | | |
| *Next to a person wearing cologne/perfume* | | | | | |
| *Shopping in an enclosed mall* | | | | | |

The questions can be repeated using a 20-min exposure if desired.

*Describe a typical reaction (if any), listing symptoms in order of onset, and describing the time frame. If your reactions are quite different from time to time, describe this also. Put "none" if no reactions.*

---

Using these questions on the clinical intake form helps avoid missing the diagnosis of irritant-exacerbated effects.

## *Using Peak Flow to Identify Current Irritant Situations*

Peak flow is safe, portable, and useful for evaluation of airway resistance (Fairbairn et al. 1962; Higgins 1957; Lal et al. 1964; Shephard 1962). Peak flow can be used as an alternative to bronchial challenge testing in evaluation of irritant asthma (Burge et al. 1979). A peak flow/symptom patient log can help identify problems exacerbating inflammation.

Peak flow can also compare effects away from work/exposure (e.g., evening, weekend, longer time off) with any changes with return to exposure. More chronic symptoms often need more time off for significant change.

| Date | Time | Peak flow | Location/situation | Symptoms |
|---|---|---|---|---|
| | | | | |

### *Avoiding Hazardous Testing*

Because of the biochemistry of their inflammatory process, reactive airway/irritant asthma patients can respond with greater risk of prolonged side effects to these commonly used tests.

1. Methacholine challenge
   Methacholine challenge can cause severe bronchoconstriction (Millqvist and Lowhagen 1998). It shows poor correlation with irritant-related asthma (methacholine for diagnosis of asthma, 1987). Results often change over time on the same patient (Muller et al. 1994) and are not a good predictor of respiratory irritant symptoms (Siwik et al. 2005; Spiropoulos et al. 1986). Prolonged exacerbation can occur lasting weeks or months.
2. Diffusing capacity
   This test often involves a prolonged breath hold of about 3,000 ppm of carbon monoxide. Carbon monoxide at even low levels greatly speeds up the nitric oxide cycle (Amitai et al. 1998; Verma et al. 1993). Prolonged exacerbation can last for months.

## Medical Treatment by Downregulating Inflammatory Biochemistry

Recent scientific advances indicate that chronic mucosal inflammation of airways is caused by a self-perpetuating biochemical cycle. This is often called the (inducible) nitric oxide/peroxynitrite cycle (Beckman and Crow 1993; Delfino et al. 2006; Mar et al. 2005). A simplified diagram is provided.

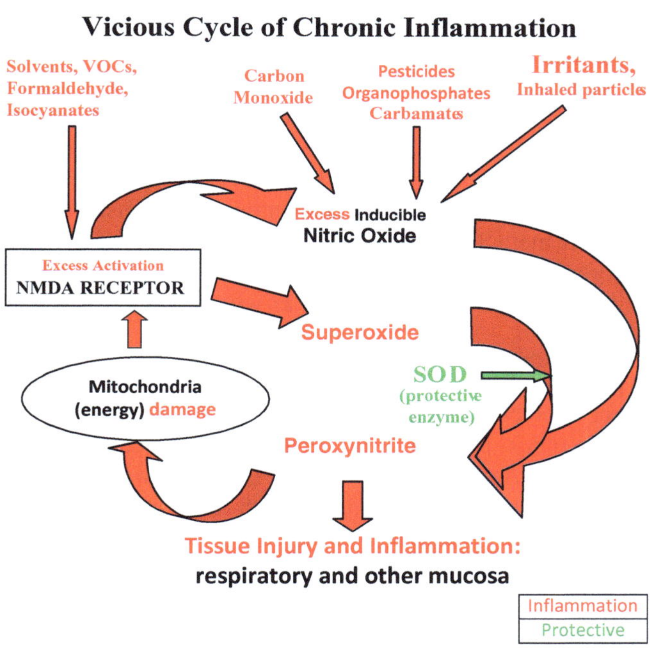

One need not delve deeply into biochemistry, however, for good treatment results. Understanding the self-perpetuating concept and thus the need to interrupt the cycle at multiple points is the key to success. Testing to guide treatment is discussed later and is available for all discussed substances.

Manufacturing "flow agents," less bioavailable forms, etc. can greatly impede absorption. These are common in most OTC brands and impede improvement. When brands are mentioned in the chapter, it is to avoid these problems. Bioactive forms often work best and are discussed below. Most oral substances to be swallowed are best absorbed and tolerated taken with food.

## *Scavenging Inducible Nitric Oxide with Methylcobalamine*

The cycle typically begins with excess inducible nitric oxide (Beckman and Crow 1993; Delfino et al. 2006; Mar et al. 2005). With many hundreds of patient users, the author has seen no adverse effects on endothelial nitric oxide. Fortunately, bioactive B12 works well for such scavenging (Wolak et al. 2001; Zheng et al. 2002). Methylcobalamine is a bioactive form and more calming than hydroxocobalamine. Cyanocobalamine is less effective than either. Daily use is essential to interrupt the biochemical cycle sufficient to control symptoms and ongoing inflammation.

It is helpful to remember that these patients can have severe inflammation and have often had adverse symptoms from many things. Some are more comfortable beginning with very small doses. This is fine. Assure them that "some is better than none." They were born with these substances, but they should proceed at a pace comfortable to them, beginning one approach at a time. Going more slowly in comfort is better than pushing the pace.

1. *Sublingual tablets for convenient, portable use.*
   For many patients, this approach is often sufficient. Methylcobalamine can be taken effectively as sublingual tablets. It is interesting to keep giving the patient two 5 mg quickly dissolving sublingual tablets, letting each dose dissolve, and watch breathing and other effects improve. Peak flow meter comparisons can be done if desired. For upper respiratory effects, patient and clinician can monitor sinus headache, earache, and nasal and throat symptoms. The author prefers Health Products methylcobalamine 5 mg, for fast dissolving, but other brands may also work.
2. *Nebulized for the entire upper and lower airway delivery*
   (a) The author uses compounded pure methylcobalamine beginning at up to 5 mg per dose. Water or saline is always put in first to avoid clogging the nebulizer filter. Nebulizing several times daily is critical.
   (b) To achieve quick, portable 5 μm particle size delivery, the author has often prescribed the AeronebGo Nebulizer. Lower airway and some systemic delivery are achieved with standard mouth breathing technique. A mask can be used for smaller children.

(c) Upper airway delivery can be achieved by creating a positive pressure in the oral–nasal cavity. *This technique delivers well to sinuses and Eustachian tubes.*

- Use a "nasal nipple" with a 1 cm cut opening in the nipple tip to fit the nostril, and stretch the nipple rim over the nebulizer mouthpiece. (We have used a Playtex baby bottle nipple with medical grade silicone, without BPA or phthalates).
- Breathe through the nasal nipple into one nostril, holding the other nostril and nebulizer slits closed while breathing in; do a 2–3-s breath hold; and then release the other nostril to breathe out.
- Switch nostrils when the mucosa of the first nostril is moist; repeat with the other nostril.
- If lower airway or systemic delivery is desired, remove "nipple" and breathe into lungs. The 5 μm particle size also allows systemic delivery.

3. *Other routes for severely inflamed patients*

(a) Injectable pure compounded methylcobalamine can be used at up to 5 or 10 mg/ml. Intramuscular can be used. Subcutaneous may be slower onset but longer lasting. Daily injections are often needed, but patients who need or prefer this approach experience enough symptom improvement that they often willingly do self-injection with proper instruction. Rotate injection sites, and avoid over 1 ml per injection.

(b) Some patients may need pure compounded methylcobalamine at 1–5 mg per drop (which they can dilute further in a 4–5 ml pharmacy bottle). This can be dropped on the surface of the *tongue*, where it will absorb systemically through the papillae (tongue surface) or diluted further for use as a *nasal spray*. The author has used up to 500 mg/ml pure compounded methylcobalamine for nasal spray. Concentration can be started lower and gradually increased as inflammation improves. More inflamed patients (worse reactions, lower test values) often need to begin more dilute. If any irritation is experienced, the patient should discontinue a day or two and then begin slightly more dilute as able. The patient is often a good judge of the amount of dilution required to feel comfortable.

## *High Gamma Tocopherol to Protect Lipid Membranes*

1. Gamma tocopherol reduces peroxynitrite damage on lipid membranes (Christen et al. 1997; Wagner et al. 2004). It complements alpha tocopherol, which activates glutathione (Pascoe et al. 1987). Roughly equal amounts of each form are needed, so "mixed tocopherols" do not function as well for inflammation control because of low gamma levels. Avoid all synthetic tocopherol: it is useless and competes for tocopherol receptors.

2. Tocopherols are lipid soluble: the author has not seen much benefit from dry forms. The author has often used Thorne Ultimate E capsules one daily, but other high gamma lipid capsule forms may also work.
3. Respiratory lipid membranes directly encounter airborne irritants, so high gamma tocopherol protection is vital. Occasionally, patients may want or prefer to puncture the capsule immediately before use, emptying contents on food or tongue, or even starting with a drop or two and slowly increasing concentration.

## *Using Glutathione to Further Control Inflammation*

Glutathione is the major antioxidant and detoxifier of the body (Gregus and Klaassen 2001; Parkinson 2001). It reduces respiratory inflammation in the lungs (Bishop et al. 2005) and upper airways (Testa et al. 1995). It also down regulates the inflammation cycle by reducing excess N-methyl-D-aspartate (NMDA) activity (Oja et al. 2000) and supports other lung defense mechanisms (Witschi and Last 2001). Glutathione helps protect B12 (cobalamine) from damage with exposure to inhaled irritants (Watson et al. 2004).

The author has not found N-acetyl cysteine (NAC) to work well as a glutathione precursor. Testing on over a thousand patients shows that cysteine is often at ample levels even when glutathione tests low.

### Oral Use of Glutathione

Glutathione, a tripeptide, taken orally is largely digested by gastric acid. Attempts to reduce this problem by micellized coating may yield some clinical benefits but do not seem sufficient.

A newer capsule form using S-acetyl glutathione (e.g., Xymogen) is intended to avoid digestion. The author has reviewed research results not yet published which seem impressive as has initial clinical response in patients. It appears worth for further use, response evaluation, and patient retesting comparison. This form is lipid soluble and is best absorbed when taken with some lipid, e.g., a small amount of fish oil, olive oil, and coconut oil. It can also be taken with a meal or a snack containing fat.

### Nebulizer Use of Glutathione

Nebulized glutathione has shown benefit in chronic lung disease (Bishop et al. 2005).

Nebulized glutathione can be tried using techniques as described above for methylcobalamine. With inhalation on inflamed airways, it is wise to use methylcobalamine and high gamma tocopherol first and then begin gradually increasing glutathione concentration. This is because glutathione used directly on inflamed airways is more irritating at higher concentrations early in treatment. Begin the patient on B12 first, because it is more gentle on inflamed airways. When it is tolerated, glutathione can then be introduced. The approach described below yields best results.

Also use pure compounded glutathione from a compounding pharmacy that protects it from oxidation by air, light, or heat in production and transport. I have used Key Compounding Pharmacy (WA) because they use bioactive, pharmaceutically pure, well-tolerated ingredients that achieve noticeable clinical progress in my patients, and improvement has been confirmed by retesting. They have accreditation by Pharmacy Compound Accreditation Board (PCAB). Any pharmacy used should meet these criteria.

**For best success, the following approach is recommended:**

1. Begin with a lower concentration prescription, e.g., 10–40 mg/ml, using the more dilute with more severely inflamed patients.
2. Add 2 ml of water first to the nebulizer (glutathione is sticky and can clog 5 μm openings in the filter).
3. Add 2 drops of glutathione to water for the first dose and then 4, 6, 8 drops, etc. in subsequent doses until full strength can be used without water. Refills can be at higher concentrations, up to 80 or even 100 mg/ml, easing up concentration gradually. If any irritation or coughing occurs, reduce dose below irritation level until more healing and gradually increase again.
4. Use immediately after putting in nebulizer to avoid oxidation.
5. Nebulizing several times daily is important for faster healing.
6. Prompt nebulizer cleaning is essential after each use to avoid clogging the 5 μm filter. Run water through the nebulizer cup plugged into electrical outlet or battery pack for ½ to 1 min to achieve good water vapor flow, and then air-dry.

## Injection of Glutathione

Glutathione can also be given by IM (or subcutaneous) injection. Because these distal sites are usually not inflamed, more concentrated initial dose can be used, e.g., 100–200 mg/ml. Compounding and shipping precautions are essential, as with nebulized glutathione, to avoid oxidation. Daily injection is important, rotating sites. Patients who experience such symptom improvement are often willing to do self-injection at home.

## Intravenous Glutathione

The author does not use intravenous glutathione. The endothelium is often inflamed in such patients, resulting in burning and even vascular changes for only a temporary benefit. (Intravenous glutathione has been used for neurologic diseases, such as Parkinson's, Alzheimer's, and others).

## *Necessary Substances for Glutathione Function and Reactivation*

At first the number of substances discussed can seem overwhelming. To ease this problem, first note that there is medically documented science behind each substance, but this does not mean that you have to memorize or recite the biochemistry. Use the chapter to remind you if you so chose. Second, doses have been suggested that are safe. Third, the test section describes how to learn which substances are needed for a specific patient. Finally, the summary describes how to start at your own comfort level. You also have a sample approach for compounded capsules that works well for most patients, and this can be started slowly if you prefer until you want to customize it more.

The dosing of these can be done more precisely with testing, discussed below.

### Selenium

*Selenium* is an essential component of the enzyme, glutathione peroxidase, which allows glutathione to function (Jayaprakash 2009; Linder 1991; Rotruck et al. 1973). Selenium also helps as a defense in scavenging inflammatory peroxynitrite (Klotz and Sies 2003). Testing can refine the dosage, but the author has used 200–400 mcg daily as bioactive selenomethionine (e.g., Thorne, Pure Encapsulations, custom compounded).

### Vitamin C

*Vitamin C (ascorbate) reactivates glutathione* in water-based body fluids (Machlin and Bendich 1987) and improves lung response to irritants (Costa 2001).

Buffered vitamin C powder in water is often best tolerated. Vitamin C needs twice-daily dosing. Capsule forms are also available. Begin slowly to avoid loose stools, and reduce dose if this occurs: the body absorbs and uses what is needed. Requirements can vary with exacerbations. The author uses testing and a gentle approach rather than inducing diarrhea and then reducing dose. Common needs range from 500 to 1,000 mg twice daily beginning slowly. The author has used Thorne buffered C, Xymogen Xcellent C, or custom compounded.

### Alpha Lipoic Acid (Dihydrolipoic Acid)

*The active dihydrolipoic acid form reactivates glutathione and other antioxidants* (Smith et al. 2004; Wagner et al. 2012), *works in lipid membranes as well as aqueous tissue*, and can increase intracellular glutathione levels (Busse et al. 1992). This substance thus helps maintain active glutathione in the many respiratory cells which directly encounter airborne inflammatory irritants, reducing respiratory membrane oxidative damage and assisting repair of past damage.

Mucosal GI inflammation can greatly affect patient tolerance of this substance. If used without compounding the author begins with small oral doses taken with food in the stomach, e.g., 100 mg twice daily, gradually increasing to a total of up to 600 mg in divided doses with food.

To ensure that the dihydrolipoic acid bioactive form is used, brand selection is important. The author has used Thorne brand or pharmaceutical grade for compounding with other substances.

Testing really helps determine need: some patients have good amounts, and others test more deficient.

#### Riboflavin

*Glutathione reductase enzyme requires riboflavin* (B2) as FAD, and even marginal reduced levels can impair enzyme function (Hustad et al. 2002; Prentice and Bates 1981). This is often low enough on testing to achieve improvement with repletion. Compounding with other deficient water-based substances often achieves best results. The author uses riboflavin-5-phosphate (the bioactive form from Thorne or custom compounded).

### *Calming NMDA to Calm the Inflammatory Nitric Oxide/ Peroxynitrite Cycle*

1. *Magnesium* calms the NMDA receptor (Akhtar et al. 2011; Miyashita et al. 2012; Nikolaev et al. 2012). This calms the self-perpetuating cycle (Oja et al. 2000). Magnesium deficiency is common in the general population (Allan and Mara 2012; Linder 1991; Mauskop and Varughese 2012) and is further depleted by buffering the acidosis of inflammation (Linder 1991).

   Magnesium is also a calcium channel blocker (Rowe 2012) and thus can help bronchoconstriction (Akhtar et al. 2011).

   In excess, magnesium can cause loose stools. When stools are looser than soft formed, use of magnesium may be delayed until inflammation improves or it should be used carefully in a well-absorbed form, such as magnesium glycinate, e.g., Pure Encapsulations brand or comparable. Other magnesium chelates can be used, but magnesium oxide is not well absorbed. Using Epsom salts (magnesium sulfate) as a foot soak or bath can also help repletion.
2. *Pyridoxal phosphate (B6)* is a cofactor for improving GABA (Linder 1991; Yoo et al. 2011), calming the inflammatory cycle (Oja et al. 2000), and helping bronchoconstriction (Prakash 2009). The author uses Thorne or custom compounded.
3. *Taurine*, an amino acid, reduces peroxynitrite changes (Kocak-Toker et al. 2005) and also relaxes GABA and respiratory smooth muscle (Gallos et al. 2012). The author uses Thorne or custom compounded.

Because Taurine is neural calming (Song et al. 2012), it can be given midevening and/or at bedtime to assist falling asleep or restless sleep, respectively. The timing is also important as an aid to sleep which is discussed below. It is best not taken with proteins because they compete for absorption.

## *Helping the Body's Protective SOD Enzyme*

Super oxide dismutase (SOD) is a natural body enzyme that helps interrupt the nitric oxide/peroxynitrite cycle (Gregus and Klaassen 2001). *Zinc* and *copper* are essential for SOD function in the cell cytosol and extracellular SOD, and *manganese* is needed for mitochondrial (energy generating) SOD protection (Fukai and Ushio-Fukai 2011; Gregus and Klaassen 2001; Linder 1991).

These three mineral nutrients are all essential but must be given in balance, best done by intracellular SpectraCell testing discussed below.

## *Improving Energy Metabolism to Promote Healing*

Every function a living person does that a corpse cannot requires energy generation. This includes repair of damaged cells and cell structures and down regulating the biochemical vicious cycle.

The author uses bioactive forms wherever possible for best effectiveness (e.g., niacinamide for niacin, riboflavin-5-phosphate, pyridoxine-5-phosphate, pantethine for pantothenate), usually Thorne or custom compounded.

### Natural Substances Required for Energy Metabolism

Not all patients need these substances, but at the discussed doses adverse effects are unusual. As mentioned above, be cautious that manganese does not lower zinc.

1. Some substances already discussed (*manganese, riboflavin, magnesium, pyridoxine* (Linder 1991)) help energy formation as well as the substances discussed below (Sun et al. 2011). *Alpha lipoic acid* helps energy by protecting mitochondria (Palaniappan and Dai 2007). Cell repair and control of the inflammation cycle require energy. Also, many patients have fatigue with chronic inflammation. Free radicals impair energy metabolism (Mailloux et al. 2007).
2. *Acetylcarnitine* is more active than L-carnitine (Liu et al. 2004). It is used in energy production (Ozaki et al. 2011), helping mitochondrial function (Patel et al. 2012; Pesce et al. 2012). It has antioxidant activity (Karalija et al. 2012; Pesce et al. 2012) and enters cells and lipid tissue better (Malaguarnera 2012). It shows neuroprotective capacity (Malaguarnera 2012; Scafidi et al. 2010; Zhang et al. 2012). Not every patient needs it. Avoid over 500 mg spread over the day. The author uses Thorne or custom compounded.

3. *Chromium* is needed to assist glucose in entering the cell to be burned for energy (Linder 1991). 200 mcg is often adequate. If you use separately (not compounded), this can be done with one Thorne Ultrachrome daily.
4. *Thiamine*, *niacin*, *pantothenate*, and *biotin* all act biochemically at different locations in energy metabolism (Chou and Tong 2011; Depeint et al. 2006; Linder 1991; Tong 2012; Tong et al. 2011). Mitochondrial nutrient addition can improve energy (Sun et al. 2011).
5. *Coenzyme Q10* functions to help energy (Lee et al. 2011). It is part of the electron transport chain (Beg et al. 2010; Lee et al. 2011; Tsai et al. 2012) and an antioxidant (Beg et al. 2010; Tsai et al. 2012) to protect the mitochondria and other tissues (Wagner et al. 2012). It is lipid soluble (Beg et al. 2010), and dry forms are poorly absorbed. The author gives it separately as lipid capsules, with dosing assisted by testing. The author has used Xymogen CoQ10 and Thorne's new CoQ Best.
6. *Pantothenate/pantethine*
   The author has noted that low tested pantothenate often correlates with poor adrenal function (cortisol) and pantethine improves this. Deficient adrenal corticosteroid levels improve with bioactive pantethine (Tarasov et al. 1985) which can reduce respiratory inflammation. This may explain some of the anti-inflammatory effect of pantethine (Cornille et al. 2010).

*Molybdenum* is essential for multiple enzymes (Mendel and Kruse 1823). For example, it is important for sulfite oxidase (Rajapakshe et al. 2012). This is needed for body compounds (e.g., proteins) that contain sulfur. Molybdenum is also needed to break down sulfur compounds (Tutuncu et al. 2012). It thus can help respiratory cell repair and detoxification.

The author has noted that patients who have difficulty with sulfur-containing foods (cabbage, broccoli, other crucifers, onion family) often need molybdenum. It is the one nutrient of all the above that is not tested on the single test panel discussed below.

## Plant-Based Antioxidants to Reduce Free Radical Damage

The author has used singly and pure compounded science-based plant-derived peroxynitrite and superoxide free radical scavengers. Both of these free radicals cause damage and inflammation, and thus scavengers of both are needed. The author uses active ingredients. The author is a conventionally trained physician, not a herbalist. However, the medical literature and the author's experience with hundreds of patients show that this approach can bring added control to the inflammatory nitric oxide/peroxynitrite cycle.

To avoid further confusion, readers may look at the listing and dose ranges used by the author for adults, dividing into BID or TID dosing when compounded together. This helps with complementary action and can reduce flow agents and other additives if the compounding pharmacy does proper sourcing and uses pharmaceutical grade. Many of these antioxidants have multiple beneficial ways of

**Table 11.1** Antioxidants of plant origin

| |
|---|
| Scavengers of peroxynitrite and its breakdown products: |
| Ginkgo biloba extract, 120 mg/day |
| Siliphos 400 mg/day |
| Bilberry extract, 300 mg/day |
| Cranberry extract, 400 mg/day |
| Carotenoid mixture (5 mg each lycopene, beta-carotene, other carotenoids: 10 mg/day each of lutein and zeaxanthine) |
| Superoxide scavengers |
| Proanthocyanidin, 400 mg/day: Activin |
| Epigallocatechin gallate (EGCG), 400 mg/d |

reducing inflammation and other damage, but I wish to spare further biochemistry stress to the reader. Children will need weight-adjusted dosing.

As with all medical treatment on inflamed patients, beginning slowly, increasing gently over 1–2 weeks, and letting patient response guide therapy yields best results. These are safe substances in the listed doses, but degree of inflammation can affect response.

## Peroxynitrite Scavengers

Peroxynitrite scavengers include *ginkgo biloba* (Hyun et al. 2006; Zizkova et al. 2010), *silimarin* (Ahmadi-Ashtiani et al. 2012; Malekinejad et al. 2012; Tong et al. 2011), anthocyanadins such as *bilberry* (Matsunaga et al. 2009; Rahman et al. 2006), flavonoids such as *cranberry* (Cheshchevik et al. 2012; Menghini et al. 2011), and other flavonoids and carotenoids (Cos et al. 2004; Kim and Yokozawa 2009). When silimarin is bound to phosphatidylcholine (e.g., siliphos), it is much more effective in helping the body produce glutathione (Kidd and Head 2005), the body's key antioxidant as discussed above.

## Superoxide Scavengers

*Grape seed* proanthocyanidins have shown superoxide and free radical scavenging activity (Bagchi et al. 1997). An extract known as *activin* demonstrated free radical scavenging (Banerjee and Bagchi 2001) and promoted cell survival (Mukerji et al. 2007).

*Green tea extract* known as epigallocatechin gallate (EGCG) has shown the ability for multiple types of free radical scavenging (Alvarez et al. 2002; Higuchi et al. 2003; Nanjo et al. 1999).

Others can also be used, but the above combination has been effective in improving cell membrane repair on testing. I have attached the doses I use for your interest (Table 11.1).

I request compounding using pharmaceutical grade pure substances into TID dosing antioxidant capsules, beginning with one daily and working up as the patient feels ready, to BID then TID. Taking with meals works best. The author has used Key Pharmacy (WA) for the reasons discussed under glutathione: correct sourcing and compounding of these substances to achieve observable, testable benefits are complex. The author has often observed improved cell membrane repair on retesting phospholipids of choline, inositol, and serine on SpectraCell testing as discussed below.

## *Sample of Compounded Protocol*

The following contains all discussed ingredients. If water is consumed through copper pipes, copper should be omitted. If the patient has frequent symptoms indicating gastric irritation, reduce lipoic acid to 200–300 mg. Ascorbic acid (vitamin C) can be added at 1,000–2,000 mg daily but less or taken separately in patients with loose stools. For best tolerance, patients should begin taking the compounded capsules 1–2 weeks after starting vitamin B12 and high gamma vitamin E supplementation. Introducing one therapy at a time works best, although the compounded substances complement each other in mode of action.

With compounded capsules always take with food in the stomach. Begin gradually: one with a meal for a few days, then one with a second meal for a few days, and then one with third meal. The goal is three times daily or more. If the patient has any stomach irritation, they can open the capsule and begin with a pinch in food, increasing gradually to a full capsule.

Slowly increase to 2 with meals, and then gradually increase further if applicable and helpful. If any irritation occurs, reduce dosage and wait for further healing before gently increasing again at a pace with which the patient feels comfortable.

Bioavailable forms are given. Do not substitute (Table 11.2).

## *Sleep*

*Sleep* is an obvious but often overlooked essential. This can be disrupted by environmental exposures (discussed below) and biochemical factors.

Relaxing substances can be given at night. *Magnesium* with the evening meal or evening Epsom salt soaks are examples. *Taurine* midevening 1–2 capsules of 500 mg for difficult sleep onset and/or at bedtime for nighttime awakening helps many. Evening use of sublingual *methylcobalamine* is calming and reduces coughing from mucosal irritant inflammation and drainage. Many patients find *glutathione* to be calming: e.g., S-acetyl-glutathione 1–2 100 mg oral capsules with the evening meal or nebulizing glutathione in the evening as well as during the day can help.

**Table 11.2** Sample of compounded protocol

| | |
|---|---|
| *Glutathione function/reactivation* | *Superoxide scavengers* |
| Ascorbic acid _______mg/day | Proanthocyanidin, 400 mg/day: activin |
| Selenomethione, 400 mcg/day | Epigallocatechin gallate (EGCG), 400 mg/day |
| Alpha lipoic acid, 600 mg/day | *GABA formation to calm NMDA activation* |
| Riboflavin-5-phosphate, 150 mg/day | Pyridoxal-5-phoshpate, 150 mg/day |
| *Components of superoxide dismutase* | *Energy metabolism for healing/ calming NMDA* |
| Zinc picolinate, 20 mg/day | Acetyl-L-carnitine, 500 mg/day |
| Copper picolinate, 0.5 mg/day without copper | Niacinamide, 100 mg/day |
| Manganese, 2 mg/day | Thiamine HCL, 100 mg/day |
| *Compounds related to peroxynitrite biochemistry* | Chromium 350 mcg/day |
| Magnesium, glycinate, mallate, 400 mg/day | Pantethine (B5), 800 mg/day |
| Betaine (trimethylglycine), 500 mg/day | Biotin, 3 mg/day |
| MTHF (bioactive folate), 1 mg/day | *Detoxification* |
| *Scavengers of peroxynitrite and its breakdown products* | Molybdenum, 200 mcg/day |
| Ginkgo biloba extract, 120 mg/day | |
| Siliphos, 400 mg/day | |
| Bilberry extract, 300 mg/day | |
| Cranberry extract, 400 mg/day | |
| Carotenoid mixture (5 mg each lycopene, beta-carotene, other carotenoids: 10 mg each lutein and zeaxanthine/day) | |

What works for sleep disruption varies with patients: since the above all help the inflammation cycle, adjusting timing per above is often enough. When the patient knows that the provider takes sleep disruption seriously, they are encouraged to seek a solution together.

Patients who cannot achieve 6 h of sleep with the above measures are unusual, but some may benefit from temporary diazepam, a GABA agonist. Usually, only 2 mg is needed: larger doses often make them groggy, perhaps reflecting detoxification difficulty. Patients sometimes come to me on 0.5–1 mg clonazepam, which seems harder to wean them off of. I always remind patients that I am not their medical dictator but will seek to get at the cause: this helps avoid longer term dependency.

Patients need methylation of norepinephrine and epinephrine through bioactive folate (methyltetrahydrofolate or MTHF). 1 mg daily is usually adequate. Trimethylglycine supports other methylation and can be given at 500–1,000 mg daily.

## Testing to Evaluate Dosing Requirements

The author has tried various testing approaches. Patients differ greatly by environmental, genetic, dietary, and cell repair needs and other factors. No single test level is able to help all or even most patients. This is analogous to fitting all men and all women with shoe sizes of 10 and 7, respectively.

Many labs measure what levels are needed to prevent scurvy, pernicious anemia and other deficiency nutritional diseases. They do not measure the need for cell repair.

The only approach which the author has found corresponds to what the patient needs for respiratory repair uses cell division (mitosis) ability. This lab uses lymphocytes, which pass through both lipid and aqueous body fluid.

Lymphocytes are involved in irritant respiratory effects (Sin and Togias 2011). Lymphocytes also show altered function with chemical toxin and irritant exposures (Anderson et al. 2008, 2012; Bao et al. 2012; Borchers et al. 2007; Dearman et al. 2003; Fukuyama et al. 2011; Gerberick et al. 2002; Godderis et al. 2012; Goutet et al. 2005; Li et al. 2012; Thompson et al. 2008).

The only US laboratory using cell division/mitosis to evaluate cell repair need also uses lymphocytes. This is the CLIA-certified SpectraCell Laboratory in Houston, Texas. This laboratory tests cell repair needs individually for every non-plant-based nutrient discussed above except molybdenum. (As with all commercial entities discussed, I have never had a financial relation with this lab.) I use their Comprehensive Nutritional Panel (Micronutrient Testing Panel) for initial and follow-up evaluation (every 6–10 months).

I have used its results to guide treatment on thousands of patients and have developed test interpretation guidelines for reactive airway patients based on this experience.

## Using the Test Results to Guide Therapy

I go directly to the diagrams (scatter plots) that compare patient results with the general population controls which consist of many who eat junk food/nutrient-depleted food but are otherwise "healthy."

For best clinical success, I have learned *where patient values need to be on the comparison diagram*:

- *B12*, because of its essential role, in the top 20 %. Top 10 % works even better.
- *B vitamins* and antioxidants (*selenium, CoQ10*), in the top third.
- *Vitamin E*—The test currently only measures alpha, not gamma tocopherol. High gamma with about equal alpha tocopherol supplementation is needed in all patients with recurring symptoms.
- *Vitamin C*—Raise slowly to top third but avoid loose stools. Buffered is better. Avoid chewable to spare tooth enamel.
- *Magnesium*—Top third is essential: balance with calcium. Remember that the US population probably has more magnesium than calcium deficiency. *D3 replacement at over 400 IU can drop magnesium by raising calcium: this can have a neuroexcitatory and bronchoconstricting effect*. This test allows you to monitor D3, magnesium, and calcium. First raise magnesium as needed, and then carefully bring calcium to average.

- *Chromium* that is not deficient or borderline deficient is okay. If insulin-glucose metabolism still looks poor, try EPA/DHA, liquid form. A 3-to-1 ratio of EPA to DHA is most physiologic. EPA/DHA also helps inflammation reduction in mucosa (Ohtsuka et al. 2011) including respiratory (Mayer et al. 2009; Mickleborough et al. 2008; Tecklenburg-Lund et al. 2010). It also helps insulin resistance (Fedor and Kelley 2009; Siriwardhana et al. 2012). The author has used Vital Nutrients ultrapure fish oil liquid, 1 tsp daily. Capsules do not have the correct EPA/DHA ratio.
- *Choline, inositol, and serine* are *membrane phospholipids* by these names. In the author's experience, dry repletion rarely works. Reducing exposure, improving antioxidant protection as per above, and proper nutrition to reduce membrane damage are better. There is a somewhat expensive supplemental phosphatidylcholine (Xymogen, Body Bio, etc.) that can be used. Adding the combination of plant-based superoxide/peroxynitrite antioxidants (see Table 11.1) with ensuring adequate other antioxidants (selenium, CoQ10, high gamma tocopherol, vitamin C, and lipoic acid) has often worked well.

As with all medical substances discussed, best success is achieved with good nutrition and requires reducing airborne irritant exposures. Both of these are discussed below using approaches that fit a busy clinician's schedule.

## Nutrition

The dietary approach that seems to work best for the author is giving a factsheet, on yellow paper to better stand out. Giving a factsheet saves clinician time and provides a frequent patient reminder. The author periodically reviews a 4-day food log to fine-tune nutritional needs and remind patients of these important principles in their food choices.

> *The Eating for Healing* factsheet (Appendix) lists basics, what to do and why. The author recommends they put this on their refrigerator with a magnet. When they can recall it, it is best taped to an inside kitchen cabinet door for easy reference. This factsheet is a basic for all patients. See appendix.

Patients can also do *blending* to get easy absorption of raw high-antioxidant food if/when desired. Cooking, drying, and canning destroy many nutrients. A blender (not juicer) can be used for raw vegetable smoothies with some fruit, for soup blended longer to warm but not "cook", etc. Leaving fiber in reduces glycemic effects and feeds normal gut flora.

There are significant benefits from *organic foods*. Organic foods have higher antioxidants (Calvert et al. 2004; Djousse and Gaziano 2007; Poulev et al. 2003; Sudha and Ravishankar 2002) and higher nutrient levels (Jacobs et al. 2007; Smith 1993). Nutrient levels will be better if foods are grown on nutrient-dense soils since neither plants nor animals can synthesize minerals.

## Reducing Environmental Exacerbation

*This is essential to success*: Medical treatment can significantly reduce inflammation, but neglecting environmental factors blocks adequate clinical progress.

A patient reference which lists safer products to avoid exacerbation is the book *Less Toxic Alternatives* (Caleta Press) by health educator, C. Gorman. The author finds that providing this reference saves clinical time and helps patients avoid spending money on things that release respiratory irritants at doses that increase symptoms and inflammation. It discusses many of the factors below in much greater detail to assist in protection, safer product/method selection, and use.

*Particles* (Penn et al. 2005; Sirivelu et al. 2006) and *VOCs* (Hudnell et al. 1992) exacerbate airway inflammation. Reducing sources is a major benefit to healing in the author's experience, and clinical progress is minimal without addressing exposure. Particles can take weeks or longer to clear from sinuses and alveoli.

*Bedroom controls* are important because 8 or more hours a day are spent sleeping and the breathing zone is on the bedding and pillow. Bedroom exposures can manifest as more respiratory or eye irritation on awakening.

*Nearby combustion products* can cause respiratory irritation (Brooks et al. 1985; Kipen et al. 1994). *Carbon monoxide* is also able even in modest amounts (lower than detected by devices designed for fire monitoring) to cause inflammation by speeding up the biochemical cycle (Lopez et al. 2009). Thus patients can have exacerbation from gas appliances, candles, and other combustion sources, with particulates or just carbon monoxide (Cormier et al. 2006; Lopez et al. 2009; Piantadosi et al. 2006; Soto et al. 2008; van Berlo et al. 2010; Zhao et al. 2006). Some gas appliances now have tight combustion chambers and can be vented to outside the home.

Many but not all patients know from past exacerbations various products to avoid. Some are not aware that *fabric softener particulate is a respiratory irritant* (Anderson and Anderson 2000; Caress and Steinemann 2009). The author has observed prolonged sinus and pulmonary exacerbation as the irritant particles are slowly degraded in the respiratory tract. The particulate contaminates and clings to furniture, bedding, vehicles, hair, and other clothing and can create ongoing chronic exposure exacerbation. Using less detergent leaves less residue which often eliminates the need for fabric softener. If not (e.g., well water in limestone areas), a water softener will pay for itself in reduced medical costs and disability.

If fabric softener were used, after discontinuing use, the residue can be removed by HEPA vacuuming the laundry, bedroom, carpet, and all porous/fabric-covered surfaces, including the car. The dryer should be wiped down and all affected clothes relaundered. Often significant symptom improvement follows this approach.

*Mold particles* and their VOC emissions can cause upper and lower respiratory inflammation (Brunekreef et al. 1989; Husman et al. 1993; Jaakkola et al. 1993; Savilahti et al. 2000). Any visible mold and mold in HVAC or air conditioning units can create ongoing respiratory and systemic exacerbation.

### *Home Environment Patient Questions*

A quick patient questionnaire can identify problems in a time-efficient manner.

| | *Check* | | |
|---|---|---|---|
| Circle all options that apply. Add any useful information | *Yes* | *No* | *Not sure* |
| *Live in mobile home/condo/apartment* | | | |
| *Live in detached home you own* | | | |
| *Live near busy road* | | | |
| *Pesticides used in building* | | | |
| *Lawn chemicals used nearby* | | | |
| *Damp basement/roof/other* | | | |
| *Mold in home* | | | |
| *Recent pesticide use* | | | |
| *Recent remodeling* | | | |
| *Gas furnace/stove/water heater/dryer* | | | |
| *Wood stove* | | | |
| *Household carpet* | | | |
| *Fabric softener used in home (liquid or dryer sheets)* | | | |
| *Symptoms with family exposures* | | | |

## Using Reasonable Accommodation as a Means of Exposure Control

Under Federal Disability Law and Regulations, a person is *entitled to reasonable accommodation* if they have a *condition that significantly affects the major life activity of breathing*. Reasonable accommodation need not be free or even cheap, as for example the common accommodations to allow access for persons in wheelchairs. Here significant does not have to be life threatening but includes irritants that trigger respiratory symptoms.

This approach can be used for *housing* (rented, condos), *schools*, and the *workplace*.

Congress wrote the law for the patient to request (giving patient signature stronger legal force), but the physician can discuss and draft the medical section and sign as well, giving vital medical backup. One need not have toxicology training to know that lowering irritant exposures will reduce respiratory inflammation. Thus the physician needs only to understand this obvious principle to request exposure controls as relevant.

## *Sample Letter*

The following sample letter lists potential factors: selecting those relevant to the patient is most effective.

Doctor Name
Address
Date

My patient, ________________, is a qualified person under Federal Disability Law and Regulations because of a medical condition that significantly affects the major life activity of breathing. The patient and I request the following medically needed and reasonable accommodations:

- Elimination of air fresheners in nearby restroom(s).
- Encourage a policy of a smoke-free, fragrance-free work area.
- Eliminate combustion product exposures from the work area, e.g., candles, incense, idling vehicles, and others.
- Frequent building inspection for water damage and mold residue.
- Frequent HVAC inspection, filter change, and mold control, using nontoxic mold control procedures. Avoid standing water in HVAC system to prevent mold growth.
- Use cleaning agents that are not respiratory irritants (not containing chlorine bleach, ammonia, other irritants).
- Educate employees in the work area that fabric softener particulate leaves an irritant respiratory residue.
- Allow ***patient name*** to leave the work area in case respiratory symptoms develop and cannot be quickly controlled.
- Allow flexitime work to reduce commuter exhaust irritation.
- Provide a less toxic work area when needed to avoid illness symptoms from irritants.
- Utilize least toxic pest control measures. See the 501(c)(3) nonprofit science-based organization, http://www.beyondpesticides.org, for expert assistance.

Please respond indicating when the above measures are in place. Thank you.

Sincerely,

| ______________________________ | ______________________________ |
| --- | --- |
| *doctor* | *patient* |

### Filters

Filters are not a substitute for reducing the above exposures but can help when adequate control is not possible. Never use devices releasing ozone or described as ion generating. Filters must be changed as needed for effectiveness. Filter devices will only be effective if proper brands and sizes are selected and used in areas for which they have adequate capacity. Thus a personal filter in a large work area is not adequate. For persons who own their homes, a whole house filter may be needed. If mold or combustion particulate is a concern, a HEPA filter is needed. For VOC control, a thicker activated charcoal bed protects far better than a thin one (e.g., an inch or less). Brands used must be those intended for reactive airways.

## Summary

The above chapter information is complex and new to many practitioners. However, *the current drug-based approach to reactive airway disease leads to patient deterioration* because it cannot address real biochemical causal factors.

Because of recent biochemical advances in understanding, it is now possible to achieve significant medical improvement in conjunction with assisting the patient in obtaining information about environmental controls and healing nutrition.

Begin by using the evaluation tools (patient questionnaire, peak flow log) and others of your choosing. If the patient has irritant exacerbations and symptoms in your office, you may wish to use sublingual methylcobalamine to watch clinical improvement. The author uses 2 at a time until symptoms clear or greatly improve.

In patients with recurring symptoms, consider the recommended test panel: the earlier the cycle is controlled, the less the ultimate disability. At the beginning, monthly follow-ups are wise, allowing for interim visits in case the patient has unexpected issues.

Use the test guidelines and select some options you are comfortable with, knowing that you are not risking dangerous side effects. Follow progress through peak flow/symptom log and a list of what they are taking with dose, brand, and duration and see if you need more medical and environmental measures. Let the patient use the Eating for Healing factsheet. Do follow-up testing in 6–10 months.

Listen to the patient at each step: I have learned that their body is wiser than any doctor on the planet. This understanding has spared them and me many difficulties.

My prediction is that you will find personal and medical gratification in watching the healing process occur. I have been practicing medicine for 45 years and never tired of observing the wisdom of the body and how it prioritizes the healing process. It is also a great joy to see the patient become healthier with a new hope of "getting their life" enjoyable again.

## Appendix. Eating for Healing

The right foods speed repair of inflammation.

- Eat fresh and organic (Baker et al. 2002; Barrett 2006; Lu et al. 2006; Smith 1993) whenever possible, reducing processed foods to get healing nutrients.
- Eat four to five serving of vegetables and fruit daily. Good antioxidant foods include berries, citrus, parsley, onions, colorful vegetables and fruits, and legumes. Eat a variety to get balanced antioxidant protection. Beans, peas, and lentils also give healthy, soluble fiber.
- Reduce carbohydrate servings to *small*, and avoid refined carbohydrates (sugars, refined grains).
- Eat free range meat/eggs/wild caught fish*, at least 1–2 times daily.
- Eat seeds/nuts daily. Refrigerate in airtight containers. These contain balanced essential fats.
- Avoid all "fake fats": margarine, hydrogenated fats, olestra, etc. Reduce canola oil and cashews because they have harmful fats. Baked, processed foods often have harmful fats: read labels.
- Balance omega 3 (flax, hemp, *and* fish*) and omega 6 (eggs, GLA, meat, sunflower seeds). If you are stiff/achy/inflamed, get some extra omega 3 and consider 1–2 tsp of good-quality fish oil. Refrigerate and keep all omega 3 products airtight.
- Don't heat or cook with any liquid oil because it forms trans fats and damages the oil. For cooking, use ghee, butter, or coconut oil. Use low temperature for all cooking to retain nutrients. Avoid chips, "French fries," and other foods cooked/fried in oils.
- Chew all food until liquid before swallowing. Sip all liquids slowly. Greatly reduce sodas and caffeine.
- Eat onion family often (onions, leeks, garlic, chives, shallots).
- Hydrate well with lots of water: avoid caffeine and diuretics when possible. "Decaffeinated" tea and coffee still contain some caffeine.
- Avoid aspartame (aka amino sweet), MSG, and Splenda. Consider stevia and/or modest amounts of honey, blackstrap molasses.

  * Scientists researching mercury in fish compared to fish benefit state that (non-farm raised) salmon, herring, trout, pollock, and tilapia were safe at up to once daily and tuna, halibut, sea bass, and lobster 1–2 times a week, avoiding shark and shellfish (Ginsberg).

Baker BP, Benbrook CM, Groth E, 3rd, Lutz Benbrook K. Pesticide residues in conventional, integrated pest management (IPM)-grown and organic foods: insights from three US data sets. Food Addit Contam. 2002; 19:427–46.

Barrett J. OP Pesticides in children's bodies: the effects of a conventional versus organic diet. Environ Health Perspect. 2006; 114:A112.

Ginsberg GL, Toal BF. Quantitative approach for incorporating methylmercury risks and omega-3 fatty acid benefits in developing species-specific fish consumption advice. Environ Health Perspect. 2009; 117:267–75.

Lu C, Toepel K, Irish R, Fenske RA, Barr DB, Bravo R. Organic diets significantly lower children's dietary exposure to organophosphorus pesticides. Environ Health Perspect. 2006; 114:260–3.

Smith B. Organic foods vs supermarket foods: element levels. J Appl Nut. 1993; 45:35–9.

## References

Ahmadi-Ashtiani H, Allameh A, Rastegar H, Soleimani M, Barkhordari E. Inhibition of cyclooxygenase-2 and inducible nitric oxide synthase by silymarin in proliferating mesenchymal stem cells: comparison with glutathione modifiers. J Nat Med. 2012;66:85–94.

Akhtar MI, Ullah H, Hamid M. Magnesium, a drug of diverse use. J Pak Med Assoc. 2011;61:1220–5.

Allan R, Mara N. Magnesium and the acute physician. Acute Med. 2012;11:3–7.

Alvarez E, Leiro J, Orallo F. Effect of (−)-epigallocatechin-3-gallate on respiratory burst of rat macrophages. Int Immunopharmacol. 2002;2:849–55.

Amitai Y, Zlotogorski Z, Golan-Katzav V, Wexler A, Gross D. Neuropsychological impairment from acute low-level exposure to carbon monoxide. Arch Neurol. 1998;55:845–8.

Anderson RC, Anderson JH. Respiratory toxicity of fabric softener emissions. J Toxicol Environ Health A. 2000;60:121–36.

Anderson SE, Ham JE, Munson AE. Irritancy and sensitization potential of glyoxylic acid. J Immunotoxicol. 2008;5:93–8.

Anderson SE, Franko J, Jackson LG, Wells JR, Ham JE, Meade BJ. Irritancy and allergic responses induced by exposure to the indoor air chemical 4-oxopentanal. Toxicol Sci. 2012;127:371–81.

Bagchi D, Garg A, Krohn RL, Bagchi M, Tran MX, Stohs SJ. Oxygen free radical scavenging abilities of vitamins C and E, and a grape seed proanthocyanidin extract in vitro. Res Commun Mol Pathol Pharmacol. 1997;95:179–89.

Banerjee B, Bagchi D. Beneficial effects of a novel IH636 grape seed proanthocyanidin extract in the treatment of chronic pancreatitis. Digestion. 2001;63:203–6.

Bao Y, Chen H, Hu Y, Bai Y, Zhou M, Xu A, et al. Combination effects of chronic cadmium exposure and gamma-irradiation on the genotoxicity and cytotoxicity of peripheral blood lymphocytes and bone marrow cells in rats. Mutat Res. 2012;743:67–74.

Beckman JS, Crow JP. Pathological implications of nitric oxide, superoxide and peroxynitrite formation. Biochem Soc Trans. 1993;21:330–4.

Beg S, Javed S, Kohli K. Bioavailability enhancement of coenzyme Q10: an extensive review of patents. Recent Pat Drug Deliv Formul. 2010;4:245–55.

Bishop C, Hudson VM, Hilton SC, Wilde C. A pilot study of the effect of inhaled buffered reduced glutathione on the clinical status of patients with cystic fibrosis. Chest. 2005;127:308–17.

Borchers MT, Wesselkamper SC, Harris NL, Deshmukh H, Beckman E, Vitucci M, et al. CD8+ T cells contribute to macrophage accumulation and airspace enlargement following repeated irritant exposure. Exp Mol Pathol. 2007;83:301–10.

Brooks SM, Weiss MA, Bernstein IL. Reactive airways dysfunction syndrome. Case reports of persistent airways hyperreactivity following high-level irritant exposures. J Occup Med. 1985;27:473–6.

Brunekreef B, Dockery DW, Speizer FE, Ware JH, Spengler JD, Ferris BG. Home dampness and respiratory morbidity in children. Am Rev Respir Dis. 1989;140:1363–7.

Burge PS, O'Brien IM, Harries MG. Peak flow rate records in the diagnosis of occupational asthma due to isocyanates. Thorax. 1979;34:317–23.

Busse E, Zimmer G, Schopohl B, Kornhuber B. Influence of alpha-lipoic acid on intracellular glutathione in vitro and in vivo. Arzneimittelforschung. 1992;42:829–31.
Calvert GM, Plate DK, Das R, Rosales R, Shafey O, Thomsen C, et al. Acute occupational pesticide-related illness in the US, 1998–1999: surveillance findings from the SENSOR-pesticides program. Am J Ind Med. 2004;45:14–23.
Caress SM, Steinemann AC. Prevalence of fragrance sensitivity in the American population. J Environ Health. 2009;71:46–50.
Cheshchevik VT, Lapshina EA, Dremza IK, Zabrodskaya SV, Reiter RJ, Prokopchik NI, et al. Rat liver mitochondrial damage under acute or chronic carbon tetrachloride-induced intoxication: protection by melatonin and cranberry flavonoids. Toxicol Appl Pharmacol. 2012;261:271–9.
Chou CY, Tong L. Structural and biochemical studies on the regulation of biotin carboxylase by substrate inhibition and dimerization. J Biol Chem. 2011;286:24417–25.
Christen S, Woodall AA, Shigenaga MK, Southwell-Keely PT, Duncan MW, Ames BN. gamma-tocopherol traps mutagenic electrophiles such as NO(X) and complements alpha-tocopherol: physiological implication. Proc Natl Acad Sci USA. 1997;94:3217–22.
Cormier SA, Lomnicki S, Backes W, Dellinger B. Origin and health impacts of emissions of toxic by-products and fine particles from combustion and thermal treatment of hazardous wastes and materials. Environ Health Perspect. 2006;114:810–7.
Cornille E, Abou-Hamdan M, Khrestchatisky M, Nieoullon A, de Reggi M, Gharib B. Enhancement of L-3-hydroxybutyryl-CoA dehydrogenase activity and circulating ketone body levels by pantethine. Relevance to dopaminergic injury. BMC Neurosci. 2010;11:51.
Cos P, De Bruyne T, Hermans N, Apers S, Berghe DV, Vlietinck AJ. Proanthocyanidins in health care: current and new trends. Curr Med Chem. 2004;11:1345–59.
Costa DL. Air pollution. In: Klaassen CD, editor. Casarett & Doull's toxicology. 6th ed. New York, NY: McGraw-Hill; 2001. p. 1003.
Dearman RJ, Betts CJ, Humphreys N, Flanagan BF, Gilmour NJ, Basketter DA, et al. Chemical allergy: considerations for the practical application of cytokine profiling. Toxicol Sci. 2003;71:137–45.
Delfino RJ, Staimer N, Gillen D, Tjoa T, Sioutas C, Fung K, et al. Personal and ambient air pollution is associated with increased exhaled nitric oxide in children with asthma. Environ Health Perspect. 2006;114:1736–43.
Depeint F, Bruce WR, Shangari N, Mehta R, O'Brien PJ. Mitochondrial function and toxicity: role of the B vitamin family on mitochondrial energy metabolism. Chem Biol Interact. 2006;163:94–112.
Djousse L, Gaziano JM. Breakfast cereals and risk of heart failure in the physicians' health study I. Arch Intern Med. 2007;167:2080–5.
Fairbairn AS, Fletcher CM, Tinker CM, Wood CH. A comparison of spirometric and peak expiratory flow measurements in men with and without chronic bronchitis. Thorax. 1962;17:168–74.
Fedor D, Kelley DS. Prevention of insulin resistance by n-3 polyunsaturated fatty acids. Curr Opin Clin Nutr Metab Care. 2009;12:138–46.
Fukai T, Ushio-Fukai M. Superoxide dismutases: role in redox signaling, vascular function, and diseases. Antioxid Redox Signal. 2011;15:1583–606.
Fukuyama T, Tajima Y, Ueda H, Hayashi K, Kosaka T. Prior exposure to immunosuppressive organophosphorus or organochlorine compounds aggravates the T(H)1- and T(H)2-type allergy caused by topical sensitization to 2,4-dinitrochlorobenzene and trimellitic anhydride. J Immunotoxicol. 2011;8:170–82.
Gallos G, Yim P, Chang S, Zhang Y, Xu D, Cook JM, et al. Targeting the restricted alpha-subunit repertoire of airway smooth muscle GABAA receptors augments airway smooth muscle relaxation. Am J Physiol Lung Cell Mol Physiol. 2012;302:L248–56.
Gerberick GF, Cruse LW, Ryan CA, Hulette BC, Chaney JG, Skinner RA, et al. Use of a B cell marker (B220) to discriminate between allergens and irritants in the local lymph node assay. Toxicol Sci. 2002;68:420–8.

Godderis L, De Raedt K, Tabish AM, Poels K, Maertens N, De Ruyck K, et al. Epigenetic changes in lymphocytes of solvent-exposed individuals. Epigenomics. 2012;4:269–77.

Goutet M, Pepin E, Langonne I, Huguet N, Ban M. Identification of contact and respiratory sensitizers using flow cytometry. Toxicol Appl Pharmacol. 2005;205:259–70.

Gregus Z, Klaassen CD. Mechanisms of toxicity. In: Klaassen CD, editor. Casarett & Doull's toxicology: the basic science of poisons. 6th ed. New York, NY: McGraw-Hill; 2001. p. 35–81.

Higgins IT. Respiratory symptoms, bronchitis, and ventilatory capacity in random sample of an agricultural population. Br Med J. 1957;2:1198–203.

Higuchi A, Yonemitsu K, Koreeda A, Tsunenari S. Inhibitory activity of epigallocatechin gallate (EGCg) in paraquat-induced microsomal lipid peroxidation—a mechanism of protective effects of EGCg against paraquat toxicity. Toxicology. 2003;183:143–9.

Hudnell HK, Otto DA, House DE, Molhave L. Exposure of humans to a volatile organic mixture. II. Sensory. Arch Environ Health. 1992;47:31–8.

Husman T, Koskinen O, Hyvarinen A, Reponen T, Ruuskanen J, Nevalainen A. Respiratory symptoms and infections among residents in dwellings with moisture problems or mold growth. In: Jaakkola JJK, Ilmarinen R, Seppanen O, editors. Proceedings of indoor air '93: the 6th international conference on indoor air quality and climate. Helsinki, Finland; 1993.

Hustad S, McKinley MC, McNulty H, Schneede J, Strain JJ, Scott JM, et al. Riboflavin, flavin mononucleotide, and flavin adenine dinucleotide in human plasma and erythrocytes at baseline and after low-dose riboflavin supplementation. Clin Chem. 2002;48:1571–7.

Hyun SK, Jung HA, Chung HY, Choi JS. In vitro peroxynitrite scavenging activity of 6-hydroxykynurenic acid and other flavonoids from Gingko biloba yellow leaves. Arch Pharm Res. 2006;29:1074–9.

Jaakkola JJ, Jaakkola N, Ruotsalainen R. Home dampness and molds as determinants of respiratory symptoms and asthma in pre-school children. J Expo Anal Environ Epidemiol. 1993;3 Suppl 1:129–42.

Jacobs Jr DR, Andersen LF, Blomhoff R. Whole-grain consumption is associated with a reduced risk of noncardiovascular, noncancer death attributed to inflammatory diseases in the Iowa Women's Health Study. Am J Clin Nutr. 2007;85:1606–14.

Jayaprakash K. Mercury vapor inhalation and its effect on glutathione peroxidase in goldsmiths exposed occupationally. Toxicol Ind Health. 2009;25:463–5.

Karalija A, Novikova LN, Kingham PJ, Wiberg M, Novikov LN. Neuroprotective effects of N-acetyl-cysteine and acetyl-L-carnitine after spinal cord injury in adult rats. PLoS One. 2012;7:e41086.

Kidd P, Head K. A review of the bioavailability and clinical efficacy of milk thistle phytosome: a silybin-phosphatidylcholine complex (Siliphos). Altern Med Rev. 2005;10:193–203.

Kim YJ, Yokozawa T. Modulation of oxidative stress and melanogenesis by proanthocyanidins. Biol Pharm Bull. 2009;32:1155–9.

Kipen HM, Blume R, Hutt D. Asthma experience in an occupational and environmental medicine clinic. Low-dose reactive airways dysfunction syndrome. J Occup Med. 1994;36:1133–7.

Klotz LO, Sies H. Defenses against peroxynitrite: selenocompounds and flavonoids. Toxicol Lett. 2003;140–141:125–32.

Kocak-Toker N, Giris M, Tulubas F, Uysal M, Aykac-Toker G. Peroxynitrite induced decrease in Na+, K+–ATPase activity is restored by taurine. World J Gastroenterol. 2005;11:3554–7.

Lal S, Ferguson AD, Campbell EJ. Forced expiratory time: a simple test for airways obstruction. Br Med J. 1964;1:814–7.

Lee JH, Jarreau T, Prasad A, Lavie C, O'Keefe J, Ventura H. Nutritional assessment in heart failure patients. Congest Heart Fail. 2011;17:199–203.

Li B, Niu Y, Liu S, Yu W, Chen J, Wu L, et al. A change in CD3gamma, CD3delta, CD3, and CD3zeta gene expression in T-lymphocytes from benzene-exposed and benzene-poisoned workers. J Immunotoxicol. 2012;9:160–7.

Linder MC. Nutritional biochemistry and metabolism with clinical applications. 2nd ed. East Norwich, CT: Appleton and Lange; 1991.

Liu J, Head E, Kuratsune H, Cotman CW, Ames BN. Comparison of the effects of L-carnitine and acetyl-L-carnitine on carnitine levels, ambulatory activity, and oxidative stress biomarkers in the brain of old rats. Ann N Y Acad Sci. 2004;1033:117–31.

Lopez IA, Acuna D, Beltran-Parrazal L, Lopez IE, Amarnani A, Cortes M, et al. Evidence for oxidative stress in the developing cerebellum of the rat after chronic mild carbon monoxide exposure (0.0025% in air). BMC Neurosci. 2009;10:53.

Machlin LJ, Bendich A. Free radical tissue damage: protective role of antioxidant nutrients. FASEB J. 1987;1:441–5.

Mailloux RJ, Beriault R, Lemire J, Singh R, Chenier DR, Hamel RD, et al. The tricarboxylic acid cycle, an ancient metabolic network with a novel twist. PLoS One. 2007;2:e690.

Malaguarnera M. Carnitine derivatives: clinical usefulness. Curr Opin Gastroenterol. 2012;28:166–76.

Malekinejad H, Rezabakhsh A, Rahmani F, Hobbenaghi R. Silymarin regulates the cytochrome P450 3A2 and glutathione peroxides in the liver of streptozotocin-induced diabetic rats. Phytomedicine. 2012;19:583–90.

Mar TF, Jansen K, Shepherd K, Lumley T, Larson TV, Koenig JQ. Exhaled nitric oxide in children with asthma and short-term PM2.5 exposure in Seattle. Environ Health Perspect. 2005;113:1791–4.

Matsunaga N, Imai S, Inokuchi Y, Shimazawa M, Yokota S, Araki Y, et al. Bilberry and its main constituents have neuroprotective effects against retinal neuronal damage in vitro and in vivo. Mol Nutr Food Res. 2009;53:869–77.

Mauskop A, Varughese J. Why all migraine patients should be treated with magnesium. J Neural Transm. 2012;119:575–9.

Mayer K, Kiessling A, Ott J, Schaefer MB, Hecker M, Henneke I, et al. Acute lung injury is reduced in fat-1 mice endogenously synthesizing n-3 fatty acids. Am J Respir Crit Care Med. 2009;179:474–83.

Mendel RR, Kruse T. Cell biology of molybdenum in plants and humans. Biochim Biophys Acta. 1823;2012:1568–79.

Menghini L, Leporini L, Scanu N, Pintore G, La Rovere R, Di Filippo ES, et al. Effect of phytochemical concentrations on biological activities of cranberry extracts. J Biol Regul Homeost Agents. 2011;25:27–35.

Methacholine for diagnosis of asthma. Med Lett Drugs Ther. 1987; 29:60.

Mickleborough TD, Lindley MR, Montgomery GS. Effect of fish oil-derived omega-3 polyunsaturated fatty acid supplementation on exercise-induced bronchoconstriction and immune function in athletes. Phys Sportsmed. 2008;36:11–7.

Millqvist E, Lowhagen O. Methacholine provocations do not reveal sensitivity to strong scents. Ann Allergy Asthma Immunol. 1998;80:381–4.

Miyashita T, Oda Y, Horiuchi J, Yin JC, Morimoto T, Saitoe M. Mg(2+) block of Drosophila NMDA receptors is required for long-term memory formation and CREB-dependent gene expression. Neuron. 2012;74:887–98.

Mukerji SS, Katsman EA, Wilber C, Haner NA, Selman WR, Hall AK. Activin is a neuronal survival factor that is rapidly increased after transient cerebral ischemia and hypoxia in mice. J Cereb Blood Flow Metab. 2007;27:1161–72.

Muller BA, Leick CA, Suelzer M, Piyamahunt A, Richerson HB. Prognostic value of methacholine challenge in patients with respiratory symptoms. J Allergy Clin Immunol. 1994;94:77–87.

Nanjo F, Mori M, Goto K, Hara Y. Radical scavenging activity of tea catechins and their related compounds. Biosci Biotechnol Biochem. 1999;63:1621–3.

Nikolaev MV, Magazanik LG, Tikhonov DB. Influence of external magnesium ions on the NMDA receptor channel block by different types of organic cations. Neuropharmacology. 2012;62:2078–85.

Ohtsuka Y, Okada K, Yamakawa Y, Ikuse T, Baba Y, Inage E, et al. omega-3 fatty acids attenuate mucosal inflammation in premature rat pups. J Pediatr Surg. 2011;46:489–95.

Oja SS, Janaky R, Varga V, Saransaari P. Modulation of glutamate receptor functions by glutathione. Neurochem Int. 2000;37:299–306.
Ozaki K, Sano T, Tsuji N, Matsuura T, Narama I. Carnitine is necessary to maintain the phenotype and function of brown adipose tissue. Lab Invest. 2011;91:704–10.
Palaniappan AR, Dai A. Mitochondrial ageing and the beneficial role of alpha-lipoic acid. Neurochem Res. 2007;32:1552–8.
Parkinson A. Biotransformation of xenobiotics. In: Klaassen CD, editor. Casarett & Doull's toxicology: the basic science of poisons. 6th ed. New York, NY: McGraw-Hill; 2001. p. 213–8.
Pascoe GA, Fariss MW, Olafsdottir K, Reed DJ. A role of vitamin E in protection against cell injury. Maintenance of intracellular glutathione precursors and biosynthesis. Eur J Biochem. 1987;166:241–7.
Patel SP, Sullivan PG, Lyttle TS, Magnuson DS, Rabchevsky AG. Acetyl-L-carnitine treatment following spinal cord injury improves mitochondrial function correlated with remarkable tissue sparing and functional recovery. Neuroscience. 2012;210:296–307.
Penn A, Murphy G, Barker S, Henk W, Penn L. Combustion-derived ultrafine particles transport organic toxicants to target respiratory cells. Environ Health Perspect. 2005;113:956–63.
Pesce V, Nicassio L, Fracasso F, Musicco C, Cantatore P, Gadaleta MN. Acetyl-L-carnitine activates the peroxisome proliferator-activated receptor-gamma coactivators PGC-1alpha/PGC-1beta-dependent signaling cascade of mitochondrial biogenesis and decreases the oxidized peroxiredoxins content in old rat liver. Rejuvenation Res. 2012;15:136–9.
Piantadosi CA, Carraway MS, Suliman HB. Carbon monoxide, oxidative stress, and mitochondrial permeability pore transition. Free Radic Biol Med. 2006;40:1332–9.
Poulev A, O'Neal JM, Logendra S, Pouleva RB, Timeva V, Garvey AS, et al. Elicitation, a new window into plant chemodiversity and phytochemical drug discovery. J Med Chem. 2003;46:2542–7.
Prakash YS. Gamma-aminobutyric acid: something old, something new for bronchodilation. Anesthesiology. 2009;110:696–7.
Prentice AM, Bates CJ. A biochemical evaluation of the erythrocyte glutathione reductase (EC 1.6.4.2) test for riboflavin status. 2. Dose–response relationships in chronic marginal deficiency. Br J Nutr. 1981;45:53–65.
Rahman MM, Ichiyanagi T, Komiyama T, Hatano Y, Konishi T. Superoxide radical- and peroxynitrite-scavenging activity of anthocyanins; structure-activity relationship and their synergism. Free Radic Res. 2006;40:993–1002.
Rajapakshe A, Meyers KT, Berry RE, Tollin G, Enemark JH. Intramolecular electron transfer in sulfite-oxidizing enzymes: probing the role of aromatic amino acids. J Biol Inorg Chem. 2012;17:345–52.
Rotruck JT, Pope AL, Ganther HE, Swanson AB, Hafeman DG, Hoekstra WG. Selenium: biochemical role as a component of glutathione peroxidase. Science. 1973;179:588–90.
Rowe WJ. Correcting magnesium deficiencies may prolong life. Clin Interv Aging. 2012;7:51–4.
Savilahti R, Uitti J, Laippala P, Husman T, Roto P. Respiratory morbidity among children following renovation of a water-damaged school. Arch Environ Health. 2000;55:405–10.
Scafidi S, Fiskum G, Lindauer SL, Bamford P, Shi D, Hopkins I, et al. Metabolism of acetyl-L-carnitine for energy and neurotransmitter synthesis in the immature rat brain. J Neurochem. 2010;114:820–31.
Shephard RJ. Some observations on peak expiratory flow. Thorax. 1962;17:39–48.
Sin B, Togias A. Pathophysiology of allergic and nonallergic rhinitis. Proc Am Thorac Soc. 2011;8:106–14.
Sirivelu MP, MohanKumar SM, Wagner JG, Harkema JR, MohanKumar PS. Activation of the stress axis and neurochemical alterations in specific brain areas by concentrated ambient particle exposure with concomitant allergic airway disease. Environ Health Perspect. 2006;114:870–4.
Siriwardhana N, Kalupahana NS, Moustaid-Moussa N. Health benefits of n-3 polyunsaturated fatty acids: eicosapentaenoic acid and docosahexaenoic acid. Adv Food Nutr Res. 2012;65: 211–22.

Siwik JP, Johnson CC, Havstad SL, Peterson EL, Ownby DR, Zoratti EM. Airway hyperresponsiveness to methacholine at age 6 to 8 years in nonasthmatic patients is not related to increased health-care utilization for asthma in the ensuing 5 years: a longitudinal study of a birth cohort. Chest. 2005;128:2420–6.

Smith B. Organic foods vs supermarket foods: element levels. J Appl Nut. 1993;45:35–9.

Smith AR, Shenvi SV, Widlansky M, Suh JH, Hagen TM. Lipoic acid as a potential therapy for chronic diseases associated with oxidative stress. Curr Med Chem. 2004;11:1135–46.

Song NY, Shi HB, Li CY, Yin SK. Interaction between taurine and GABA(A)/glycine receptors in neurons of the rat anteroventral cochlear nucleus. Brain Res. 2012;1472:1–10.

Soto KF, Murr LE, Garza KM. Cytotoxic responses and potential respiratory health effects of carbon and carbonaceous nanoparticulates in the Paso del Norte airshed environment. Int J Environ Res Public Health. 2008;5:12–25.

Spiropoulos K, Stevens J, Eigen H, Spiropoulos A. Specificity and sensitivity of methacholine challenge test in children with normal and hyperreactive airways. Acta Paediatr Scand. 1986;75:737–43.

Sudha G, Ravishankar GA. Involvement and interaction of various signaling compounds on the plant metabolic events during defense response resistance to stress factors formation of secondary metabolites and their molecular aspects. Plant Cell Tiss Org Cult. 2002;71:181–212.

Sun M, Qian F, Shen W, Tian C, Hao J, Sun L, et al. Mitochondrial nutrients stimulate performance and mitochondrial biogenesis in exhaustively exercised rats. Scand J Med Sci Sports. 2011.

Tarasov IUA, Sheibak VM, Moiseenok AG. [Adrenal cortex functional activity in pantothenate deficiency and the administration of the vitamin or its derivatives]. Vopr Pitan. 1985;51–4.

Tecklenburg-Lund S, Mickleborough TD, Turner LA, Fly AD, Stager JM, Montgomery GS. Randomized controlled trial of fish oil and montelukast and their combination on airway inflammation and hyperpnea-induced bronchoconstriction. PLoS One. 2010;5:e13487.

Testa B, Mesolella M, Testa D, Giuliano A, Costa G, Maione F, et al. Glutathione in the upper respiratory tract. Ann Otol Rhinol Laryngol. 1995;104:117–9.

Thompson CM, Subramaniam RP, Grafstrom RC. Mechanistic and dose considerations for supporting adverse pulmonary physiology in response to formaldehyde. Toxicol Appl Pharmacol. 2008;233:355–9.

Tong L. Structure and function of biotin-dependent carboxylases. Cell Mol Life Sci. 2012.

Tong S, Chu C, Wei Y, Wang L, Gao X, Xu X, et al. Preparation and effects of 2,3-dehydrosilymarin, a promising and potent antioxidant and free radical scavenger. J Pharm Pharmacol. 2011;63:238–44.

Tsai KL, Huang YH, Kao CL, Yang DM, Lee HC, Chou HY, et al. A novel mechanism of coenzyme Q10 protects against human endothelial cells from oxidative stress-induced injury by modulating NO-related pathways. J Nutr Biochem. 2012;23:458–68.

Tutuncu B, Kucukatay V, Arslan S, Sahin B, Semiz A, Sen A. Alteration of drug metabolizing enzymes in sulphite oxidase deficiency. J Clin Biochem Nutr. 2012;51:50–4.

van Berlo D, Albrecht C, Knaapen AM, Cassee FR, Gerlofs-Nijland ME, Kooter IM, et al. Comparative evaluation of the effects of short-term inhalation exposure to diesel engine exhaust on rat lung and brain. Arch Toxicol. 2010;84:553–62.

Verma A, Hirsch DJ, Glatt CE, Ronnett GV, Snyder SH. Carbon monoxide: a putative neural messenger. Science. 1993;259:381–4.

Wagner KH, Kamal-Eldin A, Elmadfa I. Gamma-tocopherol—an underestimated vitamin? Ann Nutr Metab. 2004;48:169–88.

Wagner AE, Ernst IM, Birringer M, Sancak O, Barella L, Rimbach G. A combination of lipoic acid plus coenzyme Q10 induces PGC1alpha, a master switch of energy metabolism, improves stress response, and increases cellular glutathione levels in cultured C2C12 skeletal muscle cells. Oxid Med Cell Longev. 2012;2012:835970.

Watson WP, Munter T, Golding BT. A new role for glutathione: protection of vitamin B12 from depletion by xenobiotics. Chem Res Toxicol. 2004;17:1562–7.

Witschi HR, Last JA. Toxic responses of the respiratory system. In: Klaassen CD, editor. Casarett & Doull's toxicology: the basic science of poisons. New York, NY: McGraw-Hill; 2001. p. 523.

Wolak M, Zahl A, Schneppensieper T, Stochel G, van Eldik R. Kinetics and mechanism of the reversible binding of nitric oxide to reduced cobalamin B(12r) (Cob(II)alamin). J Am Chem Soc. 2001;123:9780–91.

Yoo DY, Kim W, Kim DW, Yoo KY, Chung JY, Youn HY, et al. Pyridoxine enhances cell proliferation and neuroblast differentiation by upregulating the GABAergic system in the mouse dentate gyrus. Neurochem Res. 2011;36:713–21.

Zhang R, Zhang H, Zhang Z, Wang T, Niu J, Cui D, et al. Neuroprotective effects of pre-treament with l-carnitine and acetyl-l-carnitine on ischemic injury in vivo and in vitro. Int J Mol Sci. 2012;13:2078–90.

Zhao H, Barger MW, Ma JK, Castranova V, Ma JY. Cooperation of the inducible nitric oxide synthase and cytochrome P450 1A1 in mediating lung inflammation and mutagenicity induced by diesel exhaust particles. Environ Health Perspect. 2006;114:1253–8.

Zheng D, Yan L, Birke RL. Electrochemical and spectral studies of the reactions of aquocobalamin with nitric oxide and nitrite ion. Inorg Chem. 2002;41:2548–55.

Ziem G. Profile of patients with chemical injury and sensitivity, part II. Int J Toxicol. 1999;18:401–9.

Ziem G, McTamney J. Profile of patients with chemical injury and sensitivity. Environ Health Perspect. 1997;105 Suppl 2:417–36.

Zizkova P, Viskupicova J, Horakova L. Pycnogenol and Ginkgo biloba extract: effect on peroxynitrite-oxidized sarcoplasmic reticulum Ca-ATPase. Interdiscip Toxicol. 2010;3:132–6.

# Chapter 12
# Summary and Research Needs

**William J. Meggs**

**Abstract** Environmental exposures to noxious chemicals—both natural and synthetic—at nonlethal levels have been ubiquitous for millennia and range from hydrogen sulfide from volcanoes and hot springs to products of combustion. The harnessing of fire for human uses was a milestone in our acceptance of close proximity to irritant substances. A number of syndromes and conditions have been described that are induced or exacerbated by exposures to irritant chemicals. Irritant asthma and irritant rhinitis are now well-characterized conditions that have a solid scientific underpinning. Respiratory irritants bind to nociceptors on sensory nerve c-fibers in the airway and induce the release of inflammatory mediators, as discussed in Chaps. 1 and 3. For a normal airway, higher doses are needed to induce significant inflammation than in susceptible individuals. The pathophysiology of the increased susceptibility is now established. Inflammation leads to a pathological remodeling of airways. The remodeled airway has a decreased threshold for irritant-induced inflammation. The susceptible airway has a proliferation of nerve fibers, desquamation of epithelial barriers, and lymphocytic infiltrates.

Building on this scientific understanding, research is needed to build on our understanding of the mechanisms of other illnesses described in association with irritant exposures. Of particular importance is the need to understand the cerebral manifestations of allergy and irritant sensitivity and the relationship to neuropsychological disabilities. Environmental control units, in which subjects are housed in an environment relatively free of respiratory irritants, followed by controlled challenges with irritant chemicals while monitoring for disease exacerbations and objective parameters of disease, are needed for further research investigations.

W.J. Meggs, M.D., Ph.D., F.A.C.M.T., F.A.C.E.P. (✉)
Division of Toxicology, Department of Emergency Medicine, Brody School of Medicine at East Carolina University, 600 Moye Boulevard, Greenville, NC, USA
e-mail: meggsw@ecu.edu

W.J. Meggs (ed.), *The Toxicant Induction of Irritant Asthma, Rhinitis, and Related Conditions*, DOI 10.1007/978-1-4614-9044-9_12,

**Keywords** Neurogenic inflammation • Airway inflammation • Asthma • Rhinitis • Allergy • Respiratory irritants • Fatigue • Depression • Sleep disorders • Attention-deficit disorder

## Introduction

Environmental exposures to noxious chemicals—both natural and synthetic—at nonlethal levels have been ubiquitous for millennia and range from hydrogen sulfide from volcanoes and hot springs to products of combustion. The harnessing of fire for human uses was a milestone in our acceptance of close proximity to irritant substances. Using smoke from smoldering plants as drug delivery systems, from tobacco and marijuana to opium, further increased exposures to irritants. Progress in purifying natural substances and in synthetic chemistry added to the repertoire of materials to which we are exposed, from pesticides to organic solvents and irritant gases. That significant number of individuals report illness when exposed to environmental chemicals at levels tolerated by the public at large is well recognized, but the nature of this susceptibility has been a topic of great controversy. Science has progressed to the point that the mechanism of airway inflammation induced and/or exacerbated by irritant exposures is now well established. Respiratory irritants bind to nociceptors on sensory nerve c-fibers in the airway and induce the release of inflammatory mediators, as discussed in Chaps. 1 and 3. For a normal airway, higher doses are needed to induce significant inflammation than in susceptible individuals. The pathophysiology of the increased susceptibility is now established. Inflammation leads to a pathological remodeling of airways. The remodeled airway has a decreased threshold for irritant-induced inflammation. The susceptible airway has a proliferation of nerve fibers, desquamation of epithelial barriers, and lymphocytic infiltrates.

Irritant exposures, both acute and chronic, can induce airway inflammation that persists for years after the exposure. Reactivity to subsequent irritant exposures is a feature which is described as bronchial hyper-reactivity in asthma, which can be demonstrated by provocative challenges with methacholine, histamine, or irritants. For irritant rhinitis, there is no generally available analogue of the provocative challenges, though the capsaicin challenge test developed by Millqvist is an example of a promising avenue. Nasal washings after challenge and nasal biopsies are also promising areas to investigate. Skin reactivity to irritant injections needs to be investigated in controlled studies.

## Terminology

Terminology is a difficult area in any field of science and most particularly in medical science, with many terms for a single entity and multiple overlapping entities. In the case of illnesses induced or exacerbated by environmental chemicals at levels tolerated by the population at large, this is particularly true (see Table 12.1 for a listing). Sensory hyper-reactivity (Millqvist) is a term which closely matches the

**Table 12.1** Terminologies related to exposures to environmental chemicals

| | |
|---|---|
| Irritant asthma | Asthma induced or exacerbated by exposures to irritant chemicals |
| Irritant rhinitis | Rhinitis induced or exacerbated by exposures to irritant chemicals |
| Reactive airways dysfunction syndrome (RADS) | Onset of chronic asthma after a single exposure to an irritant chemical |
| Reactive upper-airways dysfunction syndrome (RUDS) | Onset of chronic rhinosinusitis after exposures to an irritant chemical |
| Toxicant-induced loss of tolerance (TILT) | Loss of tolerance to environment chemicals after an exposure to an environmental toxicant |
| Multiple chemical sensitivity syndrome (MCS) | Multiple organ system disease induced and exacerbated by exposures to environmental chemicals |
| Chemical sensitivity | A broad term, describing illness exacerbated or induced by environmental chemicals |
| Sick building syndrome (SBS) | Illness in those associated with working in poorly ventilated buildings that are most commonly respiratory (cough, congestion, etc.) and neurological (headaches, difficulty with concentration, etc.) |
| Sensory hyper-reactivity syndrome | Sensory nerve hyper-reactivity in individuals with intolerance to respiratory irritants |
| Reactive intestinal dysfunction syndrome (RIDS) | Irritable bowel syndrome, onset associated with a chemical exposure, exacerbated by chemical exposures |
| Reactive vocal cord dysfunction syndrome (RVCDS) | Vocal cord spasm triggered by irritant exposures |
| Office eye syndrome | A characteristic eye disease related to working in poorly ventilated buildings |
| Chemical stress syndrome | A description of the four stages of illness related to chemical exposures (see text) |
| World Trade Center syndrome | Persistent reactive airway disease in workers at the World Trade Center site |

pathophysiology of irritant sensitivity, with a biological response to stimulation of nococieptal receptors on sensory nerve fibers by irritants at lower levels than in healthy individuals. Toxicant-induced loss of tolerance (TILT) is proposed as a mechanism for the onset of sensitivity, which is what happens when the airway becomes remodeled after an irritant exposure induces inflammation (Miller). For the toxicant induction of chronic airway inflammation, reactive airways dysfunction syndrome (RADS) and reactive upper-airways dysfunction syndrome (RUDS) have been introduced. Reactive intestinal dysfunction syndrome (RIDS) describes individuals who develop irritable bowel syndrome after an infectious or a chemical insult.

Other terms for patients who have subjective complaints related to environmental chemicals include chemical sensitivity, multiple chemical sensitivity syndrome, and idiopathic environmental intolerances. Colloquial terms such as Twentieth Century Disease and Environmental Illness have been used to label individuals who complain of illness associated with environmental exposures. The introduction of such terms is unfortunate because they confuse diagnosis with etiology and obscure the fact that diagnosable medical illnesses can be induced and exacerbated by irritant exposures.

An analogue to the terminology of allergy is appropriate because allergy and irritant sensitivity have overlapping clinical manifestations, though the mechanisms by which the two classes of substances initiate inflammation in the airway and elsewhere are different. To diagnose a patient with *chemical sensitivity* is equivalent to diagnosing a patient as *allergic*. The inadequacy of a diagnosis of allergic is obvious; it leaves open to question the clinical consequences of allergy in a particular individual which can range from rhinitis and asthma to sinus headaches, urticaria, and constitutional and neuropsychological manifestations of asthma such as chronic fatigue, sleep disturbances, and depression, as discussed in Chap. 10. Further, limiting a diagnosis to *allergic* does not address to what the individual is allergic to.

The term *multiple chemical sensitivity syndrome* is problematic and equivalent to using a term such as *multiple allergic sensitivity syndrome*. Certainly, in clinical practice, highly atopic individuals with allergies to multiple pollens, danders, and foods exist. These individuals can have manifestations involving multiple organ systems (urticaria, rhinitis, asthma, gastrointestinal symptoms, cardiovascular manifestations, systemic anaphylaxis, sleep disturbances, fatigue, etc.). These individuals would not be labeled multiple allergen sensitivity syndrome. Rather, diagnoses would be rhinitis, urticaria, etc., with ragweed pollen allergy, peanut allergy, etc. The same approach should be used with irritant sensitivity. Diagnoses for a given individual would be rhinitis, asthma, airborne contact dermatitis, and so forth, with environmental tobacco smoke sensitivity, diesel exhaust sensitivity, etc., as appropriate.

The term *idiopathic environmental intolerances* is particularly unfortunate and is often used in a derogatory manner. It is also used to suggest that individuals who report illness associated with chemical exposures have a psychiatric condition such as somatization disorder, anxiety, depression, chemical phobia, or other conditions. Some individuals who complain of chemical intolerances may have a somatization disorder or chemical phobia; in such cases, the diagnosis should be somatization disorder or chemical phobia, not idiopathic environmental intolerances. It should be recognized that these disorders cannot be given until an organic cause has been ruled out. Further, cerebral manifestations of both allergy and irritant sensitivity should be recognized. Complaints such as sleep disturbances, fatigue, anxiety or depression in association with chemical exposures may be clinical manifestations of irritant sensitivity and in such cases should not be labeled idiopathic environmental intolerances.

Use of the terms multiple chemical sensitivity syndrome and idiopathic environmental intolerances obscures the fact that diagnosable medical illnesses including asthma and rhinitis can be induced and exacerbated by exposures to environmental chemicals at levels tolerated by most individuals. A derogatory attitude has been created toward individuals with irritant sensitivity that has blocked research into environmental causes of illness in the United States. The technique (Mann 2011) is similar to the approach used by commercial interests to combat the notion that smoking causes lung cancer (Davis 2009), lead exposures from leaded gasoline was lowering the IQ of children (Needleman 2005), and atmospheric carbon dioxide from burning fossil fuels is a factor in climate change (Gelspan et al. 1998). Experts are retained who challenge the science and offer alternative hypotheses. In the case of irritant sensitivity, the alternative hypothesis is that anyone who claims illness related to environmental exposures has a psychological or psychiatric condition and any physician who diagnoses chemical sensitivity is a quack. It is claimed that there is no known mechanism by which environmental chemicals can induce illness, though the mechanism by which respiratory irritants induce airway and dermal inflammation is well established (see Chap. 1 for a discussion). It is further claimed that irritant sensitivity cannot be reproduced with challenge studies, which is a claim refuted by the elegant studies such as those by Millqvist, Bascom, and Doty (Bascom 1991; Bascom et al. 1991; Doty et al. 1988, Johansson et al. 2006).

## *Adaptation to the Chemical Environment: The Chemical Stress Syndrome*

Humans are continuously exposed to sublethal concentrations of toxic chemicals and have a capacity to adapt. Adaptation was discovered in animal experiments in the 1930s by Dr. Hans Selye (Selye 1978), a medical researcher in Montreal. Seyle was trying to purify a hormone by injecting rodents with an extract of body tissues. When exposed to the tissue, the strain of rat he was working with developed stomach ulcers, joint inflammation, shrinkage of the thymus gland, and enlargement of the adrenal glands. Dr. Selye was using a medical research technique sometimes referred to as *grind and find*. The body tissue such as a gland would be ground up, made into a solution, and studied for an effect. The fluid would then be separated into two components by some property, such as a component that dissolves in alcohol, or by size of the molecule. Each component would be tested to see which one contained the sought-after ingredient.

To his dismay, Selye found that every component had the property he was trying to isolate. One day while pondering the problem, he noticed a bottle of formalin—a deadly mixture of formaldehyde and methyl alcohol used to fix tissues—on the shelf of his lab. He injected the animals with sublethal doses of formalin and found that it also produced the illness. As he continued his work, he exposed the animals to a variety of stresses, including emotional stress and surgical stress. No matter how he stressed his animals, illness resulted.

Selye continued his work by studying the reactions resulting from chronic exposure to small doses of toxins that were not sufficient to kill the animal. He found that mammals have an amazing ability to adapt to toxic exposures, but their adaptation breaks down and they become chronically ill. If they are removed from the exposure and then re-challenged, they can have a shock reaction and become extremely ill. He called his discovery the *generalized adaptation syndrome*.

Various versions of the adaptation syndrome have been described, one of which has been termed the chemical stress syndrome (Meggs 1999). In the breakdown of one's adaptation to the sublethal exposures to toxicants, there are four stages.

**Table 12.2** The stages of the chemical stress syndrome fir musculoskeletal, respiratory, and gastrointestinal systems

| | General | Musculoskeletal | Respiratory | Gastrointestinal |
|---|---|---|---|---|
| Stage 0. Normalcy | Tolerance of chemical exposures, wellness without symptoms | No symptoms | No symptoms | No symptoms |
| Stage 1. -algia | Sensory hyper-reactivity. Subjective symptoms associated with chemical exposures (arthralgias, myalgias, etc.) | Joint pains, muscle aches, pains, and spasms | Itching and or burning of nasal passages, sinus headaches, wheezing | Nausea, vomiting, diarrhea, abdominal cramps, irritable bowel syndrome |
| Stage 2. -itis | Inflammatory reactions to chemicals (arthritis, myositis, etc.) | Arthritis, myositis | Asthma, rhinitis, sinusitis | Inflammatory bowel disease, enteritis, colitis |
| Stage 3. -osis | Fibrosis. Tissue destruction (arthritic deformities, muscle atrophy and necrosis, etc.) | Deformed joints, muscle scarring | Chronic obstructive pulmonary disease (COPD), emphysema, pulmonary fibrosis | Bowel scarring, obstruction |

## *Stages 0–3:*

*Stage 0* is normal health in which there are no chemical intolerances.

*Stage 1* (-algia stage) is sensory hyper-reactivity, with symptoms related to exposures such as joint pain, headaches, burning of nasal passages, and so forth. It is termed the -algia stage because the suffix -algia in medical terminology refers to pain. For example, arthralgia means joint pain.

*Stage 2* (-itis stage) is when the substances induce inflammation. It is termed the -itis stage because the suffix -itis in medical terminology refers to inflammation. For example, arthritis means joint inflammation.

*Stage 3* (-osis stage) is when the inflammation produces tissue damage, such as joint destruction. It is the -osis stage because the suffix -osis in medicine refers to destruction. Fibrosis is the replacement of a normal tissue by scar tissue, which can be the endstage of an inflammatory process. Necrosis is the extreme of dead tissue. The end stage of arthritis is when the joints are destroyed and deformities occur.

Table 12.2 outlines the stages of the chemical stress syndrome and generalizes it from airway inflammation to other organ systems. By finding environmental factors that drive the inflammation, an afflicted individual can achieve wellness as long as the end stage 3 (-osis stage) has not been reached. At the present time, we

**Table 12.3** Intermittent stimulatory and withdrawal symptoms associated with maladaption to foods and chemicals

| | Stimulatory symptoms | Withdrawal symptoms |
|---|---|---|
| Devastating | Mania: Agitation, excitement, blackouts, seizures in extreme cases | Depression: Confabulation, hallucinosis, obsessions, delusions, transient amnesia |
| Severe | Hypomania: Hyper-responsiveness, anxiety, panic attacks, mental lapses | Brain-fag (a term used to describe fatigue, mood changes, irritability, impairment of: cognition, concentration, poor reading comprehension, memory) |
| Moderate | Hyperactivity: Restless legs, insominia, aggressive forceful behavior | Systemic physical symptoms: Fatigue, headache, myalgia, arthralgia, arthritis, edema, fast heartbeat, arrhythmias |
| Mild | Stimulation: Active, self-centered, suppression of symptoms | Localized physical symptoms: Rhinitis, bronchitis, asthma, dermatitis, gastrointestinal and genitourinary symptoms |

have no way to reverse destruction of a tissue. Stem cell research offers promise as a way to reverse destroyed tissue but unfortunately is periodically restricted in the United States for political rather than scientific reasons. Even if we achieve techniques to reverse scarring and tissue destruction, the rejuvenated tissue may be at risk if environmental factors driving the inflammation are not identified and eliminated.

Symptoms of environmental exposures have been described as having stimulatory and withdrawal phases. The stimulatory phase of illness is triggered by an exposure, while the withdrawal phase occurs after removal with exposure. Table 12.3 lists the clinically described manifestations of the two phases (Randolph 1990).

## Research Needs

### *Scientific Verification of the Brain as a Target Organ for Irritant and Allergic Exposures*

Understanding the brain as a target organ of both allergic and irritant sensitivity is a matter of great importance. There is a high burden of conditions such as depression and hyperactivity in countries with a high level of irritant exposures. Disorders of the brain that have been linked to environmental exposures—such as depression, attention-deficit hyperactivity disorder, and hyperventilation syndrome—need further investigation. Until recently, the scientific study of the inner workings of the brain in living humans has been difficult. Behavioral and subjective parameters had to be used to study cerebral reactivity to exposures. The rich clinical descriptions of behavioral and subjective symptoms related to exposures have been primarily anecdotal. Objective parameters like those that exist for asthma—for example, pulmonary function tests before and after methacholine challenges, antigen challenges, and irritant challenges—did not exist. Advances in brain imagining, including functional magnetic resonance imagining, multichannel electro- and magneto-encephalopathy, and PET and SPECT scans, allow changes in focal brain function to be monitored in real time before and after challenges.

Scientific verification of associations with environment triggers of behavior should be given high priority, given the major epidemics and increasing prevalence of hyperactivity, depression, and suicide, particularly among children and young adults. Advancing knowledge in this area could lead to improved treatment and prevention.

## *A National Laboratory to Study Environmental Effects in Diseases*

An environmental control unit is an inpatient clinical unit used to isolate individuals with specific diseases from exposures to environmental chemicals. These units allow scientific control of exposures so that factors that exacerbate disease, whether dietary or inhalational, can be studied. Several national committees sponsored by the federal government to study environmental factors in disease recommended funding of such a center to be used by researchers, similar to the national laboratories for physics and other fields. To date, these recommendations have not found fruition. Possible reasons are lack of effective leadership to advance this agenda and the political opposition to studying relationships between environmental chemicals and disease.

## *Diagnostic Modalities for Irritant Sensitivity That Can Be Used Routinely in the Clinic Need to be Developed*

The extent to which a positive methacholine or histamine challenge test correlates with irritant sensitivity needs stronger verification. Since some but not all rhinitis patients have positive methacholine challenge tests, its usefulness in irritant rhinitis patients needs to be investigated. Levels of nerve growth factor in the upper airway are increased in irritant-sensitive individuals and have been shown to rise after challenge, but this remains a research test at present. Skin reactivity to irritant injection is used by some clinicians but has not received scientific validation. Nasal biopsies in irritant-sensitive individuals have both light and electron microscopy abnormalities but is an expensive and invasive test that will be unlikely to move from the laboratory to the clinic. The capsaicin cough challenge at present does not currently have the standardization such as seen with methacholine challenges that allow its routine interpretation in the clinical setting (Milloqvist).

## *Treatments of Irritant Sensitivity Need to Be Improved*

While avoidance of irritants has been self-reported as the treatment of choice by individuals with complaints related to irritant exposures (Gibson et al. 2003), in today's world this can be difficult. Clinical experience suggests that persons with severe irritant sensitivity developing after an acute exposure have a decrease in reactivity with time if they can minimize their exposures through modifications in the home and workplace, though this has not been scientifically studied. Current pharmaceutical treatments for irritant rhinitis and asthma are not optimal. Controlled studies of alternative treatments, such as the unique proposal developed by Dr. Ziem and discussed in Chap. 11, need scientific verification.

## *Controlled Studies of the Treatment of Patients with Concomitant Rhinitis, Anxiety, and Depression*

The association that has been documented between rhinitis, whether allergic or irritant, and mental conditions such as anxiety and depression, as discussed in Chap. 10, suggests that treatment of either airway inflammation or anxiety/depression could impact the other disorder. Randomization of individuals with comorbid depression and rhinitis to treatment of one or the other could yield both improved treatments and a better understanding of the association.

## *Pathophysiological Studies Comparing Irritant and Allergic Airway Inflammation*

While many with asthma and rhinitis have both allergic and irritant triggers, some have purely allergic or purely irritant triggers. Comparative studies of these two groups has the potential to further elucidate the mechanisms involved and possibly lead to better treatment.

## *Dose–Response Curves in Experimental Models for the Toxic Induction of Asthma, Rhinitis, and Related Conditions*

There is a difference between toxicologically induced illness and hypersensitivity reactions. Toxic reactions follow a dose–response curve, with the percentage of exposed individuals who have a toxic manifestation varying with dose. A schematic

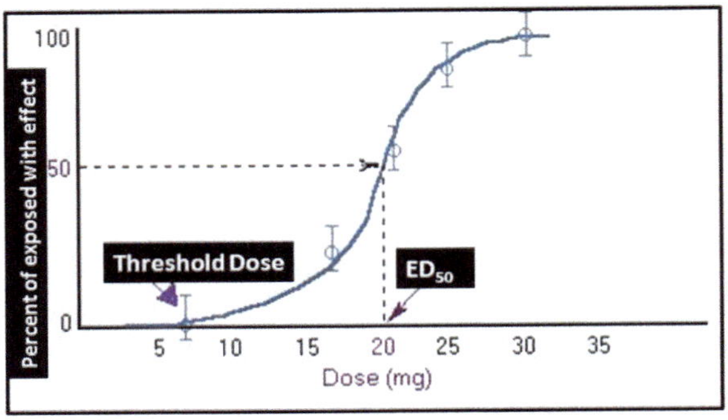


**Fig. 12.1** A typical dose-response curve is depicted, where the percentage of a population that gets an effect at a given dose is plotted against dose. The $ED_{50}$ is the dose that produces the effect in 50% of exposed subjects

depiction of the classical dose–response curve is given in Fig. 12.1. At a very low dose, no one has the toxic effect. As the dose increases, the percentage of individuals with the effect increases. At high doses, virtually all exposed individuals will have the toxic effect. The toxic dose is quoted as the ED50, the dose that will produce the toxic effect in 50 % of exposed individuals, as shown in the curve.

## References

Bascom R. Differential susceptibility to tobacco smoke: possible mechanisms. Pharmacogenetics. 1991;1(2):102–6.

Bascom R, Kulle T, Kagey-Sobotka A, Proud D. Upper respiratory tract environmental tobacco smoke sensitivity. Am Rev Respir Dis. 1991;143(6):1304–11.

Davis D. The secret history of the war on cancer. New York: Basic Books; 2009.

Doty RL, Deems DA, Frye RE, Pelberg R, Shapiro A. Olfactory sensitivity, nasal resistance, and autonomic function in patients with multiple chemical sensitivities. Arch Otolaryngol Head Neck Surg. 1988;114(12):1422–7.

Gelspan R. The heat is on: the climate crisis, the cover-up, the prescription by Ross Gelbspan. New York: Basic Books; 1998.

Gibson PR, Elms AN, Ruding LA. Perceived treatment efficacy for conventional and alternative therapies reported by persons with multiple chemical sensitivity. Environ Health Perspect. 2003;111(12):1498–504.

Johansson A, Millqvist E, Nordin S, Bende M. Relationship between self-reported odor intolerance and sensitivity to inhaled capsaicin: proposed definition of airway sensory hyperreactivity and estimation of its prevalence. Chest. 2006;129(6):1623–8.

Mann A. They're poisoning us! From the Gulf War to the Gulf of Mexico an investigative report. New York: 34th Street Press; 2011.

Meggs WJ. Mechanisms of allergy and chemical sensitivity. Toxicol Ind Health. 1999;15:331–8.

Miller CS. Toxicant-induced loss of tolerance–an emerging theory of disease? Environ Health Perspect. 1997;105 Suppl 2:445–53.

Millqvist E. The airway sensory hyperreactivity syndrome. Pulm Pharmacol Ther. 2011:24: 263–266.

Needleman H. Standing up to the lead industry: an interview with Herbert Needleman. Interview by David Rosner and Gerald Markowitz. Public Health Rep. 2005;120(3):330–7.

Randolph TG. Allergies: an alternative approach. New York: Harper Perennial; 1990.

Selye H. The stress of life. New York: McGraw-Hill; 1978.

# Index


**A**
Acetylation, 213
Acetylcarnitine, 258
Acetylcholine (Ach), 48, 110–112
Active smoking. *See also* Tobacco smoke
  asthma
    association of, 141–144, 157
    biomarkers, 147–148, 158–159
    health burden, 145–146, 158
    severity and impacts, 145–146, 158
  cohort studies, 141, 154
  upper respiratory tract
    chronic rhinosinusitis, 164
    prevalent allergic rhinitis, 172, 173
Acute lung injury (ALI), 84–85
Acute respiratory distress syndrome (ARDS), 84–85, 94
Acute toxicity. *See* Respiratory irritant exposure
Aδ fibers, 27, 35
Airborne contact dermatitis (ABCD)
  allergic and irritant, 203
  diagnosis, 202
  epidemiology, 199
  features and causes
    benzoyl peroxide, 202
    clinical manifestations, 200
    dusts, 201
    latex, 201
    parthenium dermatitis, 201
    rhus dermatitis, 199–200
    sprays, 201
  management, 202
  pathophysiology, 199
Airway inflammation
  counter regulation, 49–50
  dendritic cells, 43–44
  eosinophils, 46–47
  epithelial cells, 47–48
  inflammatory cells, 41, 42
  lymphocytes
    NK cells, 45–46
    $T_C$, 45
    $T_H$ and $T_{reg}$ cells, 44–45
  macrophages, 41, 43
  mast cells, 47
  neurons, 48–49
  polymorphonuclear leukocytes, 46
Airway sensory hyperreactivity, 75
Airway smooth muscle (ASM)
  irritant-induced asthma, 73
  respiratory tract, 39–40
Albuterol, 93
Allergic airborne contact dermatitis, 203
Allergic contact dermatitis (ACD), 194
Allergic rhinitis
  definition, 135–136
  target organ, 233, 237
  tobacco smoke
    active smoking, 172–176
    respiratory tract, 178–180
    secondhand smoke, 172, 176–177
Allergic sensitivity
  atherosclerosis, 11
  behavioral and subjective parameters, 283–284
  chemical sensitivity, 233–234, 279, 280
  chronic fatigue syndrome, 12
  environmental adjuvants, 11
  IgE antibody, 233
  initiating mechanism, 232
  irritable bowel syndrome, 12



W.J. Meggs (ed.), *The Toxicant Induction of Irritant Asthma, Rhinitis, and Related Conditions*, DOI 10.1007/978-1-4614-9044-9,

Allergic sensitivity (*cont.*)
multiple chemical sensitivity syndrome, 12–13
patholophysiological studies, 285
sick building syndrome, 11–12
site switching, 9–10
target organ (*see* Brain)
tobacco smoke, 180–181
urticaria, 233
vocal cord dysfunction syndrome, 12
Allergic-type occupational asthma, 64
Alpha lipoic acid, 256–258
Ambient and manufactured particulate matter. *See also* Particulate matter (PM) exposure
adhesion-related proteins, 116
BAL cell profiles, 114–116
leukocytes
Printex 90, 116–118
reduction, 116, 117
vehicle control, 116, 118
plasma fibrinogen and platelet, 118
alterations, 119–120
myocardial I/R injury, 120–121
Ammonia ($NH_3$), 85, 86
Aspiration reflex, 35
Asthma
brain, 234
classic description of, 3
definition, 132–134
extrinsic, 1
IgE antibodies, 2
intrinsic, 2
irritant (*see* Irritant asthma; Irritant-induced asthma)
respiratory irritants, 2, 3
tobacco smoke (*see* Tobacco smoke)
Atherosclerosis, 11
Attention-deficit disorder, 235, 238

**B**
Brain
airway inflammation, 240
allergy
chemicals, 233–234
IgE antibody, 233
initiating mechanism, 232
urticaria, 233
anxiety, 236, 285
attention-deficit disorder, 235
autonomic dysfunction, 238
behavioral disorders, 237
chemical sensitivities, 236
clinical descriptions, 232, 235
environmental control units, 241, 284
fatigue, 236–237
irritant sensitivity
airway inflammation, 234
asthma and rhinitis, 234
initiating mechanism, 232
RADS and RUDS, 235
PET scan, 239
physiological mechanisms, 238–239
pollen season, 239, 241
psychiatric evaluation, 235
pupillography, 240
seizures, 236
sick building syndrome, 237–238
Bronchial alveolar lavage (BAL), 114–116

**C**
Carbon black (CB) nanoparticles, 108
Cardiovascular inflammation
epidemiological studies, 105–106
hypothesized mechanisms
heart rate variability, 106–107
immune system, 107
metals role, 107
PM (*see* Particulate matter (PM) exposure)
Cerium oxide ($CeO_2$), 108–110
C-fibers
defensive reflexes, 33–35
lower airways, 27, 28
Chemesthesis, 223
Chemical stress syndrome
-algia stage, 282
clinical manifestations, 283
generalized adaptation syndrome, 281
grind and find technique, 281
intermittent stimulatory and withdrawal symptoms, 283
-itis stage, 282
-osis stage, 282
Chloramines, 86
Chloroacetophenone (CN), 89
Chlorobenxylidenmalononitrile (CS), 89
Chromium, 259, 264
Chronic airway inflammation, 5–6
Chronic allergic respiratory syndrome, 178, 181
Chronic fatigue syndrome, 12, 236, 237
Chronic rhinosinusitis (CRS)
active smoking, 164
secondhand smoke, 177
Coenzyme Q10, 259
Combustion products. *See* Tobacco smoke

Condensable particulate matter, 222
Cough reflex, 34–35
Cyanide, 90–91
Cynaocobalamin, 91

**D**
Defensive reflexes
  aspiration reflex, 35
  C-fibers, 33–35
  cough reflex, 34–35
  Aδ fibers, 35
  diving reflex, 35
  nasal congestion, 34
  RAR fibers, 33–35
  receptors, 35–36
  rhinorrhea, 34
  SAR fibers, 33–34
  sneezing, 34
Dendritic cells, airway inflammation, 43–44
Detergent suicides, 87
Diesel exhaust (DE), 106
Difficult asthma, 183
Dihydrolipoic acid. *See* Alpha lipoic acid
Diving reflex, 35

**E**
Electrolyte homeostasis, 37–38
Eosinophils, airway inflammation, 46–47
Epithelial cells, airway inflammation, 47–48
Exposure limits
  airborne irritants, 215–216
  chemical mixtures, 211
  definitions, 208
  environmental chemicals, 279
  genetic diversity, 213
  health effects, 209–210
  healthy conditions, 208
  human exposure, 213–214
  indoor respiratory hazards, 211–212
  inhalational exposures, 207–208
  irritant-induced airway inflammation
    Under Federal Disability Law and Regulations, 266
    filters, 268
    sample letter, 267
  permissible exposure limits, 208–209
  respiratory symptoms, 214–215
  synergistic risk, 212
  threshold limit values, 208, 210
  validity of, 209

**F**
Fatigue
  brain, 236–237
  related conditions, 12

**G**
Gamma tocopherol, 253–254
Generalized adaptation syndrome, 281
Glutathione
  exposure limits, 213
  irritant-induced airway inflammation
    alpha lipoic acid, 256–257
    description, 254
    injection of, 255
    intravenous, 255
    nebulizer use, 254–255
    oral use, 254
    riboflavin, 257
    selenium, 256
    vitamin C, 256
Grind and find technique, chemical stress syndrome, 281

**H**
Heart failure, PM, 122–123
Hydrogen chloride/chlorine, 87
Hydrogen fluoride
  acute toxicity, 86
  systemic toxicity, 92–93
Hydrogen sulfide
  acute toxicity, 87–88
  systemic toxicity, 91–92

**I**
Idiopathic environmental intolerances (IEI), 13, 280
Inhalable particulate matter (IPM), 221
Inhaled respiratory irritants. *See* Respiratory irritants
Ionic channels, 72
Irritable bowel syndrome (IBS), 12, 236, 279
Irritant airborne contact dermatitis, 203
Irritant airway inflammation
  burning sensation, 248
  downregulating inflammatory biochemistry
    chronic inflammation, 251–252
    compounded protocol, 261–262
    energy metabolism, 258–259
    gamma tocopherol, 253–254
    glutathione (*see* Glutathione)
    lipid membranes, 253–254

Irritant airway inflammation (*cont.*)
nitric oxide/methylcobalamine, 252–253
NMDA receptor, 257–258
plant-based antioxidants, 259–261
super oxide dismutase, 258
eating for healing factsheet, 269–270
environmental exacerbation, 265–266
exposure limit
Under Federal Disability Law and Regulations, 266
filters, 268
sample letter, 267
nutrition, 248, 264
organic foods, 264
progress evaluation, 248–249
exacerbation patient questions, 250
follow-up patient questions, 249–250
hazardous testing, 251
intake patient questions, 249–250
peak flow, 250
symptom-masking drugs, 248
testing approaches, 262–263
therapy, 263–264
Irritant asthma
induction of
chronic airway inflammation, 5–6
dose–response curves, 285–286
electron micrographs, 5–7
positive feedback loop, 8
RADS, 4
tumor necrosis factor, 7
mechanism of, 4, 5
sensitivity (*see* Allergic sensitivity; Irritant sensitivity)
tobacco smoke (*see* Tobacco smoke)
Irritant contact dermatitis (ICD)
*vs.* allergic contact dermatitis, 194
definition, 194
diagnosis, 198
epidemiology, 195, 196
features and causes
acids, 196–197
alkalis, 197
food-induced, 198
irritant diaper dermatitis, 197
lip-licker's dermatitis, 197
solvents, 197
water, 197
management, 198
pathophysiology, 195–196
Irritant diaper dermatitis, 197
Irritant-induced asthma
airway sensory hyperreactivity, 75
allergic-type occupational asthma, 64
etiological agents, 69–70
frequency of, 64–65
mechanisms
abnormal epithelial–mesenchymal trophic unit, 73
airway smooth muscle, 73
clinical phenotype, 74
genetic factors, 71
ionic channels, 72
neurotrophins, 72
subclinical asthma, 73–74
tachykinins, 72
odor-triggered panic attacks, 75–76
pathological features, 70–71
prognosis of, 74
repeated exposure irritant-induced occupational asthma, 64, 67–69
risk factors, 65
single exposure irritant-induced occupational asthma, 64–67
treatment, 74–75
vocal cord dysfunction, 75
work-aggravated asthma, 64
World Trade Center entities, 76
Irritant rhinitis
induction of
characteristics, 7–8
dose–response curves, 285–286
nasal airway, 7–8
positive feedback loop, 8
sensitivity (*see* Allergic sensitivity; Irritant sensitivity)
mechanism of, 4, 5
tobacco smoke (*see* Tobacco smoke)
treatment, 285
Irritant sensitivity
airway inflammation, 234
asthma and rhinitis, 234
atherosclerosis, 11
behavioral and subjective parameters, 283–284
chemical sensitivity, 279, 280
chronic fatigue syndrome, 12
diagnostic modalities for, 284
environmental adjuvants, 11
initiating mechanism, 232
irritable bowel syndrome, 12
multiple chemical sensitivity syndrome, 12–13
patholophysiological studies, 285
RADS and RUDS, 235
sick building syndrome, 11–12
site switching, 9–10

target organ (*see* Brain)
treatments, 285
vocal cord dysfunction syndrome, 12
Isocyanates, 96

**L**
Laryngopharyngitis, 177
Limulus amebocyte lysate assay, 154
Lip-licker's dermatitis, 197
Lower airways, respiratory tract, 27–29
Lymphocytes, airway inflammation
NK cells, 45–46
$T_C$, 45
$T_H$ and $T_{reg}$ cells, 44–45

**M**
Macrophages, airway inflammation, 41, 43
Magnesium, 257, 261, 263
Mast cells
airway inflammation, 47
airway smooth muscle, 39
Metal fume fever, 89–90
Methylation, 213, 262
Methylcobalamine
nebulizer, 252–253
severely inflamed patients, 253
sublingual tablets, 252
Molybdenum, 259
Mucin glycoproteins, 37, 41
Multiple chemical sensitivity syndrome (MCS), 12–13, 279, 280
Multi-walled carbon nanotube (MWCNT)
BAL cell profiles, 114, 115
lung histology, 112–114
PM (*see* Particulate matter (PM) exposure)

**N**
Neurogenic switching, 9
Neurons, airway inflammation, 48–49
Neurotrophins, 72
Nitric oxide
acute toxicity, 88
inducible cycle (*see* Irritant airway inflammation)
nebulizer, 252–253
severely inflamed patients, 253
sublingual tablets, 252
systemic toxicity, 92
tobacco smoke, 154
Nociceptors, 4

**O**
Occupational asthma (OA). *See also* Irritant-induced asthma
allergic-type, 64
repeated exposure irritant-induced, 64, 67–69
respiratory irritants, 225–226
single exposure irritant-induced, 64–67
Occupational rhinitis (OR), 226
Odor-triggered panic attacks, 75–76
Oxides of nitrogen
acute toxicity, 88–89
systemic toxicity, 92
Oxygen, 90
Ozone, 89

**P**
Pantothenate/pantethine, 259
Parthenium dermatitis, 201
Particulate matter (PM) exposure
aeroallergen challenge, 104
ambient and manufactured
BAL cell profiles, 114–116
ischemia–reperfusion injury, 116–119
serum levels, 116, 117
thrombogenic potential, 118–121
co-pollutants, 121
environmental exposure level, 104–105
epidemiological studies, 105–106
heart failure, 122–123
hypothesized mechanisms
heart rate variability, 106–107
immune system, 107
metals role, 107
impacts
carbon black nanoparticles, 108
carbon nanotubes, 109
cerium oxide, 108–110
MWCNT, 109–112
myocardial infarction, 109–110
size, 108
SWCNT, 109
thoracic aorta ACh relaxation responses, 110–112
$TiO_2$, 108
ultrafine particles, 107–108
lung histology 24 h post instillation, 112–114
Printex 90
blood leukocyte, 116–118
MWCNT, 119
platelet and fibrinogen level, 118–121

Passive smoking. *See also* Tobacco smoke
cohort studies, 141, 154
irritant rhinitis and asthma, 179
secondhand smoke, 161
Permissible exposure limits (PELs), 208–209
Phosgene, 88
Polymer fume fever, 89–90
Polymorphonuclear leukocytes (PMNs), 46
Printex 90
blood leukocyte, 116–118
MWCNT, 119
platelet and fibrinogen level, 118–121
Pyridoxal phosphate (B6), 257

**R**

Rapidly adapting (RAR) fibers, 33–35
Reactive airways dysfunction syndrome (RADS), 3, 253. *See also* Irritant-induced asthma
causative agents, 69–70
diagnostic criteria, 67
frequency of, 64–65
inhaled respiratory irritants, 225, 226
irritant asthma, 4
irritant sensitivity, 235
pathological features, 70–71
repeated exposure (*see* Repeated exposure irritant-induced occupational asthma)
single exposure irritant-induced occupational asthma, 64–67
Reactive intestinal dysfunction syndrome (RIDS), 12, 279
Reactive upper-airways dysfunction syndrome (RUDS), 7, 8, 226, 235, 279
Reflexes
defensive (*see* Defensive reflexes)
regulatory
airway smooth muscle relaxation, 33
central pattern generator, 32
inspiratory drive inhibition, 33
mechanical deformation, 32–33
$O_2$ and $CO_2$, 31–32
pharynx, 32–33
pressure changes, 33
in sleep, 32
tachycardia, 33
Repeated exposure irritant-induced occupational asthma
chlorine chemicals, 67, 69
classification, 67
diagnostic criteria, 67, 68
occurrence, 64
Respiratory irritant exposure
air pollution, 95–96
ammonia, 85
chloramines, 86
clinical manifestations, 84–85
hydrogen chloride/chlorine, 87
hydrogen fluoride, 86–87
hydrogen sulfide, 87–88
isocyanates/Bhopal, 96
metals, 89–90
oxides of nitrogen, 88–89
oxygen, 90
ozone, 89
pathophysiology, 84
phosgene, 88
polymers, 89–90
riot control agents, 89
smog, 95–96
smoke inhalation, 95
sulfur dioxide and sulfuric acid, 88
systemic toxicity
cyanide, 90–91
hydrogen fluoride, 92–93
hydrogen sulfide, 91–92
oxides of nitrogen, 92
treatment
corticosteroids, 94
emergency management, 93–94
exogenous surfactants, 95
indoors, 93
*N*-acetylcysteine, 94
neutralization therapy, 94
perfluorocarbon, 94–95
Respiratory irritants
asthma, 2, 3
definition, 220
epidemiology
allergic asthmagens, 225
non-allergic occupational asthma, 225
occupational asthma, 225–226
occupational disease mortality, 223
occupational rhinitis, 226
RADS, 225, 226
reactive upper airway dysfunction syndrome, 226
vocal cord dysfunction, 226
work-related respiratory conditions, 223, 224
health effects, 223
host-related factors, 220, 223
physical and chemical factors
fibers and fumes, 222
inhalable particulate matter, 221
particle size, 220–222

respirable particles, 221
smoke, 222
thoracic particulate matter, 221
ultrafine particles, 221–222
water, 222
worker evaluation, 227–228
worksite evaluation, 227
Respiratory tract
airborne particles
deposition, 36
mucociliary clearance, 37–38
airway musculature, 24–25
airway resistance, 38–39
airway smooth muscle, 39–40
defensive (*see* Defensive reflexes)
functional anatomy
alveolar sacs, 22–23
arteries, 24
bronchioles, 22
collagen and elastin fibers, 23
epiglottis, 21
larynx, 21
lymphatic system, 24
nasal cavity and valve, 21
olfactory region and pharynx, 21
surface tension, 23
surfactant apoproteins, 23–24
trachea, 22
upper and lower airways, 20
inflammatory response (*see* Airway inflammation)
lower airways, 27–29
mucus secretion, 40–41
regulatory reflexes
airway smooth muscle relaxation, 33
central pattern generator, 32
inspiratory drive inhibition, 33
mechanical deformation, 32–33
$O_2$ and $CO_2$, 31–32
pharynx, 32–33
pressure changes, 33
in sleep, 32
tachycardia, 33
remodeling, 51
secondhand smoke
acute rhinitis, 174–176
allergic rhinitis, 172
chronic rhinosinusitis, 177
existing allergic rhinitis, 176–177
laryngopharyngitis, 177
tobacco smoke
active smoking (*see* Active smoking)
allergic rhinitis and asthma, 178
ETS effects, 178, 179
history of, 164
irritant rhinitis and asthma, 178–180
SHS (*see* Secondhand smoke (SHS))
transient receptor potential cation channels, 28, 30–31
TRPA1, 30–31
TRPC6 and TRPV4, 31
upper airways
cranial nerves, 25, 26
preganglionic parasympathetic fiber, 26
preganglionic sympathetic fiber, 26–27
soft palate and pharynx walls, 25–26
Rhus dermatitis, 199–200
Riboflavin (B2), 257
Riot control agents, 89

**S**
Secondhand smoke (SHS)
asthma
exposure settings, 141
incident asthma, 149–152, 159–161
prevalence and usage trends, 140–141
prevalent asthma, 161, 162
upper respiratory tract
acute rhinitis, 174–176
allergic rhinitis, 172
chronic rhinosinusitis, 177
existing allergic rhinitis, 176–177
laryngopharyngitis, 177
Seizures, 236
Selenium, 256
Sensory hyper-reactivity syndrome, 278–279
Sick building syndrome, 11–12, 237–238
Single exposure irritant-induced occupational asthma, 64–67
Site switching, 9–10
Sleep, treating irritant airway inflammation, 261–262
Slowly adapting (SAR) fibers, 33–34
Smog, 95–96
Smoke inhalation
inhaled respiratory irritants, 222
respiratory irritant exposure, 95
Sulfur dioxide ($SO_2$), 88
Sulfuric acid ($H_2SO_3$), 88
Super oxide dismutase (SOD), 258

**T**
Tachykinins, irritant-induced asthma, 72
Taurine, 257–258, 261
Tear gases, 89
Thoracic particulate matter (TPM), 221

Threshold limit values (TLVs), 208–210
Tobacco smoke
on asthma
active smoking (*see* Active smoking)
definition, 132–134
difficult asthma, 183
endotypes and phenotypes, 183
ETS exposure, 183
evolution of, 137–139, 157
medical therapy, 161
passive smoking, 157
*vs.* rhinitis, 132, 135–136
SHS (*see* Secondhand smoke (SHS))
biomarkers, 156
characterization exposure, 154–155
corticosteroid therapy, 184
distribution and uptake, 155–156
epidemiologic studies, 140
health effects, 184
integrated respiratory tract
allergic rhinitis and asthma, 178
ETS effects, 178, 179
irritant rhinitis and asthma, 178–180
lexicon development, 184
mechanisms
allergy, 180–181
bacterial pathogens, 182
differential susceptibility, 182
epigenetic modulation, 181–182
mucosal structure and function, 180
prevalence and usage trends
active and passive smoking, 141
ecological analysis, 140, 141
SHS, 140
secondhand smoke exposure, 140, 154
on upper respiratory tract
active smoking (*see* Active smoking)
history of, 164–171
SHS (*see* Secondhand smoke (SHS))
vapor-phase deposition, 156
Transient receptor potential (TRP) cation channels, 28, 30–31

U
Upper airways, respiratory tract
cranial nerves, 25, 26
preganglionic parasympathetic fiber, 26
preganglionic sympathetic fiber, 26–27
soft palate and pharynx walls, 25–26

V
Vasoactive intestinal peptide (VIP), 39, 40
Vitamin B12, 91, 261
Vitamin C (ascorbate), 256, 263
Vocal cord dysfunction (VCD) syndrome
inhaled respiratory irritants, 226
irritant-induced asthma, 75

W
Work-aggravated asthma, 64

MIX
Papier aus verantwortungsvollen Quellen
Paper from responsible sources
FSC® C105338

If you have any concerns about our products,
you can contact us on
**ProductSafety@springernature.com**

In case Publisher is established outside the EU,
the EU authorized representative is:
**Springer Nature Customer Service Center GmbH**
**Europaplatz 3, 69115 Heidelberg, Germany**

Printed by Libri Plureos GmbH
in Hamburg, Germany